Infants and Hearing

A Singular Audiology Text
Jeffrey L. Danhauer, Ph.D.
Audiology Editor

Infants and Hearing

Deborah Hayes, Ph.D.
The Children's Hospital-Denver

Jerry L. Northern, Ph.D.
University of Colorado School of Medicine

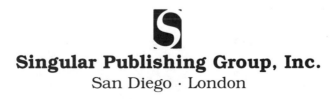

Singular Publishing Group, Inc.
San Diego · London

Singular Publishing Group, Inc.
401 West A Street, Suite 325
San Diego, California 92101-7904

19 Compton Terrace
London N1 2UN, U.K.

© 1996 by Singular Publishing Group, Inc.

Typeset in 9½/12 Bookman by So Cal Graphics
Printed in the United States of America by BookCrafters

Library of Congress Cataloging-in-Publication Data

Hayes, Deborah.
    Infants and hearing / by Deborah Hayes and Jerry L. Northern.
      p.   cm.
    Includes bibliographical references and index.
    ISBN 1-56593-191-2
    1. Hearing disorders in infants.   2. Infants (Newborn)—Medical examinations.   I. Northern, Jerry L.   II. Title.
    [DNLM: 1. Hearing Disorders—in infancy & childhood.   2. Hearing Disorders—diagnosis.   WV 271 H417i 1996]
  RF291.5.C45H29   1996
  618.92'0978—dc20
  DNLM/DLC
  for Library of Congress   96-24942
                                        CIP

Contents

Preface

Within the last decade, there has been an explosion of information about hearing and hearing loss in infants. As technology now permits measurement of auditory function in newborn babies, we have developed improved insights into the status of hearing in the newborn and the various medical conditions that affect peripheral hearing sensitivity and central auditory pathways in young infants. Because this information is not conveniently available in a single source, students and clinicians have limited access to the latest clinical and research findings. This text is written for practicing audiologists and graduate students in training. We anticipate that speech-language pathologists, neonatologists and pediatricians, nurses, and other specialists who care for infants will also find the information useful.

We chose to write *Infants and Hearing* for three reasons. First, we wanted to compile in a single volume information relevant to the clinical practice of audiology with this special population. As public awareness about the consequences of hearing loss in childhood increases, audiologists are called upon more frequently to provide professional services to infants. Audiologists in all settings should have appropriate knowledge and skills to provide adequate services to babies. Second, we wanted to compile information about the special medical considerations and genetic advances that are impacting health care of infants. Recent advances in neonatal care for critically ill babies and the rapid advances in clinical and molecular genetics are not readily available to many audiologists. With the help of our colleagues in neonatology, neonatal nursing, and clinical genetics, we have attempted to summarize this information in an accessible and useful form. Finally, with emphasis on improved education for students of audiology, we wanted to develop a comprehensive text that could serve as the foundation for an advanced course dealing with audiological services to infants. It is our goal that this text will improve the development of competent student clinicians and enhance their clinical practicum experience with babies.

The text is organized into three major sections. The first section, Perspectives on Infant Hearing, provides an overview of efforts to identify and habilitate infants with hearing loss. We discuss the rich and fascinating history of screening infants for hearing loss ranging from the observation of behavioral responses in older infants (e.g., 6 months and older) to application of sophisticated electrophysiological techniques in inpatient nursery programs. We also describe the resources necessary to mount truly comprehensive services to infants and their families.

The second major section, Clinical Aspects of Hearing in Infants, includes information useful for understanding the genetic, teratogenic, traumatic, or infectious consequences of alterations in the developmental sequence. We describe the anatomical and physiological developmental sequence and provide examples of how this sequence can be disrupted. We also explain the techniques currently available for evaluating and treating infants with significant health factors such as genetic disorders, respiratory dysfunction, and major congenital anomalies. We include discussion of the genetic techniques currently applied for evaluating genetic inheritance and how these techniques influence diagnosis of infants with hearing loss. Chapter 5, Care of Premature and Critically Ill Newborns: The Neonatal Intensive Care Unit, is a practical primer on how tertiary care units operate, the technology used in these units, and how audiologists provide services in this environment.

The final section of the text, Evaluation and Management, is devoted to issues of medical and audiological treatment within the context of the family-centered approach. We summarize the principles underlying screening theory; we also provide an overview of the sophisticated techniques currently available for the non-behavioral evaluation as well as behavioral assessment of auditory function in infants. We address amplification and aural habilitation for infants with consideration of federal and state guidelines for services to infants with disabilities.

To enhance practical application of the material, we have included a catalog of suggested readings after each chapter, listing what we consider to be some of the classic or seminal readings in specific topics. Important historical documents from a number of sources are included as appendixes. These documents are the foundation of current philosophy and practice in screening the hearing of infants. We close this text with an extensive bibliography of cited references.

We are grateful to the many colleagues who have shared their time, knowledge, and support in the completion of this text. Their unselfish contributions have enhanced our own professional development, and we hope that we have adequately represented the quality of these contributions in *Infants and Hearing.*

Foreword

*I*t has been nearly 30 years since Graham Sterrit and I organized volunteers to screen the hearing of all the babies born in
the city of Denver during a 1-year period. Some day we will look
back on these three decades as the Age of Infant Discovery—a
period of time when the potential of early infant development was
finally recognized. Out of an era of mechanistic behaviorism advocated by B. F. Skinner, there gradually grew an understanding of
the latent and hidden capabilities of the newborn human infant—
capabilities that needed to be stimulated and nurtured in certain
ways at certain times in order to develop to full maturity.

Foremost in fostering this understanding were individuals
such as Chomsky, Piaget, Lennenberg, Apgar, Spock, and, more
recently, Brazelton. The thoughts, works, and contributions of
these scientists have extended the purview of the developing
infant to other related professionals while recognizing the important roles played by the parent and family.

Nearly all professions have a stake in the human newborn
infant; hardly a specialty exists that does not claim a part of this
emergent organism. Audiologists may focus their attentions on the
hearing mechanism of the infant, but hearing does not exist in a
vacuum; it is part of a complicated, interrelated, living, breathing,
thinking organism that sustains the auditory response and, in
turn, is modified by it.

The skills that are most interrelated with hearing are linguis-
tics and speech. Both develop in the normal infant through hearing—albeit in different ways. Speech is an "overlaid" function,
dependent on auditory feedback to initiate muscular and proprio-
ceptive activity in organs created for other purposes. Normal development and production of speech is dependent on the presence of
normal hearing. Speech production intelligibility is directly propor-
tional to the degree of hearing loss in children with hearing impairment. In other words, the better the hearing, the better the speech.

Not so for language. Language skills of children with hearing
impairment appear to be fairly equally affected by almost any

degree of hearing loss between 40 and 100 dB HL. The only factor that significantly affects language abilities in young deafened children is the time of intervention. In other words, the earlier the intervention, the better the language skills.

Of course, this complex development leading to speech and language depends on normal development of the central nervous system. The brain of the newborn has more neurons than can ever be utilized, but the neurons lack the special synaptic connections that will make them functional. These connections are formed only by input from the five senses—inputs that form the synapses and link the neurons into an efficient sensory system capable of serving the needs of the developing human.

It is well known that a great deal of sensory input is effective long before birth. We know that the fetus hears, and even responds to, sound for approximately 4 months before birth. In the case of hearing, the infant emerges with many synapses already formed—enough synapses have been connected to allow a newborn to distinguish his or her mother's voice from the voices of other adult females.

One of the main tasks at birth, beyond basic survival, is combining all of the sensory inputs to develop the latent language potential that lies in every human organism. It is this potential for language that must concern us most because it is dependent on adequate functioning of the auditory system. For many years, questions have been raised as to the critical time schedule for developing normal language; only recently have the carefully controlled studies of matched young subjects been conducted to show us that the first few months of life are indeed decisive in forming basic language skills.

Based on these facts, one is struck with the realization that what we do with infants and young children during those important first 3 years of life will likely mold their futures forever. We work zealously to detect hearing loss in infants and to begin language intervention as soon as possible. Our goal is that all infants with hearing loss will achieve their full potentials and attain the best future possible.

These observations challenge us to utilize the particular skills that we acquired during our education and training. Our unique knowledge of the interrelated aspects of hearing, speech, and language is an important contribution to understanding the wonder of communication development in infants. If, with this knowledge, we can enhance and enrich the lives of infants and families, it will be a good beginning.

After 30 years of advocating for the early identification of hearing impairment in infants, I welcome this textbook for its extension of our knowledge about the newborn. It is clearly time to gather the information available about infant hearing from the many diverse and different professions working with infants, and to publish these materials in one book. The audiologist's task is to identify hearing problems and to understand auditory disorders—an especially difficult task in the infant. To this end, we must constantly hone our skills and technologies to a fine point. We will all be greatly helped through the efforts of Drs. Hayes and Northern to produce this compendium of information and insight into infant's hearing care and needs.

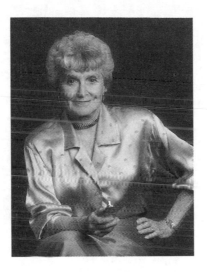

Marion P. Downs, M.A., D.H.S
Professor Emerita
University of Colorado School of
Medicine
Denver, Colorado

SECTION I

Perspectives on Infant Hearing

CHAPTER 1

The Quest for Early Identification of Hearing Loss

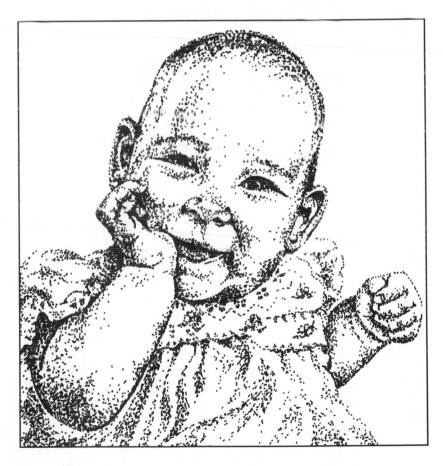

One of the most crucial factors in any child's development is the acquisition of spoken language. Spoken language is the doorway to successful communication and the social interaction which is so important to normal human development. Language is the key to the door by which we express our thoughts, needs, and feelings and by which we receive and comprehend the thoughts, needs, and feelings from others (McConnell and Liff, 1975). The acquisition and development of language, which ultimately leads to the two-way communication process that is the path to education and the full enrichment of life, is highly dependent on an adequate auditory system. Thus, it is our sense of hearing that actually opens the door to intellectual achievement. It is true, as the proverb says, "As we hear, so shall we speak."

It is this intimate relationship between speech, language, and hearing that has fascinated man since the beginning of time. Many believe that language is inherent in each child's maturation, needing only the appropriate environment to trigger the process. Speech and language are naturally and easily acquired by most children. As parents, we give little thought to its expression, except to delight as our young children mimic our vocalizations and speech patterns. We listen with awe as sounds develop into phonemes, then into words, and finally into sentences complete with meaning, intent, and significance.

However, the child with hearing loss does not automatically develop speech and may be confronted with a life of language difficulties and educational struggles. Because hearing loss in infants typically is a silent and hidden handicap, identification and treatment of the problem is often delayed. Undetected hearing loss can lead to delayed or impaired speech and language development, social and emotional problems, underachievement and academic failure.

Language develops so rapidly in the first few months of life that the longer an infant's hearing loss goes undetected, the worse the outcome is likely to be. However, many of the negative effects of hearing loss on a child's development can be prevented, or at least substantially lessened, if intervention and training are initiated early in life. Research has confirmed that early intervention with infants who have hearing impairment may result in improved language development, increased communication skills, and higher educational achievement. Although the most important period for speech and language development is generally regarded as the first 3 years of life, the average age of identification of hearing impairment in young children in the United States is nearly 3 years (NIH Consensus Statement, 1993).

Despite the advanced level of medical care in the United States, we have few programs in place to detect significant hearing loss in infants in the general newborn population. Because we do have the technology to identify hearing loss in infants at birth, this situation is truly unacceptable. Unfortunately, fewer than 5% of all newborns in the United States are screened for hearing prior to 3 months of age. In fact, all too often, identification of a child's hearing loss is delayed because parents are unaware that any child, even a newborn infant, can receive an accurate hearing test. Routine medical care seldom includes concern for hearing and a simple hearing test to identify those infants with hearing loss. Ideally, the hearing of every infant should be screened before discharge from the hospital. And, once the infant with hearing loss is identified, medical and/or audiological intervention can be initiated immediately (American Academy of Audiology, 1988). But the solution to the problem of early identification is not so simple.

The value of health screening is under constant scrutiny and criticism from science and medicine in terms of economic, political, and sociological implications. Public health experts do not agree on whether routine screening for any health problem, be it early identification of cancer, determination of cholesterol levels, or even screening for psychological depression, provides significant positive benefit in our health care system. The critics argue that health screening cannot achieve 100% accuracy, and guaranteed treatment outcomes cannot be achieved for most screened diseases. Therefore, continued focus on medical screening will result in anguish and dilemmas for the persons screened.

All screening tests include a certain error rate. The screening tests identify some false-positive cases (indications of a problem when none actually exists) and some false-negative cases (findings of no disease when disease actually is present). Economists worry that the screening of symptom-free people will bankrupt health programs because of the actual costs of the screening program and the expense of diagnostic follow-up of all screening failures. Medical scientists are developing new and more accurate health screening tests faster than they can develop and evaluate new treatments for the screened diseases. Thus, in the midst of dynamic health care reform, serious questions remain regarding the true value to our society of all public health screening programs.

And what about the hearing screening of newborns? Infant hearing screening has always generated controversy. Questions regarding the effectiveness of infant hearing screening and the value of early intervention have been discussed for nearly 40 years. Although general agreement exists that hearing impairment in infants is a serious condition that creates lifelong disability, only 14 states reported having formal infant hearing screening programs in place in the early 1990s (Blake and Hall 1990).

PREVALENCE OF CHILDHOOD HEARING LOSS

It is surprising that after nearly four decades of debating the need and value of early identification of hearing loss, few data exist regarding the actual prevalence of childhood deafness in the general population. Most research reports are based on small samples of "inadequately collected and vaguely described data which lead to conclusions that are uncertain and inaccurate" (Mauk and Behrens, 1993, p. 2). Published estimates of the incidence of childhood deafness vary widely because of different criteria for significant hearing loss used by different researchers. Differences in nonstandardized infant screening procedures, differences in the definition of hearing loss, lack of confirming follow-up of identified infants, and verification of "passed" infants to have normal hearing, as well as the inherent inaccuracies of retrospective studies, have all contributed to the inability to generalize results of specialized sample studies to the population as a whole. Further, when mild, unilateral, or conductive hearing losses are included in the statistical analysis, the estimate is considerably higher than when only permanent, bilateral hearing loss is the basis of the estimate.

For many years, 1 deaf child per 1,000 live births was the accepted and quoted prevalence of hearing loss in children. However, this 1:1000 estimate was based on the identification of newborns with congenital, profound, bilateral, sensorineural hearing loss of 80 dB HL or greater. This prevalence estimate was often questioned because it failed to include (a) the higher incidence of sensorineural hearing loss among infants with developmental disabilities and (b) well babies with a lesser degree of sensorineural hearing loss. Considering that the prevalence rate for mild-to-moderate developmental disabilities in the general population is greater than the prevalence rate of profound disabilities, 3 infants with significant hearing impairment per 1,000 may be a more realistic (although still conservative) estimate of prevalence for the well-baby population. Then, adjusting the prevalence rate to account for infants at risk for developmental disability and well babies with moderate, severe, or profound sensorineural hearing loss yields a prevalence estimate of 6 babies with significant hearing loss for every 1,000 births (Hayes and Northern, 1994).

AN HISTORICAL PERSPECTIVE

Review of the history of infant hearing screening in the United States reveals the major issues of concern that have arisen through the years. The changing emphasis in health care priorities is also represented in a review of the various attempts at establishing early identification of hearing loss programs on a national basis.

The Early Years, 1955–1970

Infant hearing testing was not given much credence prior to a report from Sir Alexander and Lady Ewing of England (1944). The Ewings used various percussion sounds and pitch pipes to elicit "aural reflex responses" in young children. They reported that auditory responses could be easily observed in infants during the first 6 months of life, but these reflexive responses to sounds were actually more difficult to observe as the infants grew older. The Ewings also reported their observation that, with their testing techniques, deaf children did not show any response to sound.

The origins of newborn hearing screening can be traced to Sweden. In 1956, Wedenberg reported that "the most easily observable response of an infant to sound is the auro-palpebral reflex, i.e., a rapid and distinctive closing of the eyelids when they are open and a screwing of them when they (eyelids) are closed" (p. 446). Wedenberg performed hearing tests on 20 infants, between 1 and 10 days of age, to pure tone stimulus presentations at 105 to 115 dB SPL (sound pressure level). He observed two infant responses to indicate the presence of normal hearing, (a) the auro-palpebral reflex threshold and (b) determination of the intensity at which the infant could be awakened from sleep. Wedenberg reported difficulties in the determination of the auro-palpebral reflex threshold and questioned the reliability of the response in both sleeping and awake infants.

A few years later, Carl-Axel Froding (1960) of Eskilstuna, Sweden evaluated the hearing of 2,000 newborns using a small gong and mallet which produced a sound of 126–133 dB SPL. His technique was to observe the auro-palpebral reflex in quiet or sleeping infants. Froding was also puzzled by the lack of consistency (reliability) in the infants' responses, stating that "Even if the child is awake, it might sometimes occur that the reflex cannot be produced at the first stroke but only after some minutes, and it is not always possible to produce another reflex directly after the first one. It will often be necessary to wait one or two

minutes" (p. 34). Nonetheless, Froding's success in eliciting positive auro-palpebral reflex responses in 96.1% of the 2,000 infants
(some of whom had positive hearing reflexes within the first half-
hour after birth) led him to conclude that "Perhaps the time has
now come for us to discuss whether an examination of the hearing
of newborn infants should not be made obligatory" (p. 40).

The initial study of newborn hearing screening in the United
States came from a research project conducted by Marion Downs,
an audiologist, and Graham Sterrit, a psychologist. Downs and
Sterrit (1964) teamed to conduct a city-wide project in Denver,
Colorado to test all the babies born during a 1-year period. Using
trained volunteers, and a specially designed, hand-held, battery-
operated infant hearing "screener" with a sudden onset stimulus
of 90 dB SPL (a noise band stimulus centered at 3000 Hz), more
than 17,000 newborns were evaluated. Their clinical screening
protocol required the volunteers to rate the presence or absence of
behavioral responses immediately following the presentation of the
stimulus (Figure 1–1). Downs and Sterrit (1964), realizing the subjective nature of this rating system, attempted to establish standard response criteria to verify that the subtle responses from the
infant were indeed reaction to the onset of the auditory stimulus.
Their protocol required teams of two trained persons to agree on
the presence or absence of infant hearing responses.

Although the Downs and Sterrit project successfully identified
nine profoundly deaf babies during the year of the study, the
researchers' review of their data raised questions concerning the
reliability and validity of newborn hearing screening based on
subjective behavioral observation. Downs and Sterrit noted a
number of false-negative results, babies who "passed" the infant
screening procedure but were identified at a later age to have significant hearing impairment. Their concerns about using trained
volunteers to note subtle behavioral responses in the infants
served as incentive to other researchers to develop specific test
protocols which would provide more objective means of identifying
infant behavioral responses to sound.

Despite numerous efforts from various researchers, none of
the studies produced an accepted protocol. Wedenberg (1971) concluded that the only reliable and valid auditory response from an
infant should be arousal from sleep. The lack of confidence in
behaviorally based mass infant hearing screening led Bergstrom,
Hemenway, and Downs (1971) to recommend the use of high-risk
factors to identify infants at risk for deafness. They argued that, if
the majority of deaf babies could be identified through a high-risk
register system, there would be no need for hearing screening of

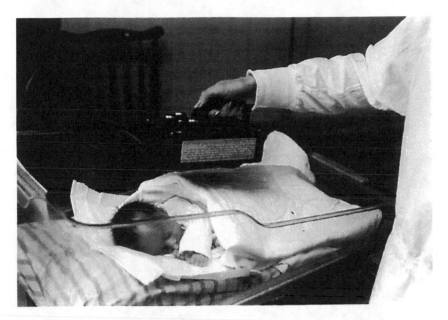

FIGURE 1-1. A specially designed battery-powered infant hearing screener used in the early 1960s known as the Apriton (from the auropalpebral reflex, the involuntary body movement and eye blink resulting from sudden sound onset). The examiner presented a sudden onset narrow-band noise stimulus of 90 dB SPL followed by observation for the presence or absence of reflexive infant responses.

the entire newborn population. Only newborns identified with a "high-risk factor for deafness" would need to be screened.

In 1969, Marion Downs approached the American Speech and Hearing Association with a request that a national joint committee, composed of representatives from professional hearing health care organizations, be formed to evaluate the status of newborn hearing screening (Downs, 1986). This group, to be known as the Joint Committee on Infant Hearing, was formed with members from the Academy of Pediatrics, the Academy of Ophthalmology and Otolaryngology, and the American Speech and Hearing Association. The Joint Committee met in early 1970 to review newborn hearing research reports including the use of auditory behavioral observation screening with calibrated noise-band stimuli as described by Downs and Sterrit (1964, 1967). The Joint Committee also discussed the concept of a high-risk register for deafness.

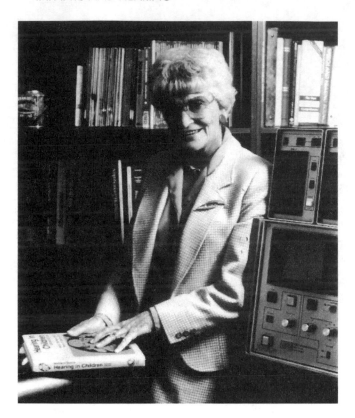

Marion P. Downs is an internationally noted audiologist who was among the first to draw attention to the need for early identification and intervention for infants with hearing loss. As an outspoken advocate for screening hearing in infants, she pioneered and developed audiometric techniques for screening hearing in infants and young children. Her numerous publications and teaching brought worldwide attention to the importance of early habilitation for deafness and alerted the medical world to the intellectual and developmental problems associated with childhood deafness.

The Formative Years, 1970–1980

The Joint Committee on Infant Hearing issued a statement early in 1970 which is reprinted in Appendix A. The statement concluded that review of data from studies of mass infant hearing screening with behavioral observation showed results that were inconsistent and confusing. Prior to reaching a decision about whether mass hearing screening of newborns should be indeed instituted, the Joint Committee recommended further study of a number of the many variables that might affect the results of infant hearing screening programs.

The 1970 Joint Committee on Infant Hearing report recommended that additional research was needed to evaluate various stimulus parameters, response patterns, environmental factors, infant status at the time of testing, and the skills of the observers. Furthermore, the Joint Committee suggested that confirmation of results obtained in the nursery must await data derived from extended follow-up studies based on quantitative assessment of the hearing status of the screened infants. In view of these concerns, the Joint Committee concluded that routine mass screening of newborn infants for hearing impairment could not be recommended without additional data.

An important conference on newborn hearing screening was sponsored jointly in 1971 by the national Maternal and Child Health Service and the California State Department of Public Health (Cunningham, 1971). A limited number of participants from a broad spectrum of disciplines was invited to represent both the proponent and the opponent viewpoints regarding newborn hearing screening. The proceedings of the conference report that, "as a result of the differences of opinion the broad spectrum of points of view represented would not be conducive to unanimity of conclusions. But the situation is not at all bleak; while we found the diversity we expected, we also found some broad areas of agreement." The conference participants drafted recommendations which suggested that a high risk for deafness in the infant population could and should be identified by prenatal history and postnatal physical assessment (see Appendix B).

During 1971, the original Joint Committee on Infant Hearing met again for further deliberations (Cunningham, 1971). In consonance with their 1970 statement, and in recognition of the facts that application of high-risk data could increase the detectability of congenital hearing impairment (Black et al., 1971), the Joint Committee established a list of five factors that would place an infant at risk for deafness. They recommended that all infants at risk for deafness should be identified by means of medical history and physical examination. Any infant identified to have one or more of the at-risk factors for deafness should be scheduled for hearing screening. Thus, in 1972, the Joint Committee issued a supplemental statement to their original 1970 position statement (see Appendix A) which listed five high-risk alerting factors for congenital deafness:

1. History of hereditary childhood hearing impairment;
2. Rubella or other nonbacterial intrauterine fetal infection (e.g., cytomegalovirus or herpes infection);
3. Defect of the ear, nose, or throat; malformed, low-set, or absent pinnae; cleft lip or palate (including submucous cleft); any residual abnormality of the otorhinolaryngeal system;
4. Birthweight less than 1500 grams;
5. Bilirubin level greater than 20 mg/100 ml serum.

The 1972 Position Statement recommended that at-risk infants were to be referred for an in-depth audiological evaluation of hearing during their first 2 months of life, and even if hearing appeared to be normal, the infant should receive regular hearing evaluations thereafter.

The 1972 Joint Committee divided the deafness risk categories into three sections: (1) factors identifiable by interview or written questionnaire with one parent (i.e., family history, rubella exposure or rash with fever during pregnancy, or parental concern for the baby's hearing); (2) factors identifiable by physical examination (i.e., abnormalities of the ears, nose,or throat); and (3) factors identifiable by review of the medical record (i.e., low birthweight or excessive bilirubin level). Downs and Silver (1972) suggested the "ABCDS" alphabetic acronym for easy recall of the high-risk register: Affected family; Bilirubin level; Congenital rubella syndrome; Defects of the ears, nose and throat; and Small at birth.

In 1974, experts from various disciplines who had familiarity with infant screening were invited to participate in an International Conference in Nova Scotia (Mencher, 1976). The conference participants presented data to compare infant hearing screening techniques and reported their results from various countries around the world. The conference proceedings were subsequently published and endorsed the use of the five-point high-risk register approach to early identification of hearing loss. The conference proceedings stated that the high-risk register approach should be supplemented with newborn behavioral observation hearing screening.

The international conference participants concluded that, by carefully defining the behavioral observation technique with specific attention to details and test variables, the number of incorrect infant passes and failures could be decreased. The Nova Scotia conference participants recommended auditory behavioral observation based on an arousal test, using a calibrated high-frequency noise-band of 90 dB SPL to awaken a sleeping baby. The protocol called for three stages: (1) a pretest observation period (15 seconds of observing the sleeping infant with eyes closed and no body movement) to determine the stage of sleep; (2) followed by a 2-second stimulus presentation; and then (3) tester observation of the infant for a response to occur within 3-seconds following cessation of the stimulus. Any infant activity before or after this specific time period was not to be considered as a response to sound. Further, the only response that was acceptable was arousal from sleep, that is (a) opening of the eyes, (b) stirring movement of the whole body, or (c) a strong and immediate eye-blink followed by a full-body response. In addition, the response must be seen and agreed on by two trained observers before the infant could be "passed" for hearing.

The Nova Scotia participants called for additional research to verify that (a) different stimuli activate different components of the auditory system; (b) different response criteria are selectively sensitive to different aspects of hearing disturbances; (c) different observers bring special sensitivities to the test procedures; and (d) different infants in different psycho-physiological states offer varying types of responses, each with different clinical meaning. To resolve these questions, these variables were to be controlled as carefully as possible (i.e., the acoustic stimulus must be specified as to its intensity and frequency [energy content], duration, rise and fall time [shape], interstimulus interval [pattern of presentation], and informational content). Response criteria must specify changes of infant behavior acceptable as a response differentiated from behavioral changes during control periods. The psycho-physiological state of the infant must be operationally defined, and the physical and physiological control of the environment must be fully described and, where possible, stabilized (Mencher, 1976). The recommendations from the Nova Scotia Conference on the Early Identification of Hearing Loss were adopted by the National Joint Committee on Infant Hearing Screening during November of 1974.

A national conference held in Ohio, sponsored by Maternal and Child Health Services in 1977, reaffirmed the 1972 Joint Committee recommendations for infant hearing screening based on the high-risk register protocol. Participants at the Ohio conference made supplementary suggestions which included (a) audiologic follow-up of the high-risk infants be made as soon as possible following identification, but certainly by 7 months of age; (b) the mother-child relationship be safeguarded by education;

(c) informed consent from a parent be obtained; (d) information regarding normal child development be provided; and (e) development and implementation of identification and diagnostic procedures related to hearing impairment be undertaken by public health agencies.

Also during the 1970s, considerable work was being conducted by a number of auditory researchers to develop objective, physiologically based hearing screening techniques which could replace the widely used subjective behavioral observation of infant responses to acoustic stimuli. Two techniques, the Crib-O-Gram and Auditory Brainstem Response Audiometry (described in Chapter 8), received attention as potentially powerful screening tools that could be used in mass infant hearing screening. Early publications of research studies on infants utilizing these two techniques had an important influence on future meetings of the Joint Committee on Infant Hearing Screening.

The Developmental Years, 1980–1989

During the early 1980s, the membership of the Joint Committee on Infant Hearing was enlarged to include the American Nurses' Association. Recognizing the need to update the position statement to meet changing high-risk criteria and incorporate new medical advances, the Joint Committee met in 1982 and issued a revised position statement relevant to the then-current practices of identifying hearing-impaired infants. The 1982 position statement expanded the risk criteria from five to seven factors. The two additional risk factors associated with deafness that were added to the list were bacterial meningitis caused by Haemophilus influenzae and severe asphyxia demonstrated by Apgar scores of 3 or lower (see Appendix C).

The 1982 Position Statement recommended that the hearing of infants who manifest any item on the list of risk criteria should be screened, under supervision of an audiologist, prior to 3 months of age, but no later than 6 months after birth. The initial screening was to be based on behavioral or electrophysiological response to sound. If consistent behavioral or electrophysiological responses were detected at appropriate sound levels, the screening process was to be considered complete except for infants who exhibited a risk factor related to late onset or progressive hearing loss. If results of the initial screening of an infant manifesting any risk criteria were equivocal, the infant was to be referred for full audiological assessment testing. The 1982 Position Statement also included, for the first time, procedures to be followed for the diagnostic work-up for infants failing the hearing screening, as well as management and habilitation recommendations for infants identified as hearing-impaired.

The Decade of the 1990s

The 1990s may well be remembered by hearing professionals as the decade of action regarding infant hearing screening. The Joint Committee on Infant Hearing did not meet again until 1990, at which time the Council on Education of the Deaf and the Directors of State Speech and Hearing Programs were added as voting members of the group. The Joint Committee was well aware that advances in science and medical technology had increased the chance of survival in markedly premature and low birthweight neonates and other severely compromised newborns. This improvement in survival rates was associated with a 2.5%–5.0% incidence of significant sensorineural hearing loss in at-risk infants. Accordingly, the 1990 Position Statement recommended that infants manifesting any of the previously noted risk criteria, warranted auditory screening. Although the Joint Committee rati fied their position statement in 1990, many of the professional groups did not actually publish the document until spring of 1991 (see Appendix D).

The 1990 Joint Committee expanded the previous position statement considerably. The document was divided into risk factors for neonates (defined as birth to 28 days) and for infants (age 29 days to 2 years). Detailed hearing screening recommendations for both groups were included. Optimally, the hearing screening was to be completed prior to the at-risk baby's discharge from the hospital, but no later than 3 months of age. Further, the Joint Committee stated that, because of the high false-positive and false-negative results related to behavioral observation screening, that the initial hearing screening should be based on the auditory brainstem response (ABR) test. With concern that the ABR technique could result in some false-positive results, ongoing assessment and observation of the infant's auditory behavior was recommended during the early intervention stages.

The 1990 Joint Committee on Infant Hearing statement reflected the influences of the two new professional society members with recommendations regarding early intervention for hearing-impaired infants and their families. These recommendations were included to bring the position statement into accordance with Public Law 99-457, enacted by Congress in 1986, known as the Education of the Handicapped Act Amendments, which required more and better services to young special-needs children and their families. Specifically, these amendments were concerned with care for handicapped children (birth through 2 years of age) and challenged professionals to reexamine existing programs and develop new services. Thus, the 1990 Joint Committee's recommendations included referral of the hearing-impaired infant to a number of specialists including a physician with expertise in the management of childhood otologic disorders; an audiologist experienced in pediatric hearing assessment techniques; and a speech-language pathologist, teacher of the hearing-impaired, or other professional with expertise in the assessment of communication skills in children with hearing impairment. Family education, counseling, and guidance, including home visits and parent support groups, represented the growing influence of the Joint Committee's concern for the adequate management of newborns with hearing loss.

The 1990 Joint Committee encouraged the continued study and critical evaluation of known and unknown risk factors and recognized that, because the recommended protocols might not be appropriate for all institutions, modifications might be appropriate to meet the specific needs of any given facility. Further, screening programs were urged to evaluate factors such as cost, availability of equipment, personnel, and follow-up services which are crucial in the development of infant hearing screening programs.

With the growing number of research reports from infant hearing screening projects based on the guidelines from the Joint Committee on Infant Hearing, it might be assumed that there would be a general proliferation of state-wide infant hearing screening programs by the early 1990s. Indeed, since the mid-1960s, infant hearing screening techniques had matured from gross behavioral observation of reflex responses to the precise electrophysiological evaluation of infants identified to be at risk for deafness. Mahoney (1986) presented a review of states in which infant hearing screening activities were under way. He reported that, in 1985, only six states had active statewide infant screening programs, three states had regional programs, and an additional seven states were "planning" statewide infant screening projects. Although eight states had a legislated mandate to implement statewide infant hearing screening, several of these states had not appropriated the financial support needed for such programs. In a later survey of states, Blake and Hall (1990) reported that, although 14 states had legislative mandates for screening, 25 other states still had no statewide policy regarding neonatal hearing screening. Blake and Hall cited reasons impeding legislative mandates as expense, state geography and population diversity, lack of consensus among professionals within the state on the most effective screening techniques, and lack of follow-up programs.

Public Awareness

The American Academy of Audiology (AAA) initiated a public awareness project in 1988 to educate the public about the importance of early identification of hearing loss in children. The AAA pointed out that routine pediatric medical care seldom includes the simple hearing evaluation that could identify children with hearing loss. In fact, according to the AAA, all too often, identification of a child's hearing loss is delayed because parents are unaware that any child, even a newborn infant, can receive an accurate hearing test. The AAA stated that "Ideally, the hearing of every infant should be screened before discharge from the hospital" (p. 1), and parents and professionals should be aware that no child is too young for a hearing test. When an infant with a hearing loss is identified, medical and audiological intervention should be initiated immediately.

The United States Public Health Service organized the Healthy People 2000 project to develop a national strategy for improving the health of the nation through a series of goals to be achieved by the turn of the century (U.S. Department of Health and Human Services, 1990). Healthy People 2000 focused on goals to reduce or prevent major chronic illnesses, injuries, and infectious diseases among Americans. Specific to solving the hearing problems of children was a goal to "reduce the average age at which children with significant hearing impairment are identified to no more than 12 months" (p. 118). C. Everett Koop, M.D., then Surgeon General of the United States Public Health Services, publicly advocated actions to reduce the delay in the average age of identification of deaf children in the United States. Dr. Koop summarized his feelings about this important issue by proclaiming himself "an optimist who could foresee a time in the near future when no child would reach his or her first birthday with an undetected hearing loss" (p. 1).

The NIDCD Consensus Conference

Another federal initiative relative to the growing awareness of the need for a national impetus for infant hearing screening came as the National Institute on Deafness and Other Communication Disorders (NIDCD) requested research proposals which addressed

The 1994 Joint Committee Position Statement

The Joint Committee on Infant Hearing convened in 1994 to reevaluate, and revise, if necessary, the 1990 Joint Committee Statement. In the intervening years, the Joint Committee membership had grown to include two additional organizations: the American Academy of Audiology and the Council for Education of the Deaf. The Council for Education of the Deaf is an umbrella organization which includes five separate societies serving the deaf: the Alexander Graham Bell Association of the Deaf, the Association of College Educators: Deaf and Hard of Hearing, the Convention of American Instructors of the Deaf, the Conference of Educational Administrators Serving the Deaf, and the National Association of the Deaf.

During their 1994 meetings, the Joint Committee gave careful consideration to the stated goals of the Healthy People 2000 initiative as well as the 1993 NIDCD Consensus Statement. Following a year of discussions and considerations, the 1994 Joint Committee on Infant Hearing endorsed the goal of universal detection of all infants with hearing loss as early as possible (Appendix F). The Joint Committee agreed that all newborns with hearing loss should be identified before 3 months of age, and all hearing impaired infants should be involved in intervention by 6 months of age.

Although the 1994 Position Statement endorsed universal infant hearing loss detection, the high-risk factors continued to be listed as "indicators" commonly associated with sensorineural and/or conductive hearing loss in newborns and infants. Other new concepts published in the 1994 Joint Committee Position Statement included identification of indicators associated with late-onset hearing loss and suggested procedures to monitor such infants. The adverse effects of fluctuating conductive hearing loss from persistent or recurrent otitis media with effusion were recognized, and monitoring procedures for such infants were recommended. The 1994 Joint Committee statement recommends provision of intervention services in accordance with Part H of the Individuals with Disabilities Education Act.

Within the procedural and technical considerations of the statement, the 1994 Joint Committee indicated that auditory brainstem response (ABR) hearing screening and otoacoustic emissions (OAE) screening each had advantages and disadvantages. The statement indicates that both of these physiological screening procedures outperform behavioral assessment for accuracy in identifying hearing impairment. In fact, the statement warns that behavioral measures cannot validly and reliably detect hearing loss of less than 30 dB HL in infants less than 6 months of age. The statement does not recommend any specific screening technique or program protocol, per se, but recognizes that infant hearing program protocols will likely vary by regional location, individual needs, and administrative structure.

Among the suggestions to facilitate establishment and maintenance of infant hearing programs, the Joint Committee recommended that a uniform state and national database be developed to enhance program evaluation. The database could be used to compare individual programs in terms of cost-benefit, quality assurance, and public policy development. The database could accompany a tracking system to insure that newborn infants identified with hearing loss, and infants identified to be at risk for hearing loss, have access to evaluation, follow-up, and intervention services. Additional research was suggested to provide systematic evaluation of techniques for identification, assessment, and intervention; refinement of the risk indicators; outcome studies to evaluate the impact of early identification of infants with hearing loss and their subsequent achievement of education and communication competence; as well as continued research into the prevention of hearing loss in newborns and infants.

IMPLEMENTATION OF INFANT SCREENING

The High-Risk Register Approach

Several methods of implementation of the high-risk register for deafness have been used in the United States. Usually, the programs are directed or supervised by a qualified audiologist. Although the hearing screening portion of the program must be carefully instituted and monitored, each program must also have a formalized strategy in place to insure that adequate follow-up of each identified child is completed. A major consideration is the requirement for personnel to conduct the many aspects of the program. Many programs depend on the utilization of trained volunteers from various community service groups. These trained volunteers are used to perform infant hearing screening, interview mothers, review hospital medical records, record test results, and ensure follow-up of failed babies as well as other administrative tasks. An obvious advantage to the use of trained volunteers is the low personnel cost; disadvantages are the attrition of volunteers over time, changes in the club's officers, or changes in direction of the service organization's activities.

Some state infant hearing screening programs depend on public health agencies to perform the administrative activities while regional audiologists conduct the actual hearing tests, determine referral patterns, and implement early intervention. The state of Utah is unique in its use of each newborn's birth certificate to record high-risk factors (Mahoney, 1984). In other states, the infant hearing screening programs are conducted through contracts developed by hospitals with community agencies (i.e., hearing, speech-language centers, group health cooperatives) or with private audiologists. These contracted services typically are provided on a fee-for-service basis as needed, especially in hospitals with a low number of annual births.

Application of the high-risk register to identify infants who would be considered at risk for hearing loss requires support from a team of professionals including the audiologist, the neonatologist, the pediatrician, the otolaryngologist, and nurses. The team cooperates to support the risk registry identification program which generally incorporates three stages: (a) face-to-face interviews with the mother of the baby; (b) visual observation of the infant specifically looking for defects such as malformation or abnormal location of the pinna, cleft lip or palate, or signs of syndromes associated with deafness; and (c) review of the medical records of the baby and the mother including the labor and delivery process.

Most of the early prevalence of hearing loss estimates were determined from high-risk register studies of newborns. By the early 1990s, however, evidence from numerous studies confirmed that use of the high-risk registry as the basis of infant hearing screening programs identified only 50% of infants with significant hearing loss (Elssman, Matkin, and Sabo, 1987; Mauk, White, Montenson, and Behrens, 1991; Pappas, 1983;). With recognition of the fact that fully one-half of the newborns with hearing impairment were being missed by the high-risk registry approach to early identification, the stage was set for consideration of new model programs and innovative technology to identify all newborns with significant hearing loss.

Numerous studies have confirmed that approximately 10% of all newborns fall within the risk factors for deafness (Galambos, Hick, and Wilson, 1984; Mahoney, 1984; Stein, Clark, and Kraus, 1983, 1990). Of the 3,700,000 live births in the United States during 1987, it was estimated that 7% to 12% were born with one or more of the risk factors associated with congenital deafness (Wegman, 1987). Of the infants at risk for deafness, 30 to 50 of every 1,000 are indeed hearing impaired (Galambos, Hick, and

Wilson, 1982; Hosford-Dunn, Johnson, Simmons, Malachowski, and Low, 1987; Simmons, 1976).

Universal Hearing Screening Programs

The Florida Universal Screening Experience

The first universal infant hearing program was formally established as a service in Winter Park Memorial Hospital in Florida in 1983 (Marlowe, 1993). This program offered automated ABR screening to every newborn as part of the routine care in the nursery. The program was designed to rely on trained volunteers to perform screenings in the newborn nursery after the parents signed a consent form. Some 15,000 infants were screened for hearing between 1983 and 1993 (approximately 80% of all births at Winter Park Memorial Hospital during this period of time). Additional benefits cited from this infant screening program include improved prenatal parent education regarding normal hearing and speech development as well as increased physician awareness that no child is ever too young for a hearing test. Success in this program is reportedly related to the overall low cost of the infant hearing screening protocol and the availability of trained volunteers to perform the testing.

The Colorado Program

Colorado has had a long and rich heritage of newborn screening aimed at the early identification of hearing loss beginning with the work of Marion Downs in the early 1960s. Currently, under the auspices of a the Colorado Department of Health, a volunteer statewide project involving some 22 hospitals is working to establish universal newborn hearing screening programs. Although no state legislative mandate exists, the project has monitored the births of some 37,000 newborns between 1993 and 1995. Of the 21,000 babies (57% of total births) who received a hearing screen with automated ABR prior to discharge, 1,500 (7%) were referred for additional audiometric evaluation. In this cohort of infants, 147 newborns were confirmed to have significant sensorineural or conductive hearing loss. These data reflect an incidence of bilateral or unilateral hearing loss of 4:1,000 births. No risk factors were present in 57% of the hearing loss group. The remaining 43% were found to have associated risk factors for congenital deafness. The Colorado experience confirms that universal infant hearing screening can identify mild to severe unilateral or bilateral hearing impairment in newborns prior to discharge from the hospital. To cite one example program from Colorado, the University Hospital has been conducting universal infant hearing screening for nearly 3 years. The program, supervised and directed by an audiologist utilizes trained volunteers who use automated ABR to screen the approximately 2,200 infants born each year. During the initial year of this hospital-based program (1992), 86% of all births received hearing screening with a 12% referral for additional audiologic testing. During the third year of the program, based on increased experience with their universal testing protocol, 93% of all births received hearing screening with a 7% referral rate. Achievement of 100% infant hearing screening is reportedly difficult to achieve because of a 12-hour discharge policy for mothers and well babies.

The Rhode Island Project

During 1990, the U.S. Office of Special Education sponsored a project in Rhode Island to evaluate the feasibility, validity, and efficiency of using the recently developed technique of transient evoked otoacoustic emissions (TEOAE) to screen the hearing of newborns. Early success of this program based on otoacoustic emission measurements led to implementation of a universal (all babies) infant screening strategy at Women and Infants Hospital of Rhode Island. By 1993, more than 12,000 infants had been screened for hearing in this research project, forming a substantial subject base from which to answer numerous research questions (White and Behrens, 1993).

Initial analysis of a subsample of 1,850 newborns from the normal nursery and the neonatal intensive care unit (NICU) accurately identified 11 infants with sensorineural hearing loss. An additional 37 infants failed the screening with conductive hearing impairment. Analysis of the results from this sample of 1,850 newborns revealed a prevalence rate of 5.9:1,000 for sensorineural hearing loss in newborns and a 20% overall rate for conductive hearing loss. As expected, the hearing loss prevalence rates of 304 NICU babies were 23% sensorineural hearing loss and 36% conductive hearing. These figures are considerably higher than noted in the well-baby nurseries (White, Vohr, and Behrens, 1993).

These results from the Rhode Island Hearing Assessment Project, and their reported success with transient otoacoustic emissions hearing screening, had considerable influence on the recommendations made by the 1993 NIDCD Consensus Development Conference on Early Identification of Hearing Impairment in Infants and Young Children. The reported success of the Rhode Island project, and the relative ease with which they incorporated otoacoustic emission measurement into universal newborn hearing screening, led the NIDCD Panel of experts to recommend the two-stage screening protocol described earlier in this chapter.

Opposition to the Early Identification of Hearing Loss

Discussions regarding infant hearing screening always generate debate. Although early identification for purposes of early intervention may seem logical to many, others are quick to voice opposing viewpoints. For example, approval of the Position Statement of the 1994 Joint Committee stalled while waiting for votes from the member organizations. During the lengthy delay period, one of the five organization members of the Council for Education of the Deaf, the National Association of the Deaf (NAD), requested the Joint Committee to delete reference to amplification devices such as hearing aids and cochlear implants which are mentioned in the document. It is suggested in the 1994 Position Statement that the parents and care providers of identified infants be made aware of all intervention options including hearing aids, personal FM systems, vibrotactile aids, and/or cochlear implants. This philosophy is in direct contrast to the Deaf Culture movement supported by the National Association of the Deaf (NAD). The deaf community holds that they are, in fact, an "ethnic" minority with a specific cultural identity, and not a handicapped group of persons with disability (Dolnick, 1993).

When the other Joint Committee member organizations opted to retain the original early intervention options language in the 1994 Position Statement, the NAD did not approve the final document. A second organization of the Council for Education of the Deaf, the Conference of Educational Administrators Serving the Deaf, stood with the NAD and did not approve the statement as written. This action from two of their member societies, thereby, eliminated endorsement of the 1994 Position Statement by the Council for Education of the Deaf.

Despite the national mandates supporting universal infant hearing screening, an editorial commentary was written in opposition by Bess, an audiologist, and Paradise, a pediatrician (1994). They characterized universal infant hearing screening as "not simple, not risk-free, not necessarily beneficial, and not presently justified" (p. 330). Bess and Paradise challenged the conclusions of the 1993 NIDCD Consensus Symposium and the expert panel recommendations for a two-stage screening protocol. This critical commentary impugned infant hearing screening and questioned the effectiveness and need for early intervention for infants with hearing loss.

The Bess and Paradise commentary ignited widespread response from professionals defending the importance of infant hearing screening and early intervention and the failure of the status quo of the high-risk register approach to identification of infants with hearing loss. In a series of Letters to the Editor (*Pediatrics*, 94:6, 948–963, 1994), most respondents indicated that ample data exist to support infant hearing screening and early intervention as an important health policy in the United States. Northern and Hayes (1994) concluded that, as advocates for children with hearing loss, professionals must improve strategies for early identification and intervention and continue open discussions and debates about the most effective protocol for screening hearing in infants.

The developmental history of infant hearing screening has covered more than 40 years. This time period has been marked by discussions and debates about recommended techniques and pro cedures, development of factors to identify newborns at risk for hearing loss, national consensus meetings and professional society statements. These activities led to four irrefutable facts about hearing impairment in early childhood summarized by Northern and Hayes (1994):

1. Sensorineural hearing impairment in infants and young children is a serious condition which results in lifelong disability.
2. Early intervention is essential for facilitating speech, language and cognitive skills, social-emotional development, and academic achievement.
3. Dependence on a high-risk registry as the means to screen infants will identify less than 50% of infants with significant hearing loss.
4. Valid screening techniques, with proven acceptable sensitivity and specificity, are available to detect significant hearing impairment in infants.

Implementation of a national universal program for infant hearing screening will undoubtedly require ongoing research and substantial commitment from a wide variety of health professionals, health agencies, third-party payers, educators, and parents. Future decisions for universal infant hearing screening will depend on results from preliminary wide-scale newborn screening programs. There can no longer be any question, however, that implementation of infant hearing screening and concomitant early intervention programs are important steps toward improving outcomes for infants and young children with hearing loss.

SUGGESTED READINGS

Cherow, E., Matkin, N., and Trybus, R. (1985). *Hearing-Impaired Children and Youth with Developmental Disabilities.* Washington, DC: Gallaudet College Press.
A multiauthored text that discusses the problems and suggests solutions for the assessment and needs of the hearing-impaired population from birth to 21 years of age.
Paul, P., and Quigley, S. (1994). *Language and Deafness* (2nd Ed.). San Diego: Singular Publishing Group.
Overview textbook on all aspects of language acquisition and assessment in hearing-impaired infants and children.

CHAPTER 2

Components of an Infant Hearing Program

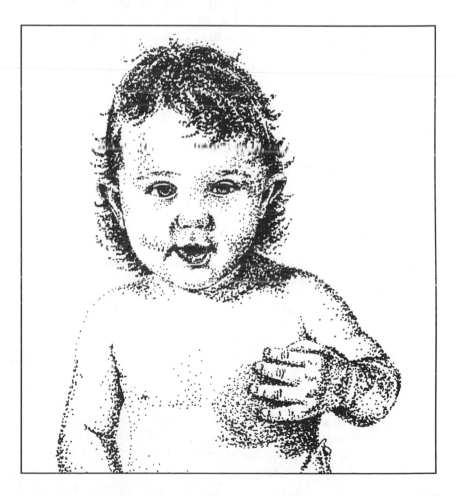

*T*here is a substantial professional literature describing results of hearing screening programs for infants and young children. Almost 50 years ago, Sir Alexander and Lady Ewing in England described a technique to test hearing of young children (Ewing and Ewing, 1947). In the 1950s, investigators in the United States applied this procedure, distraction audiometry, in public health screening of infants age 3 weeks to 1 year (Hardy, Dougherty, and Hardy, 1959). By the early 1960s, Marion Downs and her colleagues moved hearing screening of infants into newborn nurseries (Downs and Sterritt, 1964). This creative approach stimulated rapid technological development and led to innovative screening techniques such as the Crib-o-gram and the auditory response cradle. In a seminal investigation, Schulman-Galambos and Galambos (1979) described application of a newly reported auditory evoked potential, the auditory brainstem response (ABR), to hearing screening of newborn infants. Their pioneering clinical research initiated a new era of infant hearing screening and demonstrated the feasibility and practicality of identifying hearing loss in newborn and even premature infants. Today, there are more than 400 articles in the peer-reviewed literature describing hearing screening of infants, including several dozen articles on the newest approach, otoacoustic emissions (OAE). There are far fewer articles, however, describing the more complex task of developing a comprehensive infant hearing program (CIHP) of screening, diagnostic assessment, parent counseling, and aural habilitation.

In 1986, the United States Congress reauthorized and amended Public Law 94-142 (The Education of the Handicapped Act) to include mandatory special education services to preschool children age 3 to 5 years (Roush and McWilliams, 1990). This legislation, Public Law 99-457 (subsequently the Individuals with Disabilities Education Act [IDEA]), also included terms (Part H) to fund services to infants age birth to 3 years with developmental disabilities and their families. Part H of IDEA provided substantial incentives for states to develop comprehensive, multidisciplinary early identification and intervention services for infants and toddlers. Part H addresses multiple provisions of early identification and intervention including (a) eligibility criteria for early intervention; (b) guidance for identification, coordination, and referral procedures; (c) principles for comprehensive, multidisciplinary assessment; and (d) a mechanism of family-centered care, the individualized family service plan (IFSP). To receive the services specified in Part H, families typically interact with a wide spectrum of providers and agencies. A comprehensive infant hearing program provides both the range of needed services and coordination of these services for each infant and family.

COMPONENTS OF A COMPREHENSIVE INFANT HEARING PROGRAM

Because the technology used in hearing screening and evaluation of infants is sophisticated and relatively new, it is sometimes enthusiastically applied before development of a thorough follow-up and management program. Before a single infant is screened for hearing loss, an adequate program should be in place to provide appropriate diagnosis, parent counseling, and infant habilitation services.

To deliver a complete program, a CIHP is built on a foundation of the expertise and commitment of a wide variety of professionals; access to a broad spectrum of advanced technology; collaboration of health, social service, and educational agencies; and adequate funding from public and private sources. In addition to hearing screening, the program must provide hearing evaluation for infants referred from screening; medical, genetic, and developmental evaluation and diagnosis; amplification and aural habilitation; and parent support, counseling, and education.

In the classic text, *Auditory Disorders in Children A Manual For Differential Diagnosis*, Myklebust (1954) devoted an entire chapter to "Professional Specialization and Auditory Disorders in Young Children." He identified professionals in the following disciplines as important participants in the differential diagnosis of auditory disorders in young children: otolaryngology, pediatrics, neurology, child psychiatry, clinical psychology, audiology, speech pathology, and special education. Myklebust argued that the most appropriate diagnostic and therapeutic services are provided when the services provided by these specialists are integrated. To foster integration of services, Myklebust proposed changing professional training to include an orientation to the other disciplines providing services to young children with auditory disorders. He further recognized the importance of service coordination. Myklebust presented his conviction that coordination and integration of services is necessary for maximum benefit to children. More than three decades before described

(continued)

(continued)

in public law, Myklebust defined the role of multidisciplinary assessment and the importance of coordination of services to infants and young children with auditory disorders and their families.

Myklebust, H. (1954). *Auditory Disorders in Children: A Manual for Differential Diagnosis*. New York: Grune and Stratton.

Personnel

Primary Team Members

Parents.   Of course, parents are the most important members of an individual infant's team. Because parents have a unique influence on the infant's development, their roles, rights, and responsibilities, cannot be overemphasized. Parents do not anticipate the birth of a baby with disabilities. They may not be able to mobilize resources immediately to meet their infant's habilitative needs. Nonetheless, the infant hearing program team must include the full participation of parents to enable the infant's development within the family context.

Professionals with a wide variety of expertise should be available to provide diagnostic and habilitative services. Regardless of whether a CIHP is administered in a hospital, private practice, or educational setting, professionals in the disciplines of healthcare and medicine, education, and social services provide direct or consultative services. Members of the professional team who will have an ongoing commitment and continuous relationship with the infant and family include audiologists, speech-language pathologists, social workers, otolaryngologists, and pediatricians. Members whose contributions may be either ongoing or limited to a single diagnostic evaluation or consultation include healthcare, medical, and other professionals such as neurologists, neonatalogists, geneticists, nurses, occupational therapists, physical therapists, and special educators. Table 2–1 lists characteristics of expertise and education/credentials of primary professional personnel commonly associated with a CIHP.

Audiologist.   Audiologists provide diagnostic evaluation of hearing and habilitation services for hearing impairment including amplification devices and habilitative instruction. These professionals receive extensive training in psychoacoustics, electronic instrumentation, auditory development, auditory pathology and dysfunction, speech and language development, aural habilitation and rehabilitation, hearing measurement, electrophysiologic measurement, and related coursework.

Audiologists provide expertise in the evaluation of infant hearing and management of hearing loss through hearing aids and other amplification devices. Because of their extensive training in electrophysiologic measurement techniques and behavioral assessment of hearing, they can determine the degree and configuration of hearing loss, probable site of auditory dysfunction, ear symmetry, and stability of hearing loss in individual children. Audiologists will provide initial identification of hearing loss and evaluate the baby's hearing frequently during the early months following identification. They will also provide family guidance and counseling regarding amplification and, in conjunction with other team members, assist the family in making choices about the most appropriate intervention strategies. Based on ongoing observation and evaluation of the child's development, the audiologist should assist in identification of other developmental problems which require additional evaluation.

Table 2-1. Expertise and education/credentials of primary professionals who participate in a comprehensive infant hearing program.

Profession	Expertise	Education/Credential
Audiologist	Hearing evaluation and habilitation; hearing aids	Master's or doctoral degree National certification State license
Speech-language pathologist	Speech-language evaluation and habilitation; communication system development	Master's or doctoral degree National certification State license
Social worker	Psychosocial evaluation; counseling	Master's or doctoral degree State license
Otolaryngologist	Medical diagnosis; medical/surgical treatment of ear disease	Medical degree Board certification State license
Pediatrician/ Family Physician	Medical management of general health and development	Medical degree Board certification State license

Provision and monitoring of appropriate amplification is especially critical for infants with hearing loss. Audiologists often fit hearing aids on babies before comprehensive information is available on all aspects of the infant's hearing. For this reason, the audiologist must monitor frequently the baby's development, auditory responsiveness, and adjustment to hearing aids. As additional information becomes available, the audiologist can adjust the hearing aid settings to optimize amplification. Any evidence of the infant's rejection of amplification demands rapid and thorough evaluation of the appropriateness of the fitting. In addition, because successful use of hearing aids by infants is unconditionally related to parental understanding and commitment to amplification, the audiologist must provide ongoing education and training to parents.

Speech-Language Pathologist. Speech-language pathologists provide evaluation of speech and language function and intervention for disorders of speech and language development which may include auditory training; speech and language stimulation; home-based, family-centered intervention; and sign language instruction. These professionals receive extensive training in speech science, language development, normal communication processes, disorders of communication, assessment procedures, and habilitation and rehabilitation techniques for congenital and acquired disorders of speech and language, and related coursework.

Speech-language pathologists provide expertise on speech and language development and intervention for delays secondary to hearing loss. Because of their extensive training in normal communication processes, they can assess the impact of hearing loss on communication skills and speech and language development.

Early intervention through aural habilitation is essential to minimize the impact of hearing loss on communication development. By building the infant's repertoire of skills through auditory training, sound-object association, communication intent, and development of a language system, the speech-language pathologist ensures that the infant will achieve milestones in communication development at an appropriate rate. This professional will assume an essential role in parent counseling because, with the family, he or she may develop and monitor home-intervention strategies based on the family's communication style, strengths, and goals. In conjunction with the audiologist and other team members, the speech-language pathologist can assist the parents in making informed choices about the infant's communication style.

In some settings, the role of the speech-language pathologist may be assumed or supplemented by an educator with specialty training in services to infants with hearing impairment. These spe-

A valuable resource to professionals who provide services to infants with hearing impairment and their families is *The Hereditary Hearing Impairment Resource Registry* (HHIRR), a program established by the National Institute on Deafness and Other Communication Disorders (NIDCD) of the National Institutes of Health (NIH). The HHIRR disseminates information about hereditary hearing impairment and current research in this field to clinicians and their patients. In addition, the registry matches interested individuals with hearing impairment and their families to appropriate research projects. The HHIRR publishes a quarterly newsletter which includes articles on heredity, hearing loss, and related research. The newsletter is written specifically for families and professionals other than geneticists. A second quarterly publication, the *HHIRR Bulletin*, covers similar topics but is written for professionals with expertise in genetics. Reprints of articles from these publications are available at no cost as "Fact Sheets" for distribution to families, clinicians, researchers, and others interested in hereditary hearing impairment. The HHIRR has a toll-free, 24 hour, V/TTY phone number: (800) 320-1171. The e-mail address is: NIDCD.HHIRR@boystown.org; the World Wide Web site is: http://www.boystown.org.hhirr/. The Web site contains: a description of the NIDCD HHIRR, an electronic demographic survey, all current Fact Sheets, and descriptions of all current collaborating research projects.

cialists typically are state-licensed teachers with certification in early childhood special education.

Otolaryngologist. An otolaryngologist is a medical professional with specialty training in diagnosis and treatment of disorders of the ear, nose, throat, head and neck. Otolaryngologists receive extensive training in congenital and acquired disorders of the ear, nose, throat, head, and neck, medical bases of hearing loss, and medical and surgical treatment for disorders of the ear, nose, throat, head and neck, as well as disorders of hearing.

Otolaryngologists often provide diagnosis of the etiology of hearing loss in infants. Through a complete medical history, physical examination, radiographic and laboratory assessment, and integration of information from the audiologic assessment, the otolaryngologist may identify the underlying cause of hearing loss and the potential for medical and/or surgical treatment. This professional will provide ongoing assessment of the baby's middle ear status and the development of additional hearing loss from other medical causes.

Based on etiology, otolaryngologists can identify the potential for fluctuation or progression of hearing loss or genetic transmission of hearing loss. In the absence of conclusive identification of the underlying etiology, and in conjunction with audiologic assessment, he or she will monitor and treat any fluctuation and/or progression in hearing loss. If the etiology of hearing loss is genetic, the otolaryngologist can inform parents of the risk of hearing loss for future children and the risk of hearing loss in off-spring of the affected infant. Because hearing loss may be the first manifestation of syndromal disorders that affect development, the otolaryngologist will monitor many aspects of the baby's health and medical condition.

Federal regulations require that all children under 18 years of age receive medical clearance prior to hearing aid fitting. Therefore, the otolaryngologist must assess the medical status of the baby's ears prior to amplification. This ensures that infants receive medical and/or surgical treatment as appropriate, and that any medical condition contraindicating hearing aid use (e.g., draining ears) is identified and treated.

Pediatrician/Family Physician. A pediatrician is a medical professional who specializes in health and medical care of children. He or she contributes expertise in general development and knowledge about the effects of health and disease on overall child development.

In many locations, medical services to children are provided by Family Physicians. These medical specialists provide health care to individuals of all ages and are often physician to the infant, his or her siblings and parents. They receive specialty residency training in family medicine.

Pediatricians and family physicians are critical in monitoring the overall health and development of the infant. They evaluate the baby's growth and development and provide referral for additional medical and developmental assessments as required. These physicians provide important counseling and reassurance to parents about the baby's overall health and developmental progress. Because they provide frequent medical evaluation through well-baby visits, pediatricians and family physicians may be the first to identify other medical consequences of syndromal anomalies. In most managed care health plans, the pediatrician or family physician is responsible for all referrals for medical and related services. For this reason, it is essential that professionals providing diagnostic and habilitative services to infants establish a firm working relationship with this primary healthcare provider.

Social Worker.   Social workers provide assessment of family functioning and assistance in resource identification for family support services. They provide valuable insight into overall family skills and interactions that enhance or interfere with optimum services to infants. Social workers receive extensive training in family dynamics, psychosocial function, reaction to loss and death, community resources, child protection services, and related coursework.

A social worker provides expertise in assisting the family in coping with the diagnosis of hearing loss. Parents of very young children are especially vulnerable to emotions of denial, guilt, shock and depression on diagnosis of their infant's hearing loss. In conjunction with other members of the CIHP team, a social worker can support the family in the grieving process and in acceptance of their infant's hearing impairment.

The social worker may also help the family identify resources for achieving or maintaining successful family functioning. Because basic needs for housing, food, medical care, and trans portation can take priority over an infant's needs for habilitation, a social worker can help the family identify and meet basic needs. Once the family's basic needs are met, the family can concentrate more fully on meeting the infant's medical and habilitation needs.

Service Coordinator   The efforts of an infant's team should be coordinated by a single individual who helps families through the complex and often confusing evaluation and intervention process. This person is identified as the service coordinator in Part H of IDEA. He or she may be any appropriate member of the team. In many settings, the audiologist or speech-language pathologist is the service coordinator.

The service coordinator assists the team in setting goals and priorities for assessment and intervention, organizes services provided to families, assists families in gaining access to early intervention, and coordinates team communication as needed for optimum care.

Table 2–2 summarizes responsibilities of the primary professional team members to the infant and family. All members of the team must be committed to timely communication with parents and other team members.

Additional Team Members

Family Support Members.   Other individuals important to the family may assume an influential role on an infant's team. These

Table 2–2. Responsibilities of primary professionals who participate in a comprehensive infant hearing program.

Professional	Responsibilities
Audiologist	Infant hearing screening and follow-up evaluation; hearing aid fitting and monitoring amplification; parent counseling, support, and education
Speech-language pathologist	Speech-language assessment and intervention; communication system development; parent counseling, support, and education
Social worker	Psychosocial evaluation; resource identification for nonmedical/habilitation needs; parent counseling, support, and education
Otolaryngologist	Medical diagnosis of hearing loss; medical/surgical treatment of hearing loss; identification of etiology and potential for fluctuation/progression of hearing loss; parent counseling and education
Pediatrician/ Family Physician	Medical evaluation and management of overall health and development; identification of syndromal and other anomalies; parent counseling, support, and education

persons may be other family members such as grandparents, aunts and uncles, or siblings, or they may the members of the family's close community such as neighbors, clergy, or godparents. Because parents may turn to these individuals for support and understanding, their inclusion into planning services is appropriate if requested by the parents.

Other professionals are frequently needed to provide consultative, diagnostic, or intervention services to infants with hearing loss and their families or to the professional team. These individuals may provide one-time assessment or participate more fully in the process through ongoing assessment and intervention.

Physical Therapist/Occupational Therapist. Physical therapists (PTs) and occupational therapists (OTs) provide developmental assessment of motor and adaptive skills in infants. Because hearing loss often occurs as one component of a complex developmental delay, other aspects of the infant's development should be assessed as appropriate. If habilitation for motor delays is needed, the PT or OT will become an integral member of the CIHP team and may provide habilitation in conjunction with the SLP and family.

Early Childhood Educator.   An early childhood educator (ECE) may facilitate transitions between the medical diagnostic process and educational intervention process. An ECE is often employed by the state agency that provides infant-toddler intervention services (typically state department of education, health, or social services) or the local educational authority. Although an ECE may not be involved in the initial diagnostic process, he or she should be identified early in the process of planning an habilitation program to ensure that families have access to all educational ser vices available under state and federal mandate.

Other Medical Specialists.   Depending on the etiology of hearing loss and presence of additional medical and/or developmental conditions, other medical specialists such as geneticists and neurologists may be needed to provide consultation to the family and CIHP. Consultation from these individuals may influence the infant's diagnostic and habilitation services.

Developing Working Relationships

There are a variety of appropriate models for developing effective working relationships. The three most familiar approaches are the multidisciplinary, interdisciplinary, and transdisciplinary.

Multidisciplinary Approach.   The multidisciplinary approach encompasses all the professionals necessary to provide referral-based services. This model, shown schematically in Figure 2–1, is characterized by delineation of professional boundaries and independent functioning of service providers. In this approach, an infant may be seen by a medical specialist who conveys a written consultation summary of his or her diagnosis and recommendations. Typically, direct communication among professionals is limited, and coordination of services depends on self-identification of a service coordinator. In addition, there may be limited opportunity for parents to influence diagnostic and treatment decisions in the multidisciplinary model. This model is often employed in medical centers, especially during initial diagnostic process.

Without careful coordination, the multidisciplinary approach does not produce genuinely integrated services. Typically, case management conferences do not encompass all members of the assessment/intervention program. It may be especially difficult to include medical specialists or off-site care providers in team management activities because of competing or conflicting schedules. Despite this limitation, a multidisciplinary approach may be the

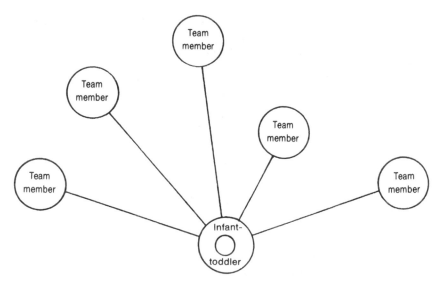

FIGURE 2-1. Representation of the multidisciplinary approach. This model of service delivery is characterized by independent functioning of various service providers. To achieve integrated services, this model requires meticulous service coordination. (From *Infant-Toddler Assessment: An Interdisciplinary Approach* by L. M. Rossetti, 1990, p. 58. Boston: College-Hill Press. Copyright 1990 by College-Hill Press. Credited to M. Briggs, 1989. Reprinted with permission.)

most appropriate model during some aspects of an infant's comprehensive program.

Interdisciplinary Approach. The interdisciplinary model strives for greater coordination of services and communication among care providers. Under this approach, represented in Figure 2–2, professionals communicate during regularly scheduled meetings about the results of assessment and intervention with individual infants and their families. Team members may work independently within their specialty or assess and intervene in conjunction with other disciplines. Typically, a service coordinator is team-appointed to assist in program development and coordination for individual infants.

Many professionals favor an interdisciplinary approach for services to infants and their families. In addition to developing a team approach for individual cases, the interdisciplinary model fosters team participation in overall program planning and service evaluation. Each member of the interdisciplinary team is responsi-

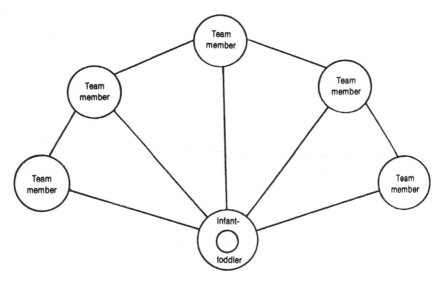

FIGURE 2-2.   Representation of the interdisciplinary approach. This model of service delivery is characterized by coordination of services and strong communication among care providers. This approach may produce highly integrated, collaborative, and interdependent team functioning. (From *Infant-Toddler Assessment: An Interdisciplinary Approach* by L. M. Rossetti, 1990, p. 60. Boston: College-Hill Press. Copyright 1990 by College-Hill Press. Credited to M. Briggs, 1989. Reprinted with permission.)

ble for overall program quality. Rossetti (1990) describes this model more fully in the context of infant-toddler assessment. He defines the interdisciplinary team as highly integrated, collaborative, and interdependent. This model is often employed in medical and educational settings.

Transdisciplinary Approach. The transdisciplinary model, represented in Figure 2-3, diminishes professional boundaries and permits coordination and delivery of services outside the traditional scope of individual professional practices. Under this model, for example, a speech-language pathologist may provide services more traditionally provided by the audiologist such as limited aspects of hearing aid/earmold services. A transdisciplinary approach depends on professionals with demonstrated expertise outside their area of primary training. This model may be encountered in educational and health care clinic settings.

Of the three approaches, the transdisciplinary model may be more difficult to achieve and maintain because of professional boundary issues and its unique dependence on strong interper-

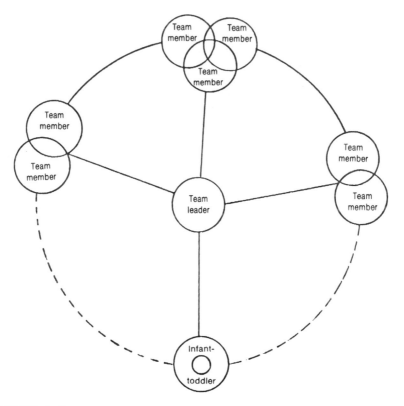

FIGURE 2-3.   Representation of the transdisciplinary approach. This model of service delivery diminishes professional boundaries and permits coordination and delivery of services outside the traditional scope of professional practice. This model depends on strong interpersonal and interprofessional interactions. (From *Infant-Toddler Assessment: An Interdisciplinary Approach* by L. M. Rossetti, 1990, p. 62. Boston: College-Hill Press. Copyright 1990 by College-Hill Press. Credited to M. Briggs, 1989. Reprinted with permission.)

sonal and interprofessional interactions. The transdisciplinary team relies on mutual understanding, acceptance, and incorporation of a unified professional philosophy in service delivery.

Any single team model or combination of team models may be successful in achieving appropriate services to infants and their families. During the initial diagnostic process, the infant hearing team may function in a multidisciplinary manner. At this time, referral to a wide variety of professionals who do not typically interact with the core CIHP team may be needed. Written reports from these consultants are often adequate to define a diagnosis and incorporate specific recommendations into the treatment plan. To be successful, however, two aspects of multidisciplinary consultants' services must be realized. First, the parents/family must have adequate communication to ensure that they understand the diagnosis and recommendations. Second, a service coordinator must be identified at a very early stage in the diagnostic process to ensure communication and follow through with specific recommendations.

During the subsequent ongoing diagnosis and intervention process, the infant hearing team may function in a more transdisciplinary manner with the disciplines of audiology, speech-language pathology, and social work most strongly represented. At this time, additional diagnostic and prognostic information is being gathered through observation of the infant's strengths and the family's skills and interactions. Individual team members gather information not solely limited to their professional boundaries. For example, the audiologist not only assesses the infant's hearing and response to hearing aids, but also discusses how factors such as how grandparent acceptance and support or parental anxiety about other developmental disabilities are affecting the family's adjustment. This information is shared in meetings with the other primary service providers and assists the team in modifying the treatment approach.

For periodic, regularly scheduled assessment services, the CIHP team frequently operates in an interdisciplinary model with the core disciplines of audiology, speech-language pathology, social work, otolaryngology, and pediatrics. Each professional assesses the infant's current status and progress from his or her professional viewpoint and shares findings at a case management conference led by the service coordinator and the infant's family. Recommendations from specific disciplines are incorporated into a total case management plan, and additional assessments from noncore member specialists may be gathered in a multidisciplinary manner. These assessments typically are provided on a scheduled basis and may be identified by specific team names such as "Infant Hearing Clinic" or "Developmental Evaluation Clinic."

Audiologic Technology

Evaluation of infants with suspected hearing loss requires a broad spectrum of complex technology. In addition to sophisticated medical technology, necessary audiological instrumentation, including equipment for nonbehavioral hearing screening and evaluation, behavioral response measurement, and assessment of amplification are required in any CIHP. Table 2–3 lists the audiologic instrumentation needed for comprehensive services to infants. Each device permits assessment of some essential component of auditory function, hearing sensitivity, or response to amplification. Chapter 8 in this text provides a comprehensive overview of audiologic technology and services required for screening, evaluation, and habilitation of infants with hearing loss.

Institutional Setting and Interagency Collaboration

Components of a CIHP may be developed and delivered in a variety of professional settings including hospitals, speech and hearing clinics, and public school programs. Because a single agency may not be able to provide all needed components and services, collaboration among the various agencies is critical for provision of effective services.

Hospital or Medical Setting

A hospital or medical center can contribute medical expertise for diagnosis and treatment of hearing loss. There is ready availability of specialists in the major disciplines of audiology, speech-language pathology, otolaryngology, pediatrics, and social work, as well

Table 2–3. Audiologic technology necessary to provide comprehensive infant hearing services.

Device	Purpose and Use	Approximate Cost (1996)
Otoacoustic emissions	Screening hearing of newborns	$8,000–$14,000
Evoked potentials	Screening hearing of newborns; diagnostic auditory assessment of newborns and infants	$10,000–$30,000
Sound field audiometry	Behavioral hearing assessment of infants; behavioral assessment of amplification	$25,000–$45,000
Acoustic immittance	Assessment of middle ear function	$4,500–$8,000
Hearing aid test system	Evaluation of hearing aid function; measures of amplification in the ear	$5,000–$13,000

as consultant specialists in genetics, neurology, and neonatology. In some centers, specialty clinical programs, such as Child Development Services and a Genetics Clinic, are available. These institutions will have technology needed for appropriate assessment and intervention.

Because hospitals negotiate reimbursement contracts with public and private funding sources, some of these institutions provide services to families who are unable to access other health-care systems.

Despite the availability of multiple services and specialists, there are disadvantages associated with designating a medical center as the primary agency in an CIHP. First, most medical centers continue to provide services on a multidisciplinary basis. Services can be fragmented among departments and professionals and lack a cohesive, coordinated approach. Despite best attempts to assemble a team in this setting, individual professional schedules may limit full participation by all consultants into the counseling/decision-making process. Second, a medical center/hospital atmosphere does not promote a normal developmental perspective about the infant. This setting promotes a subtle perspective of hearing loss as pathology or disease rather than variation in normal function. Further, it is difficult to promote a naturalized family setting in a medical-clinical environment.

Speech and Hearing Clinics

Speech and hearing clinics have two advantages as the primary site for a CIHP. First, because their mission is uniquely related to communication disorders, these settings can dedicate specific staff solely to the CIHP. An audiologist and speech-language pathologist may be assigned responsibility for infant hearing specialization without other job responsibilities. These individuals provide the core of an interdisciplinary team with time regularly scheduled for infant and family services and counseling, and program planning. Second, if the clinic is associated with a university teaching program, there is potential for student training and education.

The disadvantages of a speech and hearing clinic setting include limited access to all specialty consultations. These programs usually do not employ the medical specialists needed for assessment services resulting in fragmentation of diagnostic from intervention services. In addition, reimbursement to speech and hearing clinics may be limited from some insurance and third-party payer sources.

Public Education System

In many states, public school programs assume responsibility for services to all children with special needs, including infants with hearing impairment. There are two primary advantages to designating the public schools as the primary agency in a CIHP. First, this setting permits continuity of services from infancy throughout school age. Although service providers may change on an annual basis, there will be continuity in programming and assistance in transitions from one level to the next. Second, these services are provided at no charge to the family.

A disadvantage of public school programs may be a focus restricted to educational intervention. Services may be limited to those deemed necessary for education without incorporation of a medical perspective. Diagnostic medical evaluation and consultation typically are not available in public school programs.

Table 2–4 compares the three potential settings for CIHPs on the basis of access, cost, and primary services. As noted above, each setting has advantages and disadvantages, and the decision of where to establish a comprehensive program should recognize the potential limitations of the setting and develop mechanisms to compensate for these disadvantages.

Interagency Collaboration

Regardless of which agency assumes primary responsibility for a CIHP, all agencies must collaborate in provision of effective services to infants and their families. If professionals in either a medical setting or private speech and hearing clinic assemble the expertise and technology needed for a program, they must also

Table 2–4. Comparison of three potential settings for a comprehensive infant hearing program based on access, cost, and primary emphasis.

Setting	Access	Cost	Primary Emphasis
Hospital	Medical referral	High	Medical diagnosis and treatment
Speech and Hearing Clinic	Self- or other referral	Low to high	Rehabilitation for communication disorders
Public schools	Per state mandate	None	Education

collaborate with professionals in public health and education agencies to support funding of services and to ensure that families receive all entitled services. In addition, because infants will transition to the public education system at some point, private agencies assume responsibility for assisting in that process at a very early point in infants' programs.

Program and Service Funding

Despite federal initiatives for services to infants with disabilities and their families, families may not have access to the financial resources necessary to meet all the needs of an infant with hearing impairment. For example, families with one or two wage earners may not qualify for state-funded hearing aids even though their income is insufficient to purchase these devices. Many managed-care health insurance plans do not provide ongoing speech therapy for children, or provide only limited access to habilitation services. Identifying potential funding sources for the overall comprehensive infant hearing program and for individual infants and their families is an important responsibility for program professionals. Although individual families assume responsibility for meeting their infant's needs, a professional must be knowledgeable about community resources and provide support and assistance to families.

Health Insurance

Medical diagnostic services typically are provided under health insurance or state-funded medical services programs (e.g., Medicaid, state Department of Health programs). Insurance policies vary widely, even with the same insurance carrier, and families must become aware of the limitations of payment for services imposed by their insurance carrier. Managed-care organizations may severely limit the choice of service providers and restrict payment for specific services (e.g., speech therapy). If insurance reimbursement is an important source of revenue for the CIHP, then the program should have insurance reimbursement specialists available to negotiate contracts and payment.

Education Funds

Depending on the state, some component of early intervention may be available through Part H of IDEA at no cost to the family. This often includes a home-based, family-centered intervention program. In many cases, families opt to supplement these services with center-based intervention at public or private agencies.

Speech and hearing programs in local universities may also provide services to infants and their families, typically at substantially reduced rates. Because these institutions use clinic services as an opportunity for student training, they actively solicit referrals for audiology and speech-language pathology diagnostic and habilitation services.

Private Agencies and Foundations

Many communities participate in philanthropy programs which support services to families through community health and rehabilitation agencies. These agencies often provide services on a sliding-fee schedule related to family income and resources. Other service organizations in a community may provide hearing aids and prosthetic devices. The National Grange and Sertoma Clubs, for example, identify communication disorders and hearing loss as priorities for individual grants.

Most CIHPs will depend on a variety of sources for funding programs, services, equipment and personnel. If time-limited funding through grants or demonstration projects is utilized to initiate services, the program director must identify sources of additional funding needed to sustain the program beyond the start-up period.

DEVELOPMENT OF A PROGRAM

There are many models of successful CIHPs in the United States (Roush and Matkin, 1994). The common feature underlying each is the steadfast dedication of a core group of key individuals to family-centered comprehensive services. The commitment influences all individuals in the system, from the specialists providing services to the administrators approving budgets. At The Children's Hospital (TCH) in Denver, we established a CIHP through a process that included (a) establishing program goals and building consensus, (b) funding needed technology and staff positions, (c) marketing services, and (d) evaluating program outcome and adjusting program elements.

Establishing Program Goals and Building Consensus

The first step in development of any program is to establish program goals. Why should the program be developed and what is its intended outcome? In developing a program within an existing institution or in collaboration with professionals in multiple institutions, the new program must support the institutional mission and goals.

Institutional and Program Mission

The mission of the host institution guides development of a CIHP. By aligning the goals of a new program to the mission of the host institution, the program director can demonstrate an inherent coherence of the new program within institutional function. In fact, a program director can champion an institutional responsibility for a CIHP by carefully framing the program within the mission of the organization.

The mission of The Children's Hospital–Denver is to meet the medical needs and to improve the health of children in the Rocky Mountain region. To this end, the institution had developed a large audiology and speech-language pathology program with specialists in audiology, speech-language pathology, aural habilitation, learning disabilities, and social work. There was an active otolaryngology practice as well as child development, genetics, and neurology services available within the hospital. In addition, the hospital provided both a level II and III newborn nursery to care for premature and critically ill infants. With this breadth of professional expertise, TCH was an ideal setting to establish comprehensive hearing services to infants. The mission of the program would address the medical needs of infants through early identification of hearing loss and improve the health of identified children through prevention of secondary disabilities of speech and language delays, academic failure, and psychosocial dysfunction.

Identifying Key Individuals

Not uncommonly, the development of a new program is dependent on the commitment of an individual or a small group of professionals with a shared vision. These individuals must not only design the program and services, but also guide the program through the institutional approval process. In most settings, several groups of decision-makers need to be included at an early stage in the planning process.

At TCH, in addition to the program director, the professionals with a shared vision for expanded services to infants were the audiologists, aural habilitation specialist, and social worker. These staff enthusiastically supported efforts to enhance services to infants. They self-defined an "Infant Hearing Team" and scheduled weekly meetings to develop program goals. The program director identified other key hospital personnel for inclusion in the planning process. These were (a) hospital administrators with authority to approve expenditures for needed equipment and personnel, (b) nursery medical directors with authority to refer infants and set policy for referral standards, and (c) nurse-specialists caring for infants in the intensive care nurseries. These individuals had to understand the congruity of the proposed program with the overall institutional mission as well as with their professional goals and responsibilities. Thus, the hospital administrators needed assurance that the program would be financially viable and supported, the nursery medical director needed assurance that the program represented responsible, cost-effective standard of practice; and the nursery staff needed documentation that the program would enhance outcomes for infants and their families.

Marlowe (1993) describes development of an infant hearing screening program at a community hospital. She stresses the importance of identifying and documenting the benefits that each interested party (e.g., nursing staff, medical staff, hospital administration) will enjoy from the proposed program. These key individuals deserve regular feedback about program outcomes to affirm their role in program development, approval, and implementation.

Competing Institutional Priorities

In most organizations today, all needed programs cannot receive approval. Typically a program director competes with other directors for limited resources for equipment, personnel, and space. At TCH, we were successful in gaining approval for an expanded infant hearing program because we built on a foundation of existing services, demonstrated financially prudent outcomes, and developed other funding sources for needed technology.

Funding Technology and Staff

A CIHP needs sophisticated diagnostic and habilitative technology, and highly trained professional staff. During initial program planning, the needed technology and staff and potential funding sources should be identified. At TCH, we identified the need for evoked potential technology and increased audiologist and social worker hours. We sought funding from three sources, (a) our host institution, the hospital; (b) the hospital's fundraising arm, the hospital foundation; and (c) community philanthropic organizations.

Hospital Support

Host institutions typically assume responsibility for equipment and staff needed to support specific programs. The audiology program, for example, was already equipped for behavioral testing, immittance measures, and hearing aid measurement and evaluation. The program lacked equipment for evoked potential evaluation and loaner hearing aids. Because we determined that total program support was not possible solely from the hospital, and that support for staff positions was more critical than equipment dollars, the program director requested only partial support for capital equipment from the hospital. Additional support was requested from a local philanthropic organization. This combination of funds provided adequate support to purchase evoked potential instrumentation. In subsequent years, as we demonstrated program financial viability, the hospital additional evoked potential and otoacoustic emission equipment to serve this program.

Staff positions may be more difficult to secure than medical equipment. Because staffing represents an ongoing expense, administrators may be unwilling or unable to fund additional staff positions without clear evidence of financial or programmatic benefit. At TCH, we determined that we needed one additional audiologist to develop the nursery-based screening component and increased social worker hours to enhance follow-up services. By demonstrating expected increase in patient volume and revenue, we secured approval for additional staff from hospital administration.

Foundations and Community Organizations

Funding for ongoing equipment needs may be more difficult than funding a one-time medical technology purchase. In the case of a CIHP, funding for loaner hearing aids may prove challenging because of high maintenance and repair costs. At TCH, we received occasional donations of hearing aids from individuals in the community, but these were often in poor working condition or inappropriate for use with infants. To establish a loaner hearing aid program, we approached The Children's Hospital Foundation (TCHF), the fund-raising body associated with the hospital. Through this source, we secured occasional cash gifts from individuals who wished to donate $1,000 or less to a specific hospital project. Unfortunately, these funds did not permit purchase of the necessary numbers of loaner aids.

Unexpectedly, we received an inquiry from an estate representative who requested a proposal to fund services to children with hearing impairment. We proposed to endow a cash gift and to use the proceeds to support the loaner hearing aid program. The estate representative was especially attracted to the concept of an endowment and provided a substantial initial cash gift. Over the years, as other cash gifts have become available, they have added to the corpus of the endowment. This strategy has supported not only purchase of needed hearing aids and other amplification devices, but has also supported costs for hearing aid repair and maintenance and staff training.

Marketing Services

To attract referrals, the community must be educated that diagnostic and habilitative hearing services to infants are feasible and available. Active marketing may be necessary for institutions that do not have an established reputation for services to infants. In these programs, written referral materials should be made avail able to community neonatalogists, pediatricians, family practitioners, and public health clinics and nurses. Direct notification to parents and families is also appropriate through mechanisms such as public service announcements and community bulletin boards. The best marketing tool any program can adopt is prompt feedback to a referral once an initial referral has been made.

Notifying Referral Sources

For institutions with established reputations for services to infants, informing referral sources and collaborative institutions may achieve referral goals. To reach the TCH primary referral sources of physicians, department staff presented several inservice programs to nursing and medical personnel. The state Department of Health, Health Care Program for Children (HCP) was informed of expanded services to infants and other potential referral sources (e.g., community pediatricians and otolaryngologists, hospital-based development clinic and rehabilitation service) were contacted.

Enhancing Parent Education

A strong parent education component provides two benefits. First, it benefits the infant by improving his or her family's capacity for making informed decisions. Second, it benefits the program through community service and image enhancement. This type of program marketing can be one of the most powerful tools in developing community awareness and fostering community support for a CIHP.

At TCH, the audiology and habilitation staff identified three distinct parent education needs, (a) access to materials written for parents of children with disabilities, (b) parent discussion groups and sign language training, and (c) information about public and private educational options. To address needs for written information and in cooperation with the hospital's Family Resource Library, the staff developed a collection of published materials including books, pamphlets, and articles. These materials are available for loan to parents, families, and interested others, and are not restricted to families associated with the CIHP. Other titles in the Family Resource Library collection deal with chronic medical conditions, children with disabilities, behavior and emotions, parenting, and related topics.

The staff also developed a series of loose leaf handouts for parents that cover topics such as hearing aids and hearing aid troubleshooting, etiology of hearing loss in infants, lists of national and local parent support organizations, and local educational agency Child Find contacts. These materials are provided in a three-ring notebook for easy access and compilation.

To address parent discussion groups and sign language training, the staff developed Parent Night Programs and Sign Language Classes. Parent Night Programs are monthly educational meetings scheduled from September through May. Parents identify topics of interest, and the staff schedules appropriate speakers to address the topic. Sign Language Classes are held weekly following a therapy group for children with hearing impairment. These classes are available to parents, children, and staff. Both the Parent Night Programs and Sign Language Classes are free of charge and available to any family.

To provide more comprehensive information about educational options, the staff collaborated with other public and private agencies to present a day-long seminar on educational options for school-age children with hearing impairment. This program was attended by parents and other professionals, and included representatives from the state Department of Education, local educational authorities, the residential school for the deaf, and private agencies. In addition, the staff collaborated on development of written program descriptions with representatives of public and private educational programs.

Program Evaluation

Program evaluation is an integral part of program development and initiation. Adequate methods should be employed which permit measurement of critical aspects of the program. For example, because compliance for follow-up is a significant problem in hearing services to infants (Mahoney and Eichwald, 1987; Shimizu et al., 1990) evaluation of follow-up rates for infants who are referred from newborn hearing screening is important. Several recent publications describe management systems to facilitate program evaluation (Harrison, 1994; Margolis and Thornton, 1991).

At TCH, summary records are maintained in hard copy and electronic storage media to permit evaluation of specific aspects of the program such as number of infants tested, number of infants followed and lost-to-follow up, infants at-risk for progressive hearing loss, and other variables important to quality evaluation. These records are reviewed at 6-month intervals to monitor specific aspects of the program. All audiology staff participate in program evaluation.

Program evaluation has led to changes in referral and follow-up mechanisms. For example, we established a streamlined referral process in the nursery because program evaluation showed that infants were being discharged without referral or recommendation for hearing evaluation. We developed a house staff "Brief Communication" for inclusion in the medical chart of every patient admitted with a diagnosis of meningitis. We developed a tracking/coding system to evaluate our follow-up of infants with apparent mild conductive hearing loss. At TCH, program evaluation remains focused on patient care, although evaluation of specific management, administration, and reimbursement issues may be appropriate in other settings.

Program viability is closely linked to program evaluation. Our colleagues and administrators expect documented evidence that the CIHP is meeting its goals of early identification and intervention for infants with hearing loss and their families. Through program evaluation, we demonstrate ongoing critique and adjustment of program goals, implementation, and outcomes.

SUMMARY

A comprehensive infant hearing program involves substantial professional dedication and institutional commitment. It requires careful planning and evaluation, and continuous adjustment. Although many professionals equate infant hearing services with nursery-based hearing screening, these activities represent only one small component of a comprehensive program. In fact, before a single infant is screened, the necessary diagnostic and habilitative services must be readily available. The goal of early intervention will only be realize through a truly *comprehensive* infant hearing program.

SUGGESTED READINGS

Aylward, G. P. (1994). *Practitioner's guide to developmental and psychological testing*. In M. Gottlieb (Ed.), *Critical issues in developmental and behavioral pediatrics*. New York: Plenum Publishing Corporation.
A comprehensive overview of currently available assessment instruments.

Bess, F. H., & Hall, J. W. (Eds.). (1992). *Screening children for auditory function*. Nashville: Bill Wilkerson Center Press.
An edited textbook with contributions including principles of screening, screening newborns with ABR, screening newborns with OAEs, and habilitation services for infants.

Rossetti, L. M. (1990). *Infant-toddler assessment: An interdisciplinary approach*. Boston: College-Hill Press.
A comprehensive overview of interdisciplinary services to infants and toddlers from a speech-language pathologist's perspective.

Roush, J. & Motkin, N. D. (Eds.). (1994) *Infants and toddlers with hearing loss: Family centered assessment and intervention*. Baltimore: York Press.
An extensive overview of family centered assessment and intervention to infants and toddlers from an audiological perspective.

White, K. R., & Behrens, T. R. (Eds.). (1993). *The Rhode Island hearing assessment project: Implications for universal newborn hearing screening*. In *Seminars in Hearing, 14*. New York: Thieme Medical Publishers.
A thorough description of the Rhode Island project, the large-scale newborn hearing project using OAE technology.

SECTION II

Clinical Aspects of Hearing in Infants

CHAPTER 3

Clinical Genetics

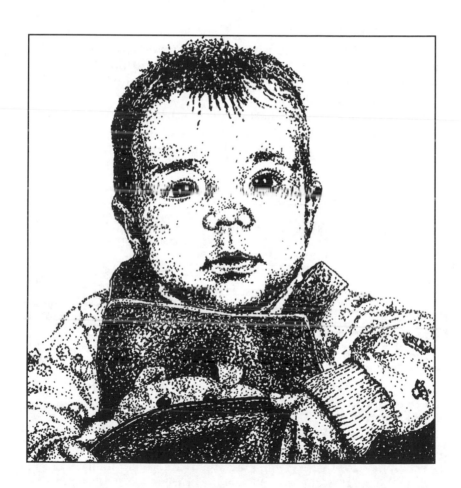

Genetics and the study of hereditary disorders are among the most rapidly evolving disciplines in medical science. Development of the Human Genome Project, an international project to identify the location of specific genes on human chromosomes and to understand their function and dysfunction, and application of sophisticated imaging techniques to genetic and chromosomal analyses have greatly enhanced knowledge of genetic disorders. To provide competent services to infants and their families, health care providers need an elementary understanding of basic genetics, cytogenetics and molecular genetics, the inheritance of hereditary disorders, specific disorders associated with genetic disease, and the process of genetic evaluation.

Although hereditary disease can become apparent at any point in an individual's lifespan, genetic and chromosomal abnormalities and associated congenital malformations are especially important in pediatric medicine. The relative contribution of these disorders to the infant mortality rate has increased as the prevalence of infectious childhood disease has decreased. In the pre-antibiotic era, most infant mortality was attributable to infectious disease; today, in developed countries, most infant mortality is attributable to genetic disorders and congenital malformations. Of

What is the difference between a *congenital, hereditary, genetic,* and *familial* condition? *Congenital* simply means present at birth; it does not imply the etiology of the condition. Infants born with hearing loss, regardless of the cause, have *congenital* hearing loss. *Hereditary* means inherited, or "passed-down" from previous generations through DNA, genes, and/or chromosomes; it implies chromosome or gene control of the condition in question. Infants with Down syndrome, a chromosomal disorder which results from an extra copy of chromosome 21 (Trisomy 21), have a *hereditary* condition. *Genetic* means caused by a gene; it may be considered a special subset of hereditary. Infants with Alport syndrome, a disorder resulting in hearing loss and progressive loss of vision, have a *genetic* condition; the gene for Alport syndrome has been identified through molecular genetic analysis. *Familial* means present in several related family members; it does not imply etiology. The families of two cousins with hearing loss of dissimilar etiology (e.g., hereditary hearing loss and post-infection hearing loss) have *familial* hearing loss.

recognized pregnancies that end in spontaneous abortion, 50% to 60% have detectable chromosomal anomalies. As many as 2.0% of all newborns demonstrate chromosomal or single-gene disorders. These abnormalities produce significant neonatal mortality and morbidity. Infants with genetic anomalies who survive into childhood require substantially greater health and educational care than nonaffected children. Study of clinical genetics allows investigators and clinicians to understand genetic transmission and to prevent and treat inherited conditions.

That humans inherit specific biologic traits from their parents has been known for centuries. How traits were inherited remained a puzzle until the 1860s when Gregor Mendel, a monk and botanist, proposed specific principles of inheritance. In his seminal paper, Mendel described inheritance of characteristics such as height and color in garden peas. His work was largely unappreciated until the early 1900s when it was rediscovered by three independent European investigators. At that time, genetics emerged as a clinical science. For traits inherited through a single gene, Mendel's principles of inheritance remain valid today, and represent a major contribution in the study of basic genetics.

Additional significant discoveries occurred slowly during the first half of the 20th century. For example, although scientists observed chromosomes in dividing cells in the late 19th century, the exact number of human chromosomes remained unknown until the second half of the 20th century. By 1960, the chromosomal bases of several important syndromes including Down syndrome were identified. The biomaterial of inheritance, deoxyribonucleic acid (DNA), was identified in the 1940s, but more than a decade passed before its physical structure and properties were deduced by Nobel laureates Watson and Crick.

More recently, new technologies for genetic investigation have led to an explosion of knowledge about genetic inheritance and disease. Significant breakthroughs in cytogenetics, high-resolution imaging techniques, and molecular genetics have resulted in identification of increasing numbers of genetic diseases. Although genetic manipulation through selective breeding has occurred for centuries, more sophisticated genetic engineering is now employed to improve disease resistance and food production in plants and animals. Application of genetic engineering techniques to reduce morbidity and mortality in individuals with genetic diseases such as cystic fibrosis and severe combined immunodeficiency is proceeding under intense investigational scrutiny. The prospect of "gene therapy" is both fascinating and frightening.

Because genetic knowledge is increasing at such a rapid pace, it is unlikely that nongeneticists will remain current with the new technologies, information, and applications of sophisticated genetics research. Nonetheless, because genetic and chromosomal abnormality account for the substantial percentage of congenital anomalies in infants, it is important for audiologists, speech-language pathologists, and other health care providers who work with infants and their families to have a basic understanding of elementary genetics.

BASIC PRINCIPLES OF GENETIC INHERITANCE

A feature article in a popular news magazine characterized the genetic instructions of human beings, the human genome, as an encyclopedia (Elmer-Dewitt, 1994). The text in the encyclopedia is composed of molecular letters (DNA) which are aggregated into sentences (genes). These sentences combine to form 23 distinct chapters or volumes (chromosomes pairs). Thus, each of the 23 chromosome pairs represents one volume in the encyclopedia which contains all the genetic information about a given individual.

DNA

DNA is the base unit of heredity, the molecular "letters" of inheritance. When changes occur in this ordered sequence of the genetic code, genetic disease may result.

DNA is a nucleic acid consisting of four nitrogen-containing bases attached to a sugar-phosphate polymer and arranged on intertwining strands, a "double helix." The four bases, adenine (A), guanine (G), cytosine (C), and thymine (T), occur in predictable pairs on complementary strands such that A on one strand always pairs with T on its complementary strand, and G on one strand always pairs with C on its complementary strand. One set of complementary bases, <AT> and <CG>, is a base-pair. Because bases occur in these invariant pairs, one strand of DNA contains all the information necessary to construct its complementary pair.

DNA stores and encodes a vast amount of information based on the sequence of base-pairs. For a segment N bases long, there are N^4 possible base pair sequences. The base-pair arrangement of DNA encodes the complete genetic information of an organism; it is called the organism's *genome*. Small viruses have genomes of only a few thousand bases pairs. It is estimated that the human genome contains 3×10^9 base pairs.

Accurate replication and transmission of the genetic code is ensured by the base-pair coding and double-helix structure of DNA. Figure 3–1 shows the double-helix structure of DNA (upper half of figure) and replication of DNA (lower half of figure). During replica-

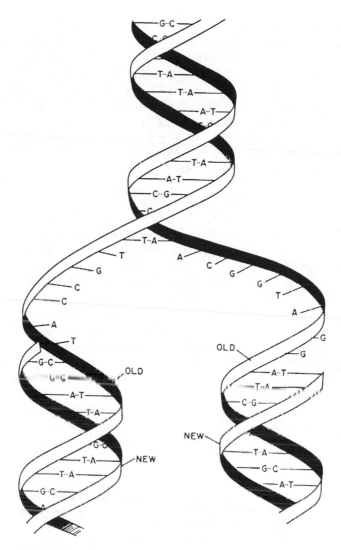

FIGURE 3-1. Schematic diagram of DNA showing base-pair arrangement on intertwining sugar phosphate strands (the double helix) and replication of the DNA code. As the double-helix unwinds and separates into single strands, each strand serves as a template for reproducing the complementary strand. (From *Clinical Genetics and Genetic Counseling*, Second Edition, by T. E. Kelly, 1986, p. 35. Chicago, IL: Year Book Medical Publishers, Inc. Copyright 1986 by Year Book Medical Publishers, Inc. Reprinted with permission.)

tion, the double helix unwinds and separates into two single strands with their associated bases. Each strand serves as the template for a new, complementary strand. For example, the unwound DNA strand at the bottom right of Figure 3–1 with bases <ATCACT> will direct synthesis of a strand with complementary bases <TAGTGA>. After replication, two "daughter" double helixes will result; each daughter will contain one original parent-strand and one newly synthesized complementary strand. In addition, if a base on one strand is lost or damaged, it can be replaced using the complementary strand to direct its repair.

Genes

Genes are sequences of DNA that direct protein synthesis. A gene may contain several hundreds or even thousands of base-pairs of DNA. A mutation in even a single base-pair may result in inaccurate synthesis of an essential protein and lead to genetic disease.

Genes are ordered in a linear fashion on uniquely identifiable structures, *chromosomes*, contained in the nucleus of all cells. Because genes occur at a specific locus on a chromosome, in some cases it is possible to identify the gene responsible for a specific genetic disorder. For example, researchers have determined that individuals with neurofibromatosis type II (bilateral acoustic neuromas) demonstrate an abnormal gene on chromosome 22, individuals with Waardenburg's syndrome demonstrate an abnormal sequence of DNA on chromosome 2, and individuals with Huntington's disease demonstrate an abnormal prolongation or repetition of a particular DNA sequence on the tip of chromosome 4.

Chromosomes

Chromosomes are long segments of DNA containing hundreds of genes. They are observed by light microscopy in nucleated cells undergoing active cell division. Chromosomes are categorized by their distinctive sizes and shapes.

Figure 3–2 is a diagrammatic representation of a chromosome during one phase of cell division. At this stage, the DNA has condensed and doubled; the chromosome appears as two longitudinal rods, called chromatids, joined at a single point, the centromere. The chromatids each contain one complete copy of the DNA. The centromere divides the each chromatid into unequal lengths, or arms; the short arms above the centromere are called the p arms (from the French *petite*) and the long arms below the centromere are called the q arms. Deletion or duplication in the p or q arm of a given chromosome results in a specific pattern of birth defect.

chromatid

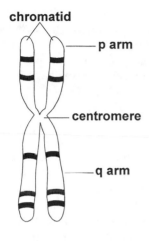

p arm

centromere

q arm

FIGURE 3-2. Diagrammatic representation of a chromosome as observed during cell division. DNA has condensed and doubled. The two longitudinal halves of the chromosome are called chromatids each of which contains a complete copy of DNA. The chromatids are joined at the centromere which divides the chromatids into unequal arms, the short, p arm and the longer, q arm.

Prior to cell division, the chromatids separate and one chromatid contributes a complete copy of DNA to each daughter cell. Chromosomes manifest this appearance only during one phase of active cell division. During other phases of the cell cycle (growth and protein synthesis), chromosomes are uncondensed, single, elongated strands.

Each species has a characteristic number of distinctly identifiable chromosomes known as the *karyotype*. The human karyotype consists of 46 chromosomes (23 distinct chromosome pairs). Of these, 44 chromosomes occur in 22 *homologous pairs (autosomes)* with one member of each pair containing the same genetic information. Autosomes are identical in both genders of the species; these chromosomes contain genes that code for and regulate somatic cell development. The 23rd pair of chromosomes differs in the two genders (sex chromosomes). The sex chromosomes determine gender and regulate some aspects of sexual development and function. Normal human females have two X chromosomes (XX); normal human males have one X and one Y chromosome (XY). One chromosome of each autosome pair and one sex chromosome are derived from each parent.

In contrast to somatic cell nuclei with their complement of 46 chromosomes (*diploid number*, or 2N), mature sex cells, or *gametes* (ova and sperm) contain 23 chromosomes (*haploid number*, or 1N). Upon fertilization of the ovum by a sperm, a single cell, the *zygote*, containing the diploid number of chromosomes (46), is formed. This single cell, with equal genetic contributions from the mother and father, contains the code necessary to develop into an unique human individual.

The principle functions of DNA, genes, and chromosomes are (a) to provide the template for protein synthesis, and (b) to direct accurate replication and transmission of the genetic code to the next generation. Protein synthesis is necessary for biologic function, and accurate replication and transmission are necessary for preservation of the species.

Protein Synthesis

The genetic code, DNA, directs synthesis of proteins. Proteins regulate cell growth and differentiation, inheritance of characteristics, and response to the environment. Errors in protein synthesis related to errors in DNA result in significant morbidity and mortality.

Proteins are comprised of amino acids, organic compounds extracted from ingested proteins or produced by the body in small quantities. The DNA code specifies the sequence of amino acids that make up a specific protein. Twenty amino acids are commonly found in proteins of the human body. A distinct set of three DNA base pairs, called a triplet or codon, codes for a specific amino acid. A gene may contain hundreds of triplets which specify the amino acid sequence of a single protein. For example, insulin, a protein necessary for sugar metabolism, consists of 51 amino acids coded by a sequence of approximately 1,430 base-pairs of DNA.

Protein synthesis is accomplished by a complex process in which a second form of nucleic acid, ribonucleic acid, or RNA, decodes and translates the DNA sequence into the constituent amino acids. This multistage process involves generation of a RNA molecule from the DNA template in the cell nucleus, transmission of this information from the cell nucleus to specific cellular bodies (ribosomes), translation of the code into the intended protein, and some intrinsic signalling mechanism to both initiate and terminate the process.

Most genes consist of protein-coding segments, exons, interrupted by nonprotein coding segments, introns, whose exact function remains unknown. During protein synthesis, RNA initially decodes the entire gene sequence, including introns. These segments are eventually spliced out of the genetic code before the final production of a protein. If splicing is inaccurate because of base-pair derangement, then no protein or an abnormal protein may be produced.

All nucleated cells have an identical genome, but only about 1% of the total genome is active in any given cell at any given time. Areas of DNA adjacent to specific protein-coding segments appear to influence decoding and synthesis of proteins. If these adjacent segments mutate, gene regulation of protein synthesis may fail.

Replication and Transmission of Genetic Information: Cell Division

Cell division is the process through which species grow and reproduce. It can result in exact replication of genetic material of the parent cell, *mitosis*, or reshuffling of and reduction in genetic material, *meiosis*. Mitosis results in preservation of the diploid number of chromosomes in somatic cells (in humans, 46). Meiosis results in reduction of chromosomes to the haploid number in gametes (in humans, 23). The processes of mitosis and meiosis are compared in Figure 3–3.

Mitosis

Mitosis occurs in somatic cells and results in two genetically identical diploid daughter cells from a single diploid parent cell. Mitosis allows a single-celled fertilized egg (zygote) to develop into a complete human being, blood and skin cells to replace dead or dying cells, and the organism to expand in size and grow.

The cycle of cell function and duplication through mitosis occurs in continuous stages. When cells are engaged in their normal, specific functions, and when they are not dividing, they are in interphase. During interphase, chromosomes are active but invisible; they are an unformed granularity in the cell nucleus.

As shown in the left half of Figure 3–3, during this stage, DNA replication results in duplication of chromosomes before cell division actually begins. Mitosis is the process of cell division which segregates this doubled DNA into two identical daughter cells.

As the parent cell enters into active cell division, the previously invisible chromosomes become visible by light microscopy. The DNA has already doubled, the membrane surrounding the cell nucleus begins to disappear, and two distinct small bodies, the centrioles, appear and migrate to opposite poles of the cell. Eventually, the cell's nuclear membrane completely disappears and the duplicated chromosomes line up side-by-side on the cell's central spindle or equator.

Next, the chromosomes separate longitudinally at the centromere and one chromatid of each chromosome pair migrates to the centrioles at opposite poles of the cell. In this manner, each pole receives a set of chromosomes identical to the original, nondividing cell prior to DNA duplication.

In the final phase of mitosis, the original parent cell divides into two identical daughter cells. The new daughter cells contain the diploid number of chromosomes which cluster at the poles of the two new cells. The chromosomes lose their distinct form and the process begins anew.

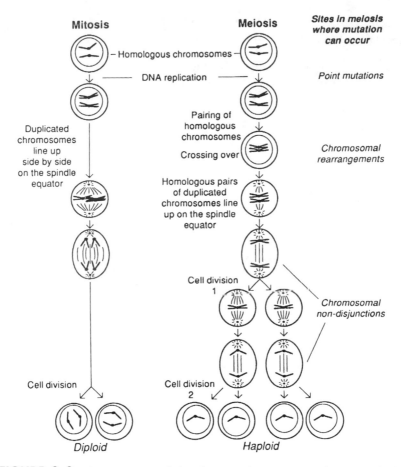

FIGURE 3–3. Comparison of the divisional processes of mitosis (*left panel*) and meiosis (*right panel*). Mitosis is the process through which a single somatic cell replicates to produce two daughter cells. Each identical daughter cell contains two complete sets of chromosomes (diploid number; 46 in humans). Meiosis is the process which produces germ cells (egg and sperm). Meiosis differs from mitosis in two important dimensions. First, "crossing over," the recombination of genetic material during meiosis produces genetic differences in germ cells. During crossing over, chromosomal rearrangements may arise which produce congenital anomalies. Second, reduction division results in germ cells which contains one complete set of chromosomes (haploid number; 23 in humans). The combination of two germ cells each with one complete set of chromosomes (haploid number) at fertilization results in a zygote with two complete sets of chromosomes (diploid number). During reduction division, chromosomal non-disjunctions may occur which produce congenital abnormalities. (From *Towards A Healthy Baby Congenital Disorders and the New Genetics in Primary Health Care* by B. Modell and M. Modell 1992, p. 37. London, England: Oxford University Press. Copyright 1992 by Oxford University Press. Used by permission of Oxford University Press.)

Meiosis

A similar process with important differences, meiosis, occurs in sex cells and results in reduction of a single diploid germ cell into four haploid gametes. As shown in the right half of Figure 3–3, the important differences during meiosis are "crossing over," or recombination of genetic material from the chromatids on a chromosome pair, and reduction in chromosome number from 46 to 23. Crossing over permits genetic material from the two parents to be shuffled into virtually infinite combinations. On the average, 30 to 40 crossing overs (one or two per chromosome) occur during meiotic division. Reduction in chromosome number results in a haploid germ cell which, when joined with the haploid germ cell from the parent of the opposite sex, produces a zygote with the species-specific diploid complement of chromosomes.

Meiosis occurs in two divisional processes; between the first and second meiotic division genetic material is not duplicated. Crossing over and recombination of genetic information occurs early in the first divisional process. During this process, chromosomal rearrangements that produce congenital abnormalities may occur. Reduction of genetic information into the haploid germ cell is the terminal meiotic event. During this process, errors in chromosomal separation and migration (chromosomal nondisjunctions) may also produce congenital anomalies.

Gametogenesis

In human males, the process of meiosis begins at puberty. The entire process takes approximately 65 days and results in four sperm cells with the haploid number of chromosomes from each original male germ cell (spermatogonia).

In human females, early germ cells in the first meiotic divisional process are present at birth and remain suspended in this stage until sexual maturity. At sexual maturity, a germ cell which has completed the first meiotic division (oocyte) is extruded each month. As it travels through the fallopian tube to the uterus, this cell undergoes the second meiotic division. In females, only one potentially fertile cell, the ovum, results from meiosis. After the first meiotic division, a major portion of cytoplasm goes to one daughter cell; the other daughter cell (polar body) contains 23 chromosomes but insignificant cytoplasm. The polar body is eventually discarded. Similarly, after the second meiotic division, another unequal division of cytoplasm occurs, and an ovum and another polar body develop. This polar body is also discarded.

LABORATORY EVALUATION OF CHROMOSOMES AND GENES

Viewing the genetic code has been an important challenge for more than a century. Although chromosomes were first observed in cells undergoing division in the late 19th century, it was more than five decades later before the actual number of chromosomes in the human karyotype was correctly identified. Today, geneticists directly view minor changes in chromosomes that lead to the identification of important hereditary disorders, and also indirectly examine DNA sequences in individual genes. In addition, diagnosis of genetic disease before birth is possible through techniques that permit examination of embryonic and fetal cells.

Cytogenetics

Cytogenetics is the branch of genetics devoted to study of chromosomes. To evaluate chromosomes, cytogeneticists must obtain body cells capable of growth and rapid division. White blood cells are easily acquired and suitable for chromosome analysis. Generally, a sample of peripheral blood is drawn and centrifuged to separate out white blood cells. These cells are placed in a tissue culture medium and cell division is stimulated by addition of a chemical agent. After a 3-day incubation, cell division is chemically arrested, the cell membrane is disintegrated, and the intact chromosomes are released. The chromosomes are fixed, mounted on slides, and stained. The prepared chromosomes are now ready for analysis.

A variety of techniques are used for chromosome staining. One common technique, G method or G-banding, requires denaturing the chromosome proteins for subsequent staining with Giemsa stain (a solution containing azure dye). G-banding results in a distinctive pattern of light and dark bands which uniquely identify specific chromosomes. Other staining methods employ different processing and compounds to illuminate the chromosomes. For example, Q-banding utilizes compounds that luminesce under fluorescence microscopy. High-resolution banding involves G-banding chromosomes in an early phase of cell division permitting visualization of subtle chromosomal aberrations such as microdeletions and small translocations.

An internationally recognized system of human chromosome classification was formulated in the early 1970s. Figures 3–4 and 3–5 show normal human chromosomes arranged in this classification system. Figure 3–4 shows the normal female karyotype (46,XX); Figure 3–5 shows the normal male karyotype (46,XY). The

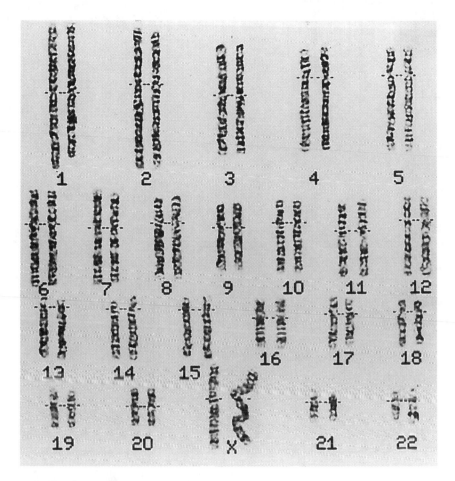

FIGURE 3–4. Karyotype of a normal human female. There are 22 pairs of autosomes arranged by size and one pair of sex chromosomes, XX. (Courtesy of Loris McGavren, Colorado Cytogenetics, Denver.)

22 autosomes are arranged according to length with the longest chromosome numbered one and the shortest numbered 22. The sex chromosomes are displayed following chromosome 22.

Recently, techniques developed for recombinant DNA research are being applied to examine chromosomes. Termed molecular cytogenetics, these techniques permit examination of specific regions of individual chromosomes. One technique, fluorescence in situ hybridization (FISH), allows detection of chromosomal aberrations through fluorescing DNA probes (segments of DNA which are labeled by radioisotopes and which contain a specific

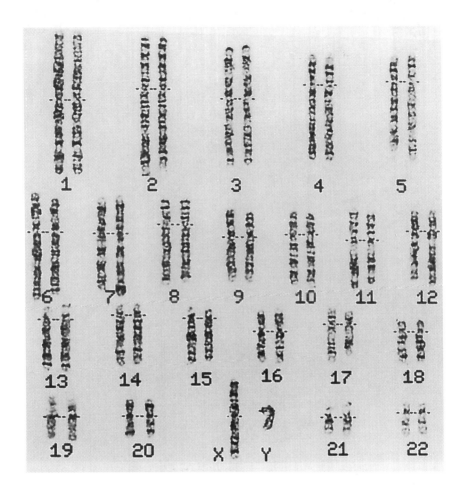

FIGURE 3–5. Karyotype of a normal human male. There are 22 pairs of autosomes arranged by size and one pair of sex chromosomes, XY. (Courtesy of Loris McGavren, Colorado Cytogenetics, Denver.)

DNA code). DNA probes will bind to complementary DNA if it is present in the sample. Molecular cytogenetics is a rapidly growing subspecialty of cytogenetics.

Molecular Genetics

Molecular genetics refers to study of the structure and function of genes through analysis of DNA. The highly sophisticated techniques used in molecular genetics have been developed primarily in the past two decades. These techniques permit detailed examination of the genetic code in both normal and abnormal genes. Molecular genetics has revolutionized understanding of human genetic disease, its inheritance, diagnosis, and treatment.

Because single genes cannot be seen directly, other methods are needed to visualize and analyze DNA. Some techniques of molecular genetic analysis include restriction endonucleases which yield restriction fragments of DNA, Southern blots, DNA probes, and polymerase chain reactions (PCR). These techniques are applied to DNA isolated from blood or tissue cells.

Restriction endonucleases are bactcrial enzymes that recognize a specific DNA base code and cleave the DNA chain each time this code is encountered. Because each individual's DNA is unique, the number and size of DNA fragments, or restriction fragments, produced by this process are unique to the individual. The fragments are sorted by molecular weight, reduced from double- to single-stranded fragments by chemical reaction, and transferred to a nylon filter membrane (Southern blot). To identify and label specific sections of DNA, single-stranded radioactive DNA probes which will bind to complementary single-stranded DNA fragments in the sample are applied to the membrane. Radioactivity from the probe-bound DNA exposes x-ray film to produce a distinct pattern of dark bands. The position and number of dark bands on the film produces the DNA "fingerprint" of the individual.

Polymerase chain reaction (PCR) permits selective amplification of a specific fragment of DNA. A fragment of interest (e.g., a segment thought to contain the DNA code for a specific hereditary disease) is isolated and bound to single-stranded complements of DNA. Under treatment with certain enzymes, these strands will double. Multiple cycles of enzyme treatment will amplify the target DNA sequence exponentially. DNA from relatively poor-quality samples, for example, saliva swabs or single embryonic cells, can be amplified quickly for molecular analysis. DNA probes can then be added to the sample to identify and label specific sections of code.

Molecular genetic analysis may be useful for assessing the probability of genetic disease in families at-risk, especially if the locus of the genetic defect is known. Through these techniques, scientists have identified the DNA abnormality in more than 125 conditions including adult polycystic kidney disease, neurofibromatosis type I and type II, hemophilia A, Usher syndrome type II, Fragile X syndrome, Treacher-Collins syndrome, and Waardenburg syndrome.

Prenatal Diagnosis

Prenatal diagnosis has been applied clinically for more than 30 years. Many conditions may be diagnosed at an early stage in fetal development through ultrasonographic imaging, cytogenetic or DNA analysis of fetal cells, or biochemical analysis of maternal serum.

Techniques for prenatal diagnosis range from indirect, non-invasive imaging by sophisticated ultrasonography to direct sampling of fetal skin or blood. Cytogenetic and molecular genetic techniques applied to fetal cells permits diagnosis of some genetic conditions and congenital malformations in utero. Major congenital abnormalities that can be accurately detected through a variety of prenatal diagnostic techniques include neural tube defects, chromosomal disorders, structural malformations, and severe hematological and metabolic disorders.

More recently, experimental techniques have been developed to assess genetic characteristics of maternal germ cells (ova) before fertilization and very early embryos (e.g., within 1 week after conception) before implantation.

Ultrasonography

Ultrasound is a sensitive and relatively risk-free approach to prenatal diagnosis. The fetus is imaged in utero by reflection of very high-frequency (e.g., above 2.0 Megahertz) energy delivered across the mother's abdominal wall. Experienced ultrasonographers can detect major central nervous system abnormalities (e.g., anencephaly, myelomeningocele, hydrocephalus), skeletal abnormalities (e.g., osteogenesis imperfecta and severe neonatal bone dysplasia), and internal abnormalities (e.g., severe congenital heart defects, renal agenesis, and fetal abdominal wall defects).

Cytogenetic or Molecular Genetic Analysis of Fetal Cells

Cytogenetic or molecular genetic analysis can be applied to fetal blood or tissue cells. As described previously, cytogenetic analysis is useful for diagnosis of chromosomal abnormalities (changes in chromosome number or alterations in chromosome structure); molecular genetic analysis is useful when the location of an abnormal gene on a specific chromosome is generally known.

Fetal cells for analysis can be obtained by several invasive procedures. The most common procedure, amniocentesis, entails removal of a small amount of the amniotic fluid, the fluid that surrounds the fetus, in mid gestation. It is typically performed under local anesthetic as an outpatient procedure. Figure 3–6 shows a schematic representation of amniocentesis. Under visualization by ultrasonographic scanning, a hollow needle is guided into the uterus through the mother's abdominal and uterine walls. A small

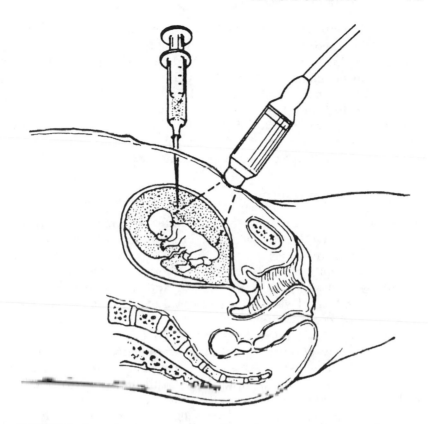

FIGURE 3-6. Schematic representation of amniocentesis, a technique by which a sample of amniotic fluid containing fetal cells and maternal scrum is withdrawn for analysis. Under ultrasonographic visualization, a hollow needle is guided through the mother's abdominal and uterine wall into the fluid-filled cavity surrounding the fetus. A small sample of fluid is then withdrawn for analysis. (From *Danforth's Obstetrics and Gynecology*, Seventh Edition, by J. R. Scott, P. J. DiSala, C. B. Hammond, and W. N. Spellacy Eds., 1994, p. 217. Philadelphia, PA: J. B. Lippincott. Copyright 1994 by J. B. Lippincott. Reprinted with permission.)

(e.g., 20 ml) sample of amniotic fluid is withdrawn for analysis. Amniotic fluid contains fetal cells, including skin cells and cells from the epithelial layer that lines the gastrointestinal, respiratory, and urinary tracts. Both the fluid itself and the fetal cells can be analyzed for fetal defects. For example, amniotic fluid can be investigated for presence of teratogenic agents such as rubella virus or specific proteins associated with neural tube defects. Viable cells obtained through amniocentesis can be cultured for cytologic, biochemical, or molecular genetic analysis. Amniocentesis is typically performed at about 15–16 weeks following the last menstrual period. Because of recent advances in ultrasonographic scanning, amniocentesis may be performed earlier in pregnancy.

Fetal cells may also be obtained by chorionic villus sampling (CVS). The chorionic villus is a fetal component of the placenta; CVS extracts a minute quantity of these fetal-placental cells for analysis. CVS may be performed either transabdominally or transcervically as early as 9 weeks following the last menstrual period.

Preimplantation Diagnosis

More recently, experimental techniques for preimplantation genetic diagnosis have been developed. Preimplantation diagnosis requires procedures developed for in vitro fertilization (fertilization outside the mother's body). Two techniques are available on an experimental basis, polar body analysis and embryo biopsy.

Polar body analysis requires retrieval of egg cells (oocytes) and their discarded by-products, polar bodies, following induced ovulation. Cytogenetic and molecular cytogenetic investigation of the first polar body permits indirect genetic diagnosis of the oocyte. Oocytes free of genetic disorder can be selected for fertilization and implantation. This technique is useful only for investigating genetic disorders inherited from the mother.

Embryo biopsy permits chromosomal and genetic analysis of the zygote before implantation. On day 3 following fertilization, when the zygote is a 6- to 10-cell mass of identical cells (see Chapter 4), one to three cells are removed for DNA analysis. Those zygotes free of genetic disease are implanted. Embryo biopsy apparently does not result in any detrimental effect to the embryo; births of normal children have been reported following embryo biopsy.

INHERITANCE OF GENETIC DISORDERS

When investigating the possibility of a genetic disorder, geneticists construct a family pedigree. A family pedigree is essentially a detailed family history of the inheritance of the trait in question. It provides a simple, universal method for recording the relevant family medical history and for illustrating familial inheritance of traits and disease.

Inherited disorders may result from a variety of factors including single-gene and chromosomal abnormalities. More recently, other means of inheritance have been identified that do not follow classically described single gene or chromosomal mechanisms. These mechanisms, "nontraditional inheritance," reveal that genetic inheritance is much more complex than previously understood. All of these mechanisms, single-gene, chromosomal abnormalities, and nontraditional inheritance, can be modeled by constructing a family pedigree.

Single Gene Defects

Single-gene defects are those which follow patterns of inheritance predicted by Mendel's famous garden pea experiments. Single-gene defects may be the result of abnormal gene or genes on one of the 22 pairs of autosomes (autosomal gene defect) or an abnormal gene on one of the sex chromosomes (X-linked defect).

Recall that, upon fertilization of the ovum by a sperm, each parent contributes one copy (allele) of each autosomal gene to the offspring. If the two alleles on the matched chromosome pair are identical, the individual is homozygous for the trait produced by that gene. If the two alleles are different, the individual is heterozygous for the trait. Mendel deduced inheritance of traits from this blending of parental gene pools.

Mendel worked with garden peas because (a) they exhibited distinct, constant, and easily recognizable traits (e.g., smooth vs. wrinkled seed; short vs. tall plant) and (b) they could be easily protected from unwanted or foreign pollen, thereby ensuring reliable breeding. By determining the nature and ratio of distinct traits in successive generations of a single parent pair, Mendel inferred inheritance of single-gene characteristics. An example from Mendel's original experiments is shown in Figure 3–7.

Mendel observed that the ripe seeds of the pea plant exhibited only two distinct forms, round and generally smooth (noted as AA, "Smooth," in Figure 3–7), or irregularly angular and deeply wrinkled (noted as aa, "Wrinkled," in Figure 3–7). To produce a first generation hybrid, Mendel cross-bred smooth seed plants with wrinkled seed plants. This crossbreeding resulted in first generation hybrids (F_1) whose seed characteristics resembled the smooth parent entirely. Mendel labeled the characteristics that were transmitted unchanged as dominant (A), and the characteristics that apparently disappeared in the process as recessive (a).

Mendel then bred a second-generation hybrid (F_2) from F_1. In this generation, he observed that the recessive trait, wrinkled seed, reappeared in an average proportion of one recessive to three dominant characteristics. Thus, among four F_2 plants, one plant developed wrinkled seeds, and three plants developed smooth seeds. He

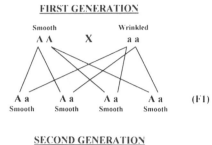

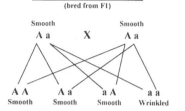

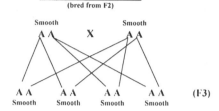

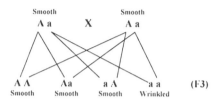

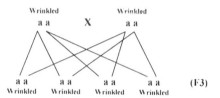

FIGURE 3–7. Representation of one of Mendel's original experiments with garden peas which elucidated inheritance of single-gene traits. In this example, inheritance of the trait of seed shape (smooth or wrinkled) is traced through three interbred generations.

expressly noted that "transitional" (e.g., semi-smooth or partially wrinkled) forms were not observed in any experiment.

Mendel continued breeding the hybrids. In the F_3 generation, Mendel noted that one third of F_2 parents always produced F_3 offspring with dominant, smooth seeds and that two thirds of those offspring of the dominant, smooth seed, F_2 parents produced F_3 plants with either dominant characteristics (smooth seeds) or recessive characteristics (wrinkled seeds) in the previously identified proportion of one recessive to three dominant. Offspring of the recessive, wrinkled seed, F_2 parents remained constant in their characteristic; they did not produce any smooth seed plants. From these experiments, Mendel deduced several principles of genetic transmission including inheritance of recessive and dominant characteristics.

Autosomal Dominant Disorders

Autosomal dominant disorders are due to an abnormality of a gene located on one of the 22 autosome pairs (chromosome numbers 1 to 22). As defined by Mendel, a disorder is dominant if one of the alleles produces the defect. In this case, the abnormal gene on one of the autosome pairs "overrides" the normal gene on its matched pair. Dominant disorders, therefore, represent an heterozygous effect. Examples of autosomal dominant disorders include Treacher Collins syndrome, Apert syndrome, and Crouzon syndrome.

The rule of inheritance of autosomal dominant includes (a) one affected parent, (b) both males and females are affected and transmit the disorder, (c) 50% risk for offspring to inherit the disorder from an affect parent, and (d) nonaffected offspring cannot transmit the disorder (no carrier state). A negative family history does not preclude presence of an autosomal dominant disorder. Reasons for a negative family history include (a) new mutation in the affected individual, (b) undiagnosed mild expression of the disorder in the parent, (c) inaccurately identified paternity, or (d) nontraditional inheritance through germ cell abnormality in one parent (gonadal mosaicism). Figure 3–8 shows a family pedigree associated with an idealized example of autosomal dominant inheritance.

An individual may inherit two copies of an abnormal autosomal dominant gene. In this relatively unusual case, the individual is homozygous for a dominant effect. For some autosomal dominant characteristics such as achondroplasia, this "double-dose" of the abnormal gene results in very severe or lethal disease. Homozygosity for dominant characteristics can occur when the prevalence of the defective gene in the general population is relatively high and its effect is relatively mild or when affected individuals preferentially marry (deaf marrying deaf).

Among the factors that may complicate diagnosis of autosomal dominant disorders is lack of penetrance and variable expression of the disorder. Lack of penetrance refers to the proportion of individuals known to carry the gene who fail to demonstrate the trait. Theoretically, all individuals who are heterozygous for an autosomal dominant trait should demonstrate the trait. In reality, a proportion of individuals known to carry the gene do not demonstrate the trait. These cases are typically detected by family pedigrees in which an unaffected individual is detected who is the offspring of an affected parent and the parent of affected offspring. This "skipped generation" is the result of a variety of mechanisms including subclinical presence of the disease, late onset, or absence of other obligatory genetic or environmental interactions in the skipped generation.

Variability in expression refers to the degree to which the disorder is manifest in the affected individual. Some autosomal dominant disorders are expressed with little variability; most demonstrate a range of expression. Individuals with Waardenburg syn-

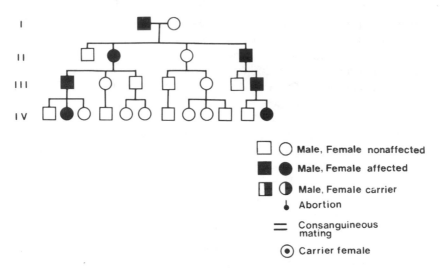

Male, Female nonaffected
Male, Female affected
Male, Female carrier
Abortion
Consanguineous mating
Carrier female

FIGURE 3–8. Diagram of an idealized example of autosomal dominant inheritance. Notice the vertical transmission and that affected individuals appear in every generation. On average, the trait is transmitted to 50% of offspring. Unaffected individuals do not transmit the trait. Equal numbers of males and females are affected. Male-to-male transmission is seen. (From *Developmental Pathology of the Embryo and Fetus* by J. E. Dimmick and D. K. Kalousek, Eds., 1992, p. 114. Philadelphia, PA. J. B. Lippincott Company. Copyright 1992 by J. B. Lippincott Company. Reprinted with permission.)

drome, a genetic syndrome including hearing loss, characteristic facial features, hair and skin pigmentary changes, ocular findings, and other symptoms, exhibit striking variability in expression of this disorder. Hearing sensitivity may range from normal to profound deafness; pigmentary changes may include none to marked areas of depigmentation.

Both lack of penetrance and variability in expression present dilemmas in the genetic evaluation. Lack of penetrance may complicate unambiguous identification of an autosomal dominant disorder; variability in expression may mislead parents into underestimating the severity of the genetic condition.

Autosomal Recessive Disorders

Autosomal recessive disorders are due to abnormalities of both alleles of a given gene. Affected individuals are thus homozygous for the effect. For an individual to exhibit an autosomal recessive disorder, he or she must inherit identical abnormal genes from each parent. Typically, the parent is heterozygous for the disorder, and because two abnormal genes must be present for the disorder to be expressed, the parent is an unaffected carrier. Examples of autosomal recessive disorders include phenylketonuria (PKU), cystic fibrosis, and Tay-Sachs disease.

The rule of inheritance of autosomal recessive transmission includes: (a) unaffected parents both of whom are heterozygous for the trait, (b) both males and females are affected, (c) 25% of offspring of two carrier parents are affected (homozygous), and (d) two thirds of unaffected offspring of heterozygous parents (carriers) are also heterozygous (carriers). Figure 3–9 shows family pedigrees associated with idealized autosomal recessive inheritance.

In autosomal recessive disorders, lack of penetrance is rarely encountered, and variability in expression is less pronounced than in autosomal dominant disorders. A important factor influencing successful diagnosis of an autosomal recessive condition is often lack of a positive family history (example C, Figure 3–9). In some rare autosomal recessive disorders, consanguinity (marriage/mating of close relatives) may be a factor (example A, Figure 3-9). The risk of inheritance of abnormal traits in consanguinous marriages is related to the proportion of shared genes. Table 3–1 summarizes the degree of family relationship and proportion of shared genes. The higher the proportion of shared genes, the greater the risk of inheritance of abnormal traits.

X-linked Disorders

X-linked disorders are caused by an abnormal gene or genes on the X sex chromosome. Most X-linked disorders are recessive. In these cases, females are unaffected because they have two X chromosomes with at least one normal gene. If a female is heterozygous for the defect, 50% of her male offspring will be affected (each male offspring will inherit one X chromosome; those who inherit the X chromosome with the abnormal gene will exhibit the disorder). Female offspring of the same heterozygous mother will have a 50% chance of being a carrier for the trait. Examples of X-linked inheritance include hemophilia.

The rule of inheritance for X-linked disorders includes: (a) inheritance through the maternal line, (b) no male-to-male (father-to-son) inheritance, (c) 50% male offspring of a carrier female affected, (d) 50% of female offspring of a carrier female are also carriers, and (e) absence or milder form of the disorder in the car-

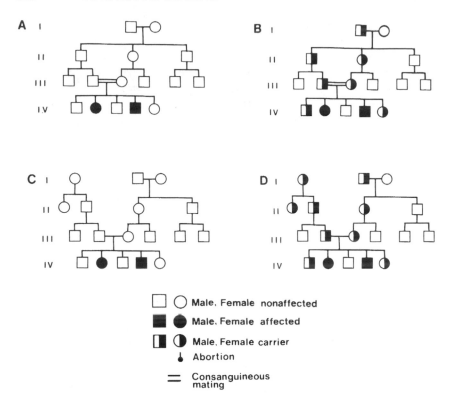

FIGURE 3-9. Diagram of idealized examples of autosomal recessive inheritance. Notice the horizontal distribution of affected individuals. Carriers are present among parents, siblings, offspring, and other relatives. On average 25% of the offspring of two carriers will be affected, and 50% will be carriers (i.e., two-thirds of the unaffected children). The number of affected individuals or carrier individuals who are male and female are equal. (A) and (C) do not show carrier status, whereas (B) and (D) indicate carriers. (A) and (B) demonstrate a family with consanguinity and the inheritance of the abnormal gene from thje common ancestor, the grandfather. (From *Developmental Pathology of the Embryo and Fetus* by J. E. Dimmick and D. K. Kalousek, Eds. 1992, p. 114. Philadelphia, PA. J. B. Lippincott Company. Copyright 1992 by J. B. Lippincott Company. Reprinted with permission.)

rier female. Figure 3-10 shows idealized examples of the variations in family pedigrees associated with both recessive and dominant X-linked inheritance.

Table 3-1. Degree of family relationships and proportion of shared genes.

Degree	Proportion of Shared Genes
First	One-half
Siblings	
Dizygotic twins	
Parents	
Children	
Second	One-fourth
Half siblings	
Uncles, aunts	
Nephews, nieces	
Third	One-eighth
First cousins	
Half uncles, aunts	
Half nephews, nieces	

Abnormalities Related to Gene/Environment Interaction

Many common congenital anomalies do not exhibit classic Mendelian inheritance and are not associated with a chromosomal abnormality. Although exact cause of these anomalies remains largely unknown, it is believed that birth defects such as congenital heart defects, cleft lip and palate, and neural tube defects are inherited through the interaction of multiple genes with environmental influences (multifactorial inheritance). Similar to single-gene defects, multifactorial disorders often cluster in families. Unlike single gene defects, which exhibit predictable patterns of familial inheritance, these disorders demonstrate no predictable pattern of family inheritance.

Risk for multifactorial inheritance is often described by the liability model with a threshold effect. By this model, all individuals in a population are at risk (liable) for a specific disorder but only individuals who exceed an imaginary threshold will exhibit the disorder. For example, consider a case in which there are seven conditions that influence development of a defect: three gene pairs (six alleles) and one environmental condition (e.g., prenatal nutrition). An individual may exhibit normal function with as many as four unfavorable conditions (e.g., three abnormal alle-

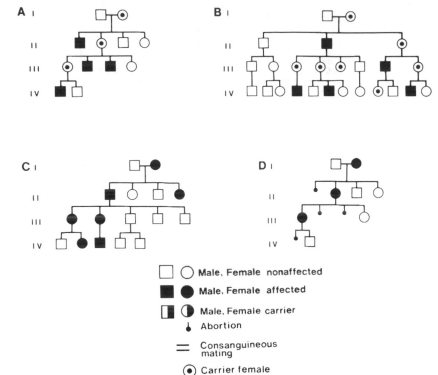

FIGURE 3–10. Diagram of idealized examples of X-linked inheritance: (A) X-linked recessive inheritance, with lethality or absence of reproduction in males; (B) X-linked recessive inheritance with fertility in males; (C) X-linked dominant inheritance; (D) X-linked dominant inheritance with lethality in utero to affected males, who are seen as spontaneous abortions. Note there is no male-to-male transmission. Carrier females do not ordinarily manifest disease in X-linked recessive disorders. In X-linked dominant disorders there are twice as many affected females as males. (From *Developmental Pathology of the Embryo and Fetus* by J. E. Dimmick and D. K. Kalousek, Eds., 1992, p. 114. Philadelphia, PA: J. B. Lippincott Company. Copyright 1992 by J. B. Lippincott Company. Reprinted with permission.)

les and inadequate prenatal nutrition). If five unfavorable conditions exist (e.g., four abnormal alleles and inadequate prenatal nutrition), however, the individual will exhibit the disorder; the imaginary threshold has been passed.

Recurrence risk for multifactorial disorders cannot be predicted by mathematical rules based on population studies. Factors influencing risk include number of family members affected, degree of relatedness to those affected (e.g., first-degree vs. second-degree relatives), severity of the disorder, and frequency of the disorder in specific populations (e.g., neural tube defects are more prevalent in Irish and English populations).

Chromosomal Abnormalities

Two basic defects result in chromosomal abnormalities: changes in chromosome number (chromosomal nondisjunctions) and changes in chromosome structure (chromosomal rearrangements).

Changes in Chromosomal Number

Recall that the human karyotype contains 46 chromosomes, 22 autosomal pairs and 1 sex pair. During meiosis, the diploid cell with its 46 chromosomes replicates and reduces into four haploid cells with 23 chromosomes each. Nondisjunction, or failure of chromosomes to separate during this process (see Figure 3–3), results in development of at least one gamete with 24 chromosomes and one gamete with 22 chromosomes. The other two gametes may either be normal haploid cells with 23 chromosomes, or abnormal with 24 and 22 chromosomes respectively, depending on when nondisjunction occurred. If one of these abnormal gametes fertilizes or is fertilized, the resulting zygote will have trisomy (2N + 1 chromosomes) or monosomy (2N − 1 chromosomes). Trisomy 21 (three copies of the 21st chromosome), Down syndrome, is a common birth defect occurring with an overall frequency of 1 in 600 live births. Figure 3–11 shows a human karyotype with a extra copy of chromosome 21 (trisomy 21).

Few monosomies are compatible with life; monosomy of the X chromosome results in Turner syndrome.

Changes in chromosome number typically result in marked physical abnormalities including dysmorphism (unusual appearance), congenital malformations, and mental retardation.

Changes in Chromosome Structure

Changes in chromosome structure, chromosomal rearrangements, are relatively common. Depending on the location of the abnormality, there may be little or no effect, or a severe disorder. The major types of chromosome rearrangements are deletions, duplications,

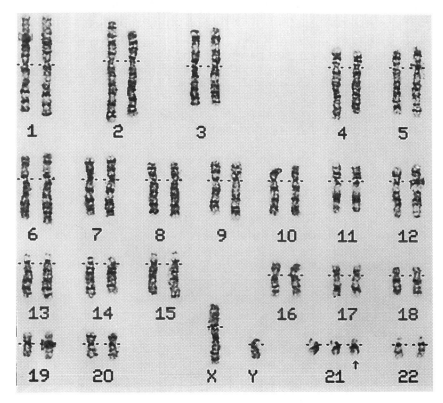

FIGURE 3–11. Karyotype of a male infant with trisomy 21 (Down syndrome). Note the presence of an extra copy of the 21st chromosome. (Courtesy of Loris McGavren, Colorado Cytogenetics, Denver.)

inversions, and translocations. These chromosomal rearrangements occur during the crossing over phase of meiosis (see Figure 3–3).

Deletions occur when a portion of the chromosome is missing. Deletions may occur at the ends of long (q-) or short arms (p-), or as an interstitial deletion. Interstitial deletions result when the chromosome breaks in two locations and the distal portion reattaches to the remaining chromosome fragment. Genes located on the deleted portion of the chromosome are missing. Because a portion of the genetic code in lost in chromosome deletions, individuals with this chromosomal abnormality are often severely affected. Cri-du-chat syndrome with associated profound psychomotor retardation is the result of deletion of the short arm of the fifth chromosome (5p-).

Duplications occur when a segment of a chromosome occurs more than the normal number of times within a given chromosome. The process of duplication results in extra copies of specific genes on the chromosome which may or may not result in noticeable characteristics. Some individuals with Cornelia de Lange syndrome have been identified with duplication in a segment of the long arm (q) of chromosome 3.

Inversions occur when a portion of a chromosome is rearranged in reverse order. When this occurs, the chromosome breaks in two locations, and the portion of the chromosome intermediary to the breaks rotates 180° and reattaches.

Translocations occur when one segment of a chromosome transfers to another chromosome following breakage. During translocation, all genetic information may be transferred unaltered (balance translocation) or genetic information may be added or lost (unbalanced translocation). Persons with balanced translocations appear normal but are at risk for transmitting unbalanced translocations to their offspring. Person with unbalanced translocations may demonstrate specific disorders.

Nontraditional Inheritance

Nontraditional inheritance is a recent concept which explains genetic inheritance by mechanisms other than mendelian principles or chromosomal abnormalities.

Uniparental Disomy

Uniparental disomy refers to the phenomenon of inheriting both chromosomes of a pair from a single parent. In this case, the child inherits both copies of a specific chromosome (either both copies of a specific autosome or the sex chromosomes) from one parent with no representation of that chromosome from the other parent. This atypical form of genetic transmission has been described in cases of cystic fibrosis, Prader-Willi syndrome, and hemophilia A. The frequency of uniparental disomy is unknown and may be undetected if an abnormal gene is not involved. It may account for the unexpected presence of autosomal recessive disorders in patients with only one carrier parent or for an unusual presentation of a disorder.

Genomic Imprinting

Genomic imprinting refers to the differential expression of a genetic disorder related to the gender of the transmitting parent. In this case, the expression of inherited traits depends on whether the specific gene for that trait was inherited from the mother or the father.

Two of the most striking examples of genomic imprinting are Prader-Willi syndrome and Angelman syndrome. These two syndromes are clinically distinct. Prader-Willi syndrome is a dysmorphic syndrome characterized by obesity, short stature, small hands and feet, hypogonadism, and mental retardation. Angelman syndrome is characterized by severe mental retardation, microcephaly, seizures, electroencephalogram (EEG) abnormalities, mild hypotonia, ataxic gait, and eye abnormalities.

Both Prader-Willi and Angelman syndrome result from abnormalities in inheritance of chromosome 15. Approximately 70% of individuals with Prader-Willi syndrome exhibit a deletion in a portion of the long arm of chromosome 15 inherited from the father; the genomes of these patients have genetic information on a portion of chromosome 15 that is derived solely from their mother (the other 30% of affected individuals exhibit maternal uniparental disomy for chromosome 15). In contrast, individuals with Angelman syndrome exhibit a deletion in the same region of the long arm of chromosome 15 inherited from the mother. The genomes of these patients have genetic information that is derived solely from their father.

Genomic imprinting has been studied in laboratory-bred mice. In these experiments, mouse development has been shown to be strikingly affected by parental origin of specific DNA. These experiments, as well as the clinical observations in Prader-Willi and Angelman syndrome, suggest that, at least for some traits, (a) difference in parental origin of DNA is somehow recognized in the developing organism, and (b) a complement of both maternal and paternal DNA is necessary for normal development.

Mitochondrial Inheritance

Mitochondria are small spherical bodies found in the cytoplasm of cells. They are the principle energy source for the cell. Mitochondria are believed to have evolved from microorganisms that formed a symbiotic relationship with the progenitors of animal cells many millennia ago. Because these bodies evolved from separate biologic material, they contain their own DNA which replicates independently of nuclear DNA.

Similar to nuclear DNA, mutation of mitochondrial DNA can produce inherited disorders. Typically, these disorders affect muscle and nervous tissue. Several specific disorders associated with mitochondrial DNA mutation have been identified including disorders with associated hearing loss (Elverland & Tobergsen, 1991; Hutchin & Cortopassi, 1995). In most cases, onset of dysfunction associated with mitochondrially inherited disorders is observed after infancy.

Mitochondria are transmitted exclusively through the maternal egg cell. Maternal mitochondrial inheritance is similar to autosomal dominant inheritance with two important differences. First, in mitochondrial inheritance, 100% of offspring are affected rather than the 50% in highly penetrant autosomal dominant inheritance. Second, traits inherited through mitochondrial DNA are never transmitted through a male. Although males and females are affected at equal rates, males do not transmit mitochondria to future generations.

Triplet Repeat Disorders

Some inherited disorders present in more severe forms or at an earlier age in successive generations. Until recently, this phenomenon, anticipation, was thought to reflect diagnostic bias rather than a true biologic event. Molecular genetic methods, however, have revealed that anticipation is associated with an abnormal number of DNA repeats on specific chromosomes. For example, Fragile X syndrome, the most common cause of mental retardation in males, involves multiple replications of the DNA sequence <CGG> at a particular location on the X chromosome in affected males. In nonaffected individuals, this sequence may be repeated up to 50 times; in affected individuals, as many as 1000 <CGG> repeats may be present. Individuals with more severe expression of Fragile X syndrome tend to demonstrate greater numbers of triplet repeats. Other disorders exhibiting triplet repeats include Huntington's disease, spinobulbar muscular atrophy, and spinocerebellar ataxia type 1.

In all clinical conditions in which a triplet expansion has been found, anticipation is present; that is, there is a correlation between the number of triplet repeats and the severity of the disorder or its age of onset. DNA expansion and anticipation do not account for all variability in expression of these disorders, however.

Nontraditional inheritance represents one of the new frontiers of genetics that have been revealed by molecular genetics. Expansion of the human genome project will undoubtedly disclose even more unexpected patterns of human genetic inheritance.

HEARING LOSS ASSOCIATED WITH GENETIC ABNORMALITY

The hereditary basis of hearing impairment has been investigated for more than 100 years. In the mid 1800s, an Irish physician, Sir William Wilde, described inheritance of deafness through various modes of genetic transmission. His descriptions distinguished between transmission by "hereditary taint" (dominant) and by "too close consanguinity" (recessive). He also observed a higher proportion of deaf male versus deaf female offspring from congenitally deaf parents suggesting X-linked transmission. Wilde has been credited with describing indirectly the three forms of single-gene (mendelian) inheritance of deafness a decade *before* Mendel published his treatise on inheritance of traits in garden peas. In the late 1800s, by evaluating the families of children in schools for the deaf, investigators confirmed and extended Wilde's pioneering findings.

Hereditary hearing impairment may be categorized by a variety of schemes including (a) type of inheritance (single-gene, chromosomal, multifactorial), (b) onset (congenital, acquired, early onset, late onset), (c) degree (mild through profound), (d) affected structures (external ear, middle ear, inner ear, neural), and (e) associated with other abnormalities (syndrome delineation). In working with infants and families, audiologists and speech-language pathologists are most often interested in congenital or early onset hearing loss occurring in isolation or associated with other abnormalities. Syndromes most commonly observed in infants are discussed below. In addition, some hereditary disorders with onset later than infancy are included because of their relatively high frequency (e.g., Alport syndrome).

Congenital or Early-Onset Hearing Loss with No Associated Abnormalities

Twenty-three forms of hereditary hearing loss with no other abnormalities have been described (Gorlin, Toriello, & Cohen, 1995). These forms of hereditary hearing loss are characterized as separate genetic entities on the basis of mode of inheritance (dominant, recessive, or X-linked), age of onset, degree of hearing loss, and audiometric configuration. Among persons with hereditary hearing loss, it is estimated that autosomal dominant transmission is present in 22%, autosomal recessive transmission is present in 77%, and X-linked transmission is present in 1% (Morton, 1991). At least three genes responsible for autosomal recessive hearing loss and two genes for autosomal dominant hearing loss have been located.

Hereditary Hearing Loss with Associated Abnormalities

One of the most useful systems for classifying hereditary hearing impairment is syndrome delineation. Through this approach, the major clinical features of the syndrome are identified (e.g., hearing impairment with central nervous system abnormalities). This approach permits identification and comparison of syndromes with similar characteristics. A recent comprehensive text (Gorlin, Toriello, and Cohen, 1995) provides an exhaustive description of more than 400 hereditary syndromes that include hearing impairment with associated abnormalities. Some of the syndromes more commonly identified in infants are described below.

Hearing Loss with Associated Craniofacial Disorders

It is not unexpected that hearing impairment is commonly associated with congenital craniofacial disorders. Because the external and middle ear arise from tissues associated with development of other head and face structures, alteration in normal tissue development during the embryonic period may result in disorders of craniofacial and auditory mechanisms. Infants with hearing impairment associated with craniofacial disorders are especially vulnerable to delay in oral speech and language development. These babies should receive prompt evaluation and management by a team of specialists in genetics, otolaryngology, audiology, speech-language pathology, child development, and other disciplines as needed.

Aural Atresia and Microtia. Although frequently associated with syndromal anomalies, aural atresia with microtia and conductive hearing loss often occurs in isolation. It is not unusual for an audiologist to encounter an infant in the newborn nursery who is normal in all respects except for an isolated atresia and microtia. Typically, the defect is unilateral although bilateral forms can occur. Males are affected twice as often as females (2M:1F); the right side is more often affected than the left (65% right, 35% left). Hearing loss is typically conductive and ranges from moderate-to-severe; unilateral or bilateral in unilateral atresia and bilateral in bilateral atresia. Both autosomal dominant and autosomal recessive transmission of congenital aural atresia, microtia, and conductive hearing loss have been identified.

Mandibulofacial Dysostosis (Treacher Collins Syndrome). Treacher Collins syndrome is one of the more widely recognized hereditary hearing impairment syndromes. Individuals with Treacher Collins syndrome demonstrate a variety of craniofacial abnormalities including narrow face, downward-sloping palpebral fissures (lateral junction of the upper and lower eyelid), malformed pinnae, aural atresia, anomalies of the auditory ossicles, and mandibular hypoplasia. Bilateral, conductive hearing loss secondary to external and middle ear anomalies is frequently present. Typically, children with Treacher Collins syndrome have normal intelligence although mild mental retardation has been reported. This syndrome is characterized by autosomal dominant transmission with variable expression. The genetic locus has been mapped to the long arm of the fifth chromosome (5q). Approximately 60% of individuals with Treacher Collins syndrome are thought to represent new mutations.

Oculo-Auriculo-Vertebral (OAV) Spectrum (Goldenhar Syndrome). This syndrome is diagnosed in infants who demonstrate unilateral involvement of structures that evolve from the first and second branchial arches. Infants with OAV spectrum may show a wide range of anomalies including mandibular hypoplasia and unilateral aural atresia and microtia. Abnormalities may also be observed in ocular, central nervous, pulmonary, cardiovascular, gastrointestinal, and renal systems. Infants with OAV spectrum usually have unilateral or bilateral conductive hearing loss. Mental retardation has been reported in as many as 15% of cases. OAV spectrum appears to be sporadic in most families although an autosomal dominant form has been identified in some families (less than 2% of cases).

Branchio-Oto-Renal (BOR) Syndrome (Ear-Pit Hearing Loss Syndrome). BOR syndrome refers to identification of branchial cleft cysts, fistulas or sinuses (cysts, fistulas or sinuses in the lower third of the neck), otologic abnormalities including malformed pinnae, preauricular pits (ear pits) and hearing loss, and renal abnormalities including renal agenesis, polycystic kidneys, and other structural anomalies. Hearing impairment may be conductive, mixed, or sensorineural. Children with BOR syndrome usually have normal intelligence. Studies of multiple generations of several families support an autosomal dominant inheritance with variability in expression. Deletions and rearrangements of the long arm of chromosome 8 (8q) have been implicated in BOR syndrome.

CHARGE Association. CHARGE is an acronym for a group of anomalies that often appear together. These include: c = coloboma (defect of the iris, retina, or optic disc), h = congenital heart disease, a = atresia of the choanae (bony obstruction of nasal passages), r = growth retardation, g = genital defects, and e = ear anomalies. Infants with CHARGE association frequently have abnormally formed external ears, and up to 85% have some degree of conductive, mixed, or sensorineural hearing loss. Mental retardation is reported in most children. Typically, CHARGE association arises sporadically but both autosomal dominant and, less commonly, autosomal recessive transmission have been inferred from multigeneration family studies. Many of the characteristics observed in CHARGE association are also observed in infants exposed to teratogens in utero (rubella, thalidomide) and to infants of diabetic mothers.

DiGeorge Sequence. DiGeorge sequence represents a pattern of abnormalities which includes absence or hypoplasia of the thymus and/or parathyroid glands, cardiovascular abnormalities, craniofacial anomalies, and middle and inner ear developmental defects. Many of these abnormalities are associated with developmental anomalies of the branchial arches in the early embryonic period. Conductive hearing loss is often present secondary to multiple middle ear abnormalities, but bilateral Mondini anomaly of the inner ear (one and one-half turns of the cochlea rather than the normal two and one-half turns) has also been reported. Severe cardiac, metabolic and/or immunologic compromise may lead to early death in infants with DiGeorge sequence; infants who survive with less severe manifestations are usually mentally retarded. Although both autosomal dominant and autosomal recessive inheritance of DiGeorge sequence have been reported, new cases are usually considered sporadic. In addition, DiGeorge sequence may arise from chromosomal (22 q-) and teratogenic effects.

Hearing Loss with Associated Visual Abnormalities

Babies use both hearing and vision to monitor their environment. For infants with hearing loss, visual learning and reinforcement are important sensory experiences. The double loss of hearing and vision is a dreaded complication of some congenital conditions (e.g., congenital rubella syndrome) and one that substantially complicates early language-learning and socialization. In many hereditary conditions that include hearing impairment and visual abnormalities, sensory loss is progressive allowing some period of normal development. Usher syndrome is an example of congenital hearing impairment associated with progressive visual impairment.

Retinitis Pigmentosa and Sensorineural Hearing Loss (Usher Syndrome). Among children with profound hereditary deafness, Usher syndrome is considered the most common, single, identifiable cause. Three forms of Usher syndrome have been identified; type I—congenital severe-to-profound sensorineural hearing loss, absent vestibular responses, and development of retinitis pigmentosa (progressive degeneration of photoreceptors in the eye leading to blindness) by age 10 years; type II—congenital moderate-to-severe sensorineural hearing loss, normal vestibular responses, and development of retinitis pigmentosa in late teens/early 20s; and type III—progressive hearing impairment with variable onset of retinitis pigmentosa (to date, reported only in families in Finland). Children with Usher syndrome have normal intellectual and neurological function. Usher syndrome is an autosomal recessive disorder with marked genetic heterogeneity; at least five different Usher genes have been identified. Three different genes have been identified as being responsible for Usher syndrome type I (a gene localized to chromosome 14, and two different genes linked to chromosome 11), and two different genes for Usher syndrome type II (a gene on the chromosome 1, and a gene of unknown locus).

Hearing Loss with Associated Musculoskeletal Abnormalities

Cohen and Gorlin (1995) describe more than 85 disorders that include hearing impairment and musculoskeletal abnormalities. These disorders may affect development of the skull, axial skeleton, limbs, hands, and/or feet. In common with disorders in other systems, both congenital and late-onset musculoskeletal effects may be observed.

Cervico-Oculo-Acoustic Syndrome (Klippel-Feil Anomaly; Wildervanck Syndrome). Cervico-oculo-acoustic syndrome refers to a con-stellation of disorders that include fused cervical vertebrae, paralysis of the VIth cranial nerve (prevents abduction, or external rotation, of the affected eye), and sensorineural and/or conductive hearing loss. Klippel-Feil anomaly is encompassed within this broader category of congenital disorders.

Hereditary hearing loss may be part of a *syndrome, sequence,* or an *association.* As defined by Toriello (1995), a *syndrome* is a pattern of anomalies with a specifically defined cause such as Down syndrome (trisomy 21). A *sequence* is a constellation of anomalies that result from a primary abnormality. For example, in Pierre Robin sequence, the primary abnormality is mandibular hypoplasia (failure of the mandible to grow in utero) which results in displacement of the tongue, obstruction of palate closure, and ultimately cleft palate. The etiology of the primary abnormality in a sequence may not necessarily be identified. Finally, an *association* is an often unrelated group of anomalies that occur together with greater-than-chance frequency. Similar to a sequence, the etiology of the various anomalies may not be established. In a child with evidence of one of these anomalies, presence of the other anomalies should be investigated.

Infants with this anomaly frequently demonstrate facial asymmetry, fusion of one or more cervical vertebrae, short and thick neck with severe restriction in mobility of the neck, unilateral microtia and atresia, middle ear anomalies, and conductive, sensorineural, and/or mixed hearing loss. In children with Klippel-Feil anomaly intelligence is typically normal although a few cases mental retardation have been reported. All cases of this disorder are sporadic. Although autosomal recessive inheritance of Klippel-Feil syndrome has been proposed, a specific genetic mechanism has not been identified. In addition, nongenetic causes may influence development of this disorder. Because other identified syndromes include features of cervico-oculo-acoustic syndrome, there is considerable overlap in syndromes that include these major characteristics.

Achondroplasia. Achondroplasia is a form of short-limbed dwarfism. Individuals with this disorder demonstrate an enlarged head with characteristic facial features. Musculoskeletal defects include short limbs with the upper limbs more severely affected, marked lordosis (ventral-dorsal bowing) of the lumbar spine, bowing of the legs, and protuberant abdomen. Infants with achondroplasia often have recurrent otitis media with conductive hearing loss although sensorineural hearing impairment has also been reported. Intelligence in infants with achondroplasia is usually normal. Achondroplasia is inherited through autosomal dominant transmission; as many as 80% of cases represent new mutations. The gene associated with achondroplasia has been mapped to 4p.

Apert Syndrome. Apert syndrome is one of several inherited disorders associated with craniosynostosis (abnormal closure of the sutures of the skull). Infants with Apert syndrome demonstrate midfacial malformations with a characteristic appearance; low-set external ears; complete syndactyly (fusion) of the second, third, and fourth digits and toes; and mild-to-moderate conductive hearing loss. Most children with Apert syndrome have some degree of mental retardation. Apert syndrome is inherited by autosomal dominant transmission but most cases represent new mutations.

Crouzon Syndrome. Crouzon syndrome, also called craniofacial dysostosis, is characterized by craniosynostosis with substantial variability in expression among affected family members. Skull deformities range from no detectable abnormality to severely deformed (e.g., cloverleaf) skull. Ocular proptosis (prominent protrusion of the eyes) is the most invariant feature of Crouzon syndrome. Conductive hearing loss is a frequent finding and atresia is infrequently present. Children with Crouzon syndrome usually have normal intelligence. Crouzon syndrome is inherited through autosomal dominant transmission with substantial variability in expression; the gene has been localized to the long arm of chromosome 10. Up to 50% of cases of Crouzon syndrome represent new mutations; increased paternal age is statistically significant in new mutations.

Pfeiffer Syndrome. Pfeiffer syndrome is characterized by craniosynostosis, ocular proptosis, broad thumbs and broad great toes, and soft tissue syndactyly of the hands. Cloverleaf skull deforming may be present in severe forms of Pfeiffer syndrome. Hearing impairment secondary to middle ear anomalies or aural atresia may be present. Typically, children with Pfeiffer syndrome have normal intelligence. Inheritance is autosomal dominant with markedly variable expressivity.

EEC Syndrome (Ectrodactyly-Ectodermal Dysplasia—Clefting Syndrome). This syndrome is characterized by ectrodactyly (defects in the midportion of the hands and feet ranging from fusion of the digits to absence of digits; clawlike fusion), cleft lip and palate, and obstruction of the nasolacrimal gland. Individuals with EEC syndrome may have conductive hearing loss related to middle ear anomalies; sensorineural hearing impairment has been occasionally reported. Although most children have normal intelligence, microcephaly and mental retardation have been reported in as many as 10% of cases. Studies of multiple families suggest transmission by autosomal dominant inheritance with low penetrance and variability in expression. Many cases may represent new mutations. The gene for EEC syndrome is mapped to 7q.

Stickler Syndrome.   Patients with Stickler syndrome may present with midface hypoplasia, cleft palate, joint hypermobility, alteration in ossification, myopia and retinal detachment, and conductive and/or progressive sensorineural hearing loss. It is estimated that 30% of infants with Pierre Robin sequence (mandibular hypoplasia with cleft palate secondary to posterior displacement of the tongue) have this syndrome. Children with Stickler syndrome usually have normal intelligence. Stickler syndrome is inherited through autosomal dominant transmission. Two genes for Stickler syndrome have been identified. One is localized to the long arm of chromosome 12 and the other is localized to the short arm of chromosome 6. Both genes are thought to contribute to the code for a type of collagen (a protein necessary for connective tissue formation and function).

Hearing Loss Associated with Integumentary Disorders

The integumentary system consists of the skin, nails, hair, scalp, and sweat glands. Congenital disorders affecting this system can result in highly visible, painful, and disabling conditions. Toriello (1995) describes 55 disorders involving genetic hearing loss associated with integumentary disorders.

Waardenburg Syndrome.   Waardenburg syndrome is certainly the most well-known and common disorder of hearing and the integumentary system. It is estimated that 2% to 5% of individuals with congenital hearing impairment have Waardenburg syndrome.

Two types of Waardenburg syndrome have been defined. Type I always includes lateral displacement of the medial canthi (inner corner of the eye); type II never includes this characteristic. Other effects variably observed in both type I and type II Waardenburg syndrome include: broad nasal root and hyperplasia of the median portion of the eyebrow. Integumentary effects may include presence of a white forelock (20% to 40% of cases) or premature greying and a variety of skin pigmentary changes. Abnormal eye color has also been observed, including heterochromia (two colors of the eyes), or brown sections of pigment in a predominantly blue eye and vice versa. Hearing is variably affected in individuals with Waardenburg syndrome, ranging from normal hearing through profound unilateral or bilateral sensorineural loss. Progressive loss has been reported in type II Waardenburg syndrome. Children with this syndrome usually have normal intelligence. Waardenburg syndrome is inherited by autosomal dominant transmission. Expression of the syndrome is markedly variable. Some forms of type I Waardenburg syndrome have been mapped to 2q; location of the second gene for Waardenburg syndrome is mapped to chromosome 3p. Both genes are thought to control some aspect of development of the face and/or ear.

Hearing Loss Associated with Renal Disorders

Hearing loss is closely associated with disorders of the renal system. The association between ototoxicity and kidney dysfunction is well established. A relatively more common hereditary hearing loss syndrome, Alport syndrome, is characterized by progressive hearing impairment and kidney failure. Gorlin, Wester, and Carey (1995) describe more than 20 hereditary hearing impairment syndromes associated with renal disorders.

Alport Syndrome.   This syndrome is characterized by progressive kidney disease and sensorineural hearing loss. Changes in the visual system may also be present which lead to myopia in affected individuals. Onset of end-stage renal disease may be early (during childhood) or late (in adulthood). As a rule, females are less severely affected than males. Hearing is typically normal through childhood with onset of progressive, high-frequency sensorineural hearing impairment in the second decade of life. Children with Alport syndrome usually have normal intelligence. Several genetic types of Alport syndrome have been identified including X-linked dominant inheritance, autosomal dominant, and autosomal recessive inheritance. The gene for X-linked Alport syndrome has been identified; it codes for one type of collagen which forms part of the connecting structure within the inner ear and kidney. Changes in two other collagen genes, located on the long arm of chromosome 2 are responsible for autosomal recessive Alport syndrome. The gene associated with autosomal dominant Alport syndrome has not been localized. Expression of Alport syndrome is variable; some affected individuals shows mild disease with minimal effects, others demonstrate severe disease leading to kidney failure and death despite aggressive intervention including transplantation.

Hearing Loss Associated with Metabolic/Endocrine Disorders

Metabolic and endocrine disorders are especially important in infancy because they affect overall growth and development. In some cases, progressive metabolic deterioration leads to severe disability and death. More than 50 disorders with hearing impairment and associated metabolic and endocrine abnormalities have been described (Gorlin, 1995).

Mucopolysaccharidoses (MPS).   Several related diseases comprise the disorders encompassed within the diagnosis of MPS. These disorders arise from deficiency in specific lysosomal enzymes responsible for degrading mucopolysaccharides. As a consequence, cellular accumulation of mucopolysaccharides results in systemic disease. In severe forms of MPS, progressive deterioration leads to childhood death.

Seven forms of MPS, designated MPS I through MPS VII, have been identified. Characteristics of MPS range from severe growth deficiency after infancy, severe mental retardation, characteristic facial features with full lips, flared nostrils and low nasal bridge, skeletal, joint, and cardiac abnormalities, and death within the first decade of life secondary to cardiac or respiratory complications (MPS I-II, Hurler syndrome) through normal growth and intelligence, broad face with mandibular prognathism and full lips, joint limitations, aortic stenosis, and normal or near-normal lifespan (MPS I-S, Scheie syndrome). In most reported types of MPS, hearing impairment is variably present, typically mild, and conductive or mixed. Progressive loss may be present and children with MPS often exhibit chronic otitis media. MPS is inherited through autosomal recessive transmission except for MPS II (X-linked Hunter syndrome). The gene for each type of MPS has been mapped permitting prenatal diagnosis by molecular genetic techniques.

Hearing Loss Associated with Goiter (Pendred Syndrome).   Goiter is enlargement of the thyroid gland in response to dietary deficiency or metabolic dysfunction. In the case of Pendred syndrome, goiter appears around age 8 to 10 years secondary to metabolic dysfunction. Children with Pendred syndrome frequently have congenital, symmetrical, sensorineural hearing loss ranging from mild to severe with more than 50% of affected children showing severe hearing loss. Hearing loss may progress after head trauma or resemble progressive loss associated with round window fistula. Bony changes in the cochlea resemble Mondini dysplasia. Pendred syndrome is thought to account for as many as 5% of cases of congenital sensorineural hearing loss. Children with this syndrome usually have normal intelligence. Pendred syndrome is probably transmitted by autosomal recessive inheritance although autosomal dominant inheritance with incomplete penetrance and variable expression cannot be ruled out.

Genetic Hearing Loss Associated with Chromosomal Disorders

Hearing loss is a frequent component of chromosomal disorders. In most chromosomal disorders, a complex of physical and behavioral effects is present which results in multiple disabilities.

Trisomy 21 (Down Syndrome).   Down syndrome represents one of the most common congenital disorders occurring with an overall frequency of 1:600 births. It results when an extra copy of chromosome 21 (trisomy 21) is present in the individual's karyotype (see Figure 3–11). There is a well-established association between frequency of Down syndrome and maternal age; as maternal age increases, risk for Down syndrome also increases. Down syndrome was first described in the latter half of the 19th century; its chromosomal etiology was first identified in the latter half of the 20th century.

The features of Down syndrome include characteristic facial appearance with flat face; protrusion of the tongue; upper slant of the palpebral fissures; fine, straight hair; hypotonia; small hands with short fingers and characteristic palmar fold (Simian crease); small, unusually shaped auricles with very narrow external auditory meati; and mild to severe mental retardation. Hearing impairment is a common feature of Down syndrome including conductive hearing loss secondary to frequent otitis media and sensorineural and mixed hearing loss. Disproportionate language delay has also been reported in children with Down syndrome and may be compounded by mild, fluctuant conductive hearing loss.

Trisomy 13.   Infants with trisomy 13 (extra copy of chromosome 13) demonstrate severe disability including growth retardation, congenital microcephaly, microphthalmia with coloboma (small eyes with defect of the iris), cleft lip and palate, polydactyly of fingers and toes (extra digits), congenital heart disease, and renal defects. All infants with trisomy 13 exhibit profound development delay; many exhibit sensorineural and conductive hearing loss. Survival beyond 2 years of age is unexpected.

Trisomy 18. Trisomy 18 also results in severe congenital disabilities. Similar to trisomy 13, infants with an extra copy of chromosome 18 exhibit severe growth retardation, congenital microcephaly, abnormalities of hands and feet, heart, and renal defects. Profound developmental delay is universal, and hearing impairment is very common in trisomy 18. Infants with this disorder rarely survive until 2 years of age.

Hearing Loss and Miscellaneous Disorders

There are many conditions which include congenital hearing impairment and other disorders which have not been defined as a syndrome or whose transmission and inheritance is unknown. Several of these conditions important in infancy are described below.

Congenital Sensorineural Hearing Loss and Electrocardiographic Abnormalities (Jervell and Lange-Nielsen Syndrome). A constellation of anomalies which include severe, congenital sensorineural hear-ing loss, electrocardiographic abnormalities, and fainting spells was described in the mid-1950s. At that time, individuals demonstrating this disorder often died unexpectedly in childhood, apparently secondary to cardiac arrhythmias. Children with Jervell and Lange-Nielsen syndrome typically have normal intelligence. This syndrome is present in less than 1.0% of persons with congenital sensorineural loss. Jervell and Lange-Nielsen syndrome is transmitted through autosomal recessive inheritance.

de Lange Syndrome (Cornelia de Lange Syndrome; Brachmann-de Lange Syndrome). This syndrome is characterized by low birthweight and growth retardation; typical facial appearance including thin eyebrows that meet at midline (synophrys), long eyelashes, and short upturned nose; limb abnormalities and small hands and feet; heart defects; and cleft palate. Most infants with de Lange syndrome exhibit moderate to severe mental retardation; hearing loss is variably present and ranges from mild to severe. De Lange syndrome is thought to represent new mutation of a gene, possibly located on chromosome 3.

SUMMARY

The hereditary hearing loss syndromes presently identified will un-doubtedly be reclassified, renamed, redefined, or expanded as new information becomes available. In addition, new syndromes are being identified at a rapid rate. Through the Human Genome Project, it is estimated that new syndromes of human genetic disease are being identified at the rate of one per week. In their work with infants and families, audiologists and speech-language patholo-gists will benefit from the rapid expansion in knowledge about genetic hearing loss. Genetic evaluation of infants and families is discussed in detail in Chapter 9.

The explosion of knowledge in medical genetics will continue to expand our understanding of disease and its prevention and treatment. Human genetics is challenging the frontiers of medical science and bioethics with its capacity to alter the genetic charac-teristics of individuals. It is important for audiologists and speech-language pathologists to continually update their knowledge of human genetics, hereditary disease, and treatment for congenital disorders.

SUGGESTED READINGS

Gorlin, R. J., Toriello, H. V., & Cohen, Jr., M. M. (1995). *Hereditary Hearing Loss and Its Syndromes.* New York: Oxford University Press.
The definitive, current text detailing hereditary hearing loss.
Jones, K. L. (1988). *Smith's Recognizable Patterns of Human Malformation (4th ed.).* Philadelphia: W. B. Saunders.
The standard *pediatric guide to congenital malformations.*
Mueller, R. F., & Young, I. D. (1995). *Emery's Elements of Medical Genetics (9th ed.).* New York: Churchill Livingstone.
A comprehensive text explaining current concepts in medical genetics.

CHAPTER 4

Human Development Before Birth

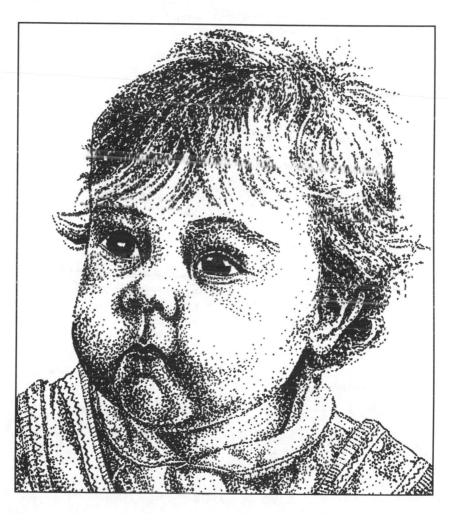

*D*uring the 38 weeks between fertilization of an ovum by a sperm and the birth of a human baby, a remarkable and highly intricate sequence of development results in an unique human individual. Knowledge of the developmental sequence, the critical periods of development, and the conditions that affect development will aid in understanding many congenital birth defects.

HUMAN PRENATAL DEVELOPMENT

Human prenatal development is defined in three stages, pre-embryonic development encompassing the period from fertilization through 3 weeks, embryonic development from 4 through 8 weeks postfertilization, and fetal development from 9 weeks through term.

The 40 weeks of a normal pregnancy (gestation) encompass the time span from the first day of the mother's last menstrual period (LMP) until birth. Although few women can be certain of when they conceived, most women can remember the date of their LMP. For this reason, physicians use the LMP to date the pregnancy. Of course, in most cases, the ovum was not fertilized by the sperm until about 2 weeks after the LMP. A term pregnancy is 40 weeks or 10 lunar months (approximately 9 calendar months). Premature birth is any birth that occurs before the completion of the 37th week.

Pre-embryonic Stage

The pre-embryonic stage consists of the first 2 to 3 weeks following fertilization. The female gamete, or ovum, is fertilized by the male gamete, or sperm, in the fallopian tube near the ovary. Fertilization of the ovum creates a diploid cell called a zygote with 22 autosomes and 1 sex chromosome from each parent (46 chromosomes in total). At the moment of fertilization, the genetic characteristics of the future individual are determined; this unique human's genetic code is encoded within this single cell.

The zygote increases in size by mitosis, the cell division process that results in genetically identical cells (see Chapter 3). At about day 3, a solid ball of approximately 12 to 16 cells reaches the uterus. This cell mass evolves into a blastocyst, a structure with three distinct components: (a) an inner cell mass, or embryoblast, which develops into the embryo, (b) a large, central fluid-filled cavity into which the embryoblast projects, and (c) a thin outer layer of cells which encloses the embryoblast and central cavity and contributes to formation of the placenta.

Between the sixth and seventh day following fertilization, the blastocyst superficially implants into the wall of the uterus. It is estimated that approximately 45% of fertilized ova fail to develop and implant, or abort shortly after implantation.

During the second week of development, the blastocyst becomes firmly implanted. Maternal blood supply to the embryoblast is established and nourishes the embryoblast prior to development of the placenta. The embryoblast differentiates into a flattened, circular embryonic disk with two layers. By the end of the second week, a slight thickening indicates the future cranial region of the embryo, and the location of the future mouth.

During the third week of development, rapid proliferation and growth results in evolution of the bilaminar embryonic disk into a trilaminar disk. This phenomenon, termed gastrulation, is one of the most important events in prenatal development. It marks the beginning of rapid development of the embryo. The germ cell layers which are established during this process, the ectoderm, mesoderm, and endoderm, will eventually give rise to all fetal organs and tissues.

Table 4–1 reviews the primary germ layers and their derivatives, the tissue and organ systems. **Ectoderm** gives rise to skin,

Table 4–1. Derivatives of the three primary germ layers: ectoderm, mesoderm, and endoderm.

Germ Layer	Tissues	Organ Systems
Ectoderm	Epidermis (skin)	Central nervous system
	Hair	Brain
	Nail	Spinal cord
	Sensory epithelia	Autonomic ganglia
	Lens	Meninges
	Inner ear	Peripheral nervous system
	Olfactory	
	Teeth enamel	
	Mammary glands	
	Pituitary gland	
	Subcutaneous glands	
Mesoderm	Cartilage	Heart
	Bone	Kidneys
	Connective tissues	Gonads
	Striated and smooth muscles	Spleen

(continued)

Table 4–1. *(continued)*

Germ Layer	Tissues	Organ Systems

Endoderm	Epithelia membranes which line:
	    Digestive and
	    respiratory systems
	    Eustachion tube and
	    middle ear cavity
	Thyroid and parathyroid
	    glands
	Thymus
		Liver
		Pancreas

hair and nails; sensory epithelia of the ear, eye, and nose; teeth enamel; the mammary glands; pituitary gland; and subcutaneous glands. Organ systems derived from ectoderm include the central and peripheral nervous systems. **Mesoderm** gives rise to cartilage, bone, connective tissues, and striated and smooth muscles. Organ systems that develop from mesoderm include the heart, kidneys, gonads, and spleen. **Endoderm** gives rise to epithelial lining of the digestive and respiratory tracts including the eustachian tube and tympanic cavity, the thyroid and parathyroid glands, and the thymus. Organ systems associated with endoderm include the liver and pancreas.

During this important third week of development, the notochord, the structure that evolves into the bony axial skeleton (vertebral column, ribs, sternum, and skull), develops. The notochord induces development of the primitive nervous system. As shown in Figure 4–1 ectoderm overlying the notochord thickens to form the neural plate. The neural plate ultimately develops into the central nervous system. It invaginates to form the neural groove at about day 18 with edges (neural folds) that approach each other and fuse to form an enclosed neural tube. As the neural folds join, neuroectodermal cells lying lateral to the folds separate into cells which will evolve into spinal ganglia and ganglia of the autonomic nervous system. Fusion of the neural tube begins in the middle of the embryo and progresses to the cranial and caudal end. By the end of the fourth week of development, closure of the neural tube is complete. Disruption in fusion of the neural folds and incomplete closure of the neural tube results in severe congenital abnormalities of the brain and spinal cord (see Chapter 6).

The primitive cardiovascular system also begins to form during the third week of human development. This important organ

(A)

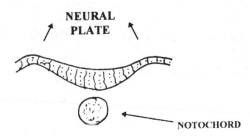

NEURAL
PLATE

NOTOCHORD

(B)

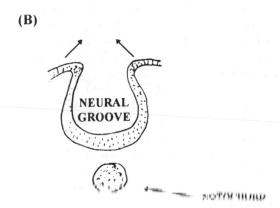

NEURAL
GROOVE

NOTOCHORD

(C)

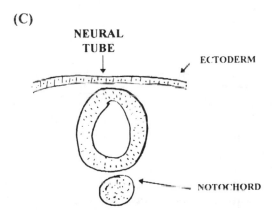

NEURAL
TUBE

ECTODERM

NOTOCHORD

FIGURE 4-1. Development of the neural plate, folding of the neural groove, and fusion of the neural tube. Disruption of this process and/or incomplete closure of the neural tube results in severe congenital abnormalities of the brain and spinal cord.

system is the first system to become functional in the embryo. The heart begins to develop at the end of the third week; during the same period, primitive blood is forming. The primitive heart has only one atrium and one ventricle. It begins to beat by the 22nd day.

Summary of the Pre-embryonic Stage

During the first 3 weeks following fertilization, the single, diploid cell (zygote) resulting from the union of ovum and sperm rapidly evolves from a dividing cell mass into an embryo with well-defined cell layers and the primitive beginnings of major organ systems (bony axial skeleton, nervous system, cardiovascular system). The first week of development is marked by rapid mitosis of the zygote into a ball of identical cells. Upon entering the uterus, this cell mass develops into a blastocyst with structures that ultimately evolve into the embryo and the extraembryonic tissues of conception. By the end of the first week, the blastocyst is superficially implanted into the uterine wall. The second week of development is marked by differentiation of the inner cell mass of the blastocyst into a bilaminar disc. A localized thickening in this bilaminar disc marks the position of the future mouth. Finally, rapid cell proliferation and differentiation during the third week of development generates a trilaminar embryonic disc with well-defined germ layers. Precursors to the axial skeleton (notochord) and central nervous system (neural plate, groove and tube) arise, and a primitive cardiovascular system is developing. Although the first 3 weeks of development are traditionally viewed as the pre-embryonic period, events in the third week signal rapid development of the embryo.

Embryonic Development

The embryonic period of development continues from about the beginning of the fourth week through the end of the eighth week following fertilization. During this period, all major organ systems begin and/or undergo critical development and the embryo achieves a human-like appearance. This period of development is crucial; exposure to teratogens (drugs, infections, or toxins that cause birth defects) during this period results in either death of the developing embryo or major congenital anomalies affecting multiple organ systems.

Development of External Characteristics

Early in the embryonic period, the flat trilaminar embryonic disk folds into a more cylindrical appearing embryo. Brisk growth of the embryo, especially of its central nervous system, and differences in relative growth rate of the sides of the embryo vs. its long axis, are responsible for development of the characteristic C-shaped appearance of the embryo at the end of the fourth week.

Major events during the fourth week include appearance of structures destined to become principal components of the face and ear. Figure 4–2 shows a representation of an embryo at this time. By the end of this week, four pairs of branchial (from the Greek *branchia* for gill; at this stage the embryo resembles a fish at a similar stage of development) or pharyngeal arches are discernible. The first, or mandibular arch, which is visible early in the fourth week, will evolve into the mandible (lower jaw), the maxilla (upper jaw), and other structures of the face. Otic pits, which will develop into the sensory structure of the inner ear, are

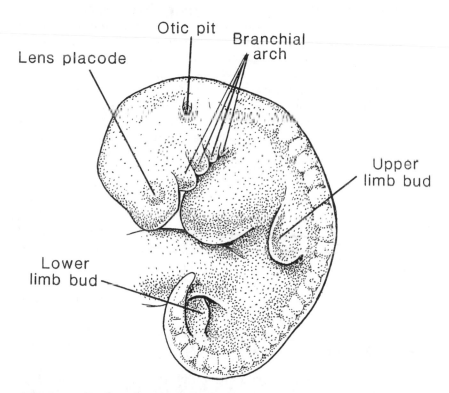

FIGURE 4–2. An embryo at the end of the fourth week of development. The lens placode which will develop into the eye, the otic pit which will develop into the inner ear, and the branchial arches which will contribute to development of the ear and face, are all clearly visible. Both upper and lower limb buds are also apparent.

visible as thickenings on the lateral surface of the head. Lens pla-codes, which will develop into the lenses of the eyes, are also apparent on the lateral surface of the head. Earlier in the fourth week, upper limb buds appear; by the end of the fourth week, lower limb buds are also visible.

Major external features apparent during the fifth week of devel-opment include enlargement of the head and differentiation of struc-tures in the limbs. Head growth is secondary to increase in brain size. On the upper limbs, hand plates develop and elbows become evident. On the lower limbs, foot plates appear. The major features of the face develop primarily during the fifth through eighth weeks.

During the sixth week, structures important to future develop-ment of the external ear emerge. Several small swellings (auricular hillocks) develop around the groove between the first and second branchial arches; these auricular hillocks will eventually fuse and form the external ear. The first branchial groove will deepen to become the external auditory meatus. The eye is especially apparent during the sixth week because it has become pigmented. Both the upper and lower limbs continue to differentiate. In the upper limbs, both elbow and wrist regions can be observed and condensation of mesenchymal tissue in the hand plates (digital rays) marks the beginnings of future fingers. In a 6-week-old embryo, increase in head size is substantial relative to increase in trunk size.

A major external feature of the seventh week is further differen-tiation of the limbs. On the upper limbs, notches between the digital rays clearly mark the future fingers and thumb. Lower limb devel-opment parallels upper limb development but lags by a day or two.

The eighth week marks the final week of embryonic develop-ment. As shown in Figure 4–3, by the end of this week, the embryo has a distinctly human appearance. Differentiation of the limbs produces clearly recognizable structures with distinct joints, fingers, and toes. The head remains disproportionately large; it comprises one-half the length of the embryo. Facial features are clearly distinguishable with well-formed eyes, nose, and mouth. The ears remain low-set but show both external auditory meati and auricles.

Organogenesis

The embryonic period is critical for differentiation and develop-ment of the major organ systems.

As described previously, the nervous systems initiates devel-opment during the third week (pre-embryonic period). The central nervous system (brain and spinal cord) arise from the neural tube;

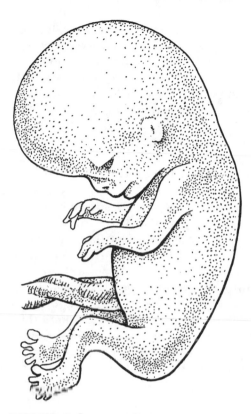

FIGURE 4-3. An embryo at the end of the eighth week of development. The embryo has a distinctly human-like appearance. Well-formed extremities with distinct joints, fingers and toes are clearly recognizable and the face has well-formed eyes, nose, and mouth. The ears are low-set but show both external auditory meati and auricles.

the peripheral nervous system evolves from the neural crest. The neural tube closes by the fourth week of development; failure of the neural tube to close results in severe congenital malformation. Failure of the neural tube to close at the caudal end (the most common neural tube defect) results in spina bifida. Failure of the neural tube to close at the cranial end results in severe malformations of the brain, most commonly anencephaly (see Chapter 6).

The cardiovascular system, which also begins to develop during the pre-embryonic period, continues to evolve during the embryonic period. During the fourth week, for example, differentiation of the primitive heart into two ventricles begins; by about the end of the seventh week, communication between the two ventricles is eliminated with closure of the intraventricular foramen. Incomplete closure into two ventricles results in the most common congenital heart defect, ventricular septal defect (see Chapter 6). The critical period for development of the heart is encompassed within the embryonic period.

The respiratory system begins to develop during the fourth week with formation of the precursor to the trachea and larynx, the laryngotracheal tube. This structure arises from the primitive pharynx which will develop into the esophagus. Incomplete separation of the laryngotracheal tube from the primitive pharynx results in tracheoesophageal fistula, a congenital abnormality which occurs in about 1 in 2,500 births (see Chapter 6).

During weeks 5 through 8, important structures of the respiratory system evolve from rapid development of the laryngotracheal tube. The bronchi emerge and lung development ensues. It is not until well into the fetal period (weeks 9 through 38), however, that the critical interface between the respiratory and circulatory systems develops.

The primitive gut also begins to develop during the fourth week. The foregut consists of the esophagus, stomach, liver, and pancreas; it communicates through the stomodeum (future mouth) with the amniotic cavity. The midgut consists of the small intestines, ascending colon, and substantial portions of the transverse colon. During the embryonic period, portions of the midgut develop in the umbilical cord because the mass of the developing liver and kidneys limits space in the abdominal cavity.

The hindgut consists of portions of the colon, the rectum, and cloaca (Latin for drain or sewer; the embryologic common terminus of the urologic, reproductive, and intestinal systems). Initially, the rectum is isolated from the exterior by an anal membrane which breaks down by the beginning of the eighth week of development. Failure of normal development of the hindgut results in a variety of congenital malformations including persistent cloaca, imperforate anus, anal stenosis or atresia, and anorectal agenesis.

The urinary system, consisting of the kidneys, ureters, bladder, and urethra, begins to develop in the early embryonic period. The kidney appears in the fifth week and begins to produce urine at about the 11th week of development.

A baby's gender is determined at the moment of fertilization based on the presence of an X or Y chromosome in the sperm. Without chromosomal analysis, however, male and female embryos cannot be distinguished before about the seventh week when the gonads (testes or ovaries) begin to develop. The external genitalia do not become distinctly male or female until the fetal period.

Summary of the Embryonic Period

During the embryonic period, the three germ layers differentiate into the major tissue and organ systems. By the end of the eighth week, all major organ systems have become established, at least in a primitive state. During this period of rapid differentiation, major congenital anomalies may arise from exposure to terato- gens, or from genetic or chromosomal abnormalities.

Fetal Development

The interval from approximately 9 weeks to birth represents the period of fetal development. During this period, the human- appearing *fetus* (Latin for offspring) undergoes rapid growth of body structures, and growth and differentiation of tissues and major organ systems. Because the major organ systems were estab- lished during the embryonic period, the fetus is less susceptible to death or major deformity from teratogens, although these agents may interfere with growth and normal functional development.

At the beginning of the ninth week of development, a major external characteristic of the fetus is its relative head size. At this time, the head constitutes almost one-half of the length of the fetus as measured from crown to rump. However, during the ninth week, acceleration in growth of the body alters the relationship of head size to body length. By the end of the twelfth week, overall fetal length has more than doubled primarily due to growth in body length. Lower limb growth continues to lag upper limb growth. By the end of the twelfth week, the upper limbs have almost achieved their final relative length (length relative to body length) but the lower limbs remain somewhat shorter than their final relative length.

During the thirteenth through sixteenth weeks of development, growth is very brisk. Similar to the previous 3 weeks, growth in body length outpaces growth in head size; by the end of the six- teenth week, head-to-body ratio is relatively small compared to a 12-week-old fetus. The external ears become repositioned through growth of the head and lie closer to their final birth position.

During the next 3 weeks of fetal development, weeks 17 through 20, the rate of growth slows. The very thin fetal skin becomes pro- tected by a mixture of fatty secretions and dead skin cells (vernix caseosa). In addition, a fine, downy-like hair, lanugo, covers the body of the fetus. Eyebrows as well as head hair become apparent on a 20-week-old fetus. Fetal movements (quickening) become noticeable to the mother.

During weeks 21 through 25 of development, the fetus gains substantial weight. Blood in peripheral vessels is visible giving the fetal skin a pink-to-red appearance. At about 24 weeks, gas-exchange sites (alveoli) in the fetal lungs are apparent and begin to produce surfactant, a substance necessary to maintain alveolar patency at birth (see below and Chapter 6).

During weeks 26 through 29, further development of the lungs and alveoli improve the fetus's chance of extrauterine survival. Head hair and lanugo are well-developed, and the fetus has developed substantial subcutaneous fat resulting in smoother skin appearance. The fetus may rotate into an head-down orientation in the uterus due to uterine shape and relative weight of the fetal head.

During the final 9 to 10 weeks of gestation, the fetus is preparing for extrauterine life by rapid development of the respiratory system, and by adding subcutaneous fat. Prior to approximately 24 weeks of development, the fetus is incapable of survival outside the womb due to immaturity of the respiratory system. After approximately 25 weeks of intrauterine development, the fetus may survive in an extrauterine environment with sophisticated medical care available in the NICU.

Summary of the Fetal Period

The fetal period, from approximately 9 weeks after fertilization until birth, is characterized by rapid body growth and completion of organ system differentiation. As shown in Figure 4–4, relative head size of the fetus decreases from almost one-half fetal crown-to-rump length at 8 weeks to one-quarter fetal length at 38 weeks. In addition to growth in body length, the fetus gains substantial weight during this period, much of it in the form of subcutaneous fat. Fetuses less than 30 weeks appear thin with wrinkled skin; fetuses close to term appear relatively plump with smooth skin. Although changes during the fetal period are less dramatic than changes during the embryonic period, they are essential for preparing the infant for independent, extrauterine survival.

FETAL RESPIRATORY AND CIRCULATORY SYSTEMS

The major pathology affecting the premature infant is dysfunction of the respiratory system. As described above, prior to about 24–25

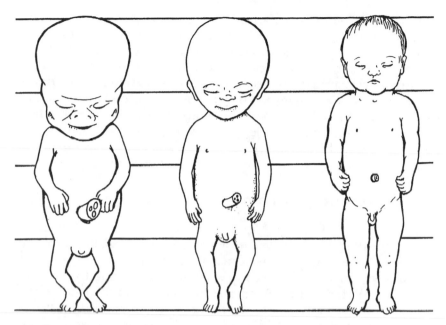

FIGURE 4–4. Representation of a fetus at about 8, 16, and 38 weeks. Relative head size of the fetus decreases from approximately one-half fetal length at 8 weeks to one-quarter fetal length at 38 weeks.

weeks, extrauterine survival is improbable because gas-exchange sites and surfactant production in the lungs are insufficient to support respiration. Survival of infants born after about 25 weeks is possible with sophisticated NICU care.

Fetal Respiratory System

The purpose of respiration is to introduce oxygen to blood hemoglobin molecules for circulation to all body tissues. At the tissue level, oxygen is exchanged with carbon dioxide and transported back to the lungs for elimination. Oxygen/carbon dioxide gas exchange occurs in mature lungs in the alveoli. In the developing fetus, gas-exchange occurs in the placenta; compromise of maternal-fetal circulation results in fetal distress due to decreased oxygenation to the developing tissues and organ systems. At birth, the infant must rapidly convert from a placental-based oxygenation system to a lung-based oxygenation system.

Prior to about 24–25 weeks, the fetal respiratory system is not sufficiently mature to support extrauterine life. The fetal lungs exhibit no functional gas-exchange mechanisms to oxygenate blood. From approximately 24 through 28 weeks, the oxygen/carbon dioxide gas exchange system of capillary-surrounded alveoli begins to develop and gas-exchange sites form. Infants born at 24 weeks of development may survive if the lungs can be expanded, respiration sustained, and gas exchange maintained. From 29 through 35 weeks, mature, vascularized gas exchange sites form. Babies born during this period have adequate anatomy to support gas exchange, but may develop alveoli collapse and compromised gas exchange. From 36 weeks through term, there is a marked expansion of gas-exchange surface area and production of surfactant, a surface tension-reducing biocompound that prevents alveoli collapse at expiration.

Fetal Circulatory System

Blood circulation in fetal life is markedly different from blood circulation after birth. Because blood is oxygenated by placental-based mechanisms in the fetus, a fetal circulatory pattern is developed which shunts blood away from the dormant fetal lungs (fetal circulatory pattern). In the newborn infant, blood is oxygenated by gas exchange in the lungs; the fetal pattern of circulation must rapidly change to shunt blood into the now active lungs (extrauterine circulatory pattern).

The simpler of the two circulatory patterns, extrauterine circulation, is summarized in Figure 4–5 by a schematic diagram of the adult heart. In this situation, the heart acts as a double pump. The first pump, the right chambers of the heart, is responsible for delivering poorly oxygenated blood to the lungs. Following gas-exchange in the lungs, the well-oxygenated blood is returned the second pump of the heart, the left atrium and ventricle. From these chambers, the oxygen-rich blood is pumped through the aorta for distribution to all parts of the body. Oxygen is exchanged with carbon dioxide at the tissue level in the body and the oxygen-depleted blood is returned to the right atrium of the heart to begin the cycle anew.

The more complex circulatory pattern, fetal circulation, is summarized in Figure 4–6. It is often described in two parallel circuits which interact in the right atrium. In one circuit, blood from the placenta flows into the fetus through the umbilical vein. About one-half of this blood enters the fetus's liver and the other half flows directly into the inferior vena cava. In the inferior vena cava, the well-oxygenated blood mixes with less well-oxygenated blood returning from the fetus's gastrointestinal tract, lower extremities, and liver. This mixture enters the right atrium where more than half of it flows through the foramen ovale, an opening which closes shortly after birth, into the left atrium. Blood in the left atrium flows into the left ventricle where it is pumped into the ascending aorta to perfuse the heart and brain.

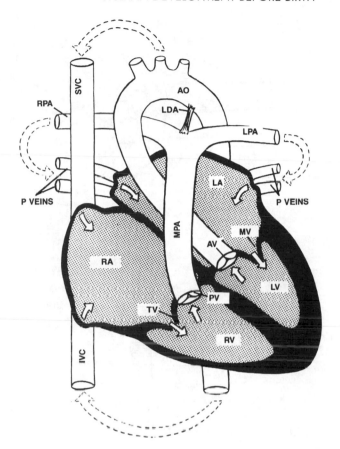

The normal heart.

AO	Aorta	**MV**	Mitral valve
AV	Aortic valve	**PV**	Pulmonary valve
IVC	Inferior vena cava	**P VEIN**	Pulmonary vein
LA	Left atrium	**RA**	Right atrium
LDA	Ligamentum ductus arteriosus	**RPA**	Right pulmonary artery
LPA	Left pulmonary artery	**RV**	Right ventricle
LV	Left ventricle	**SVC**	Superior vena cava
MPA	Main pulmonary artery	**TV**	Tricuspid valve

FIGURE 4–5. Schematic representation of extrauterine blood circulation as revealed by the normal adult heart. The heart acts as a double pump. The first pump, the right chambers of the heart, is responsible for delivering poorly oxygenated blood to the lungs. Following gas-exchange in the lungs, the well-oxygenated blood is returned the second pump of the heart, the left atrium and ventricle. From these chambers, the oxygen-rich blood is pumped through the aorta for distribution to all parts of the body. Oxygen is exchanged with carbon dioxide at the tissue level in the body and the oxygen-depleted blood is returned to the right atrium of the heart to begin the cycle anew. (Courtesy of Ross Laboratories, Clinical Education Aid.)

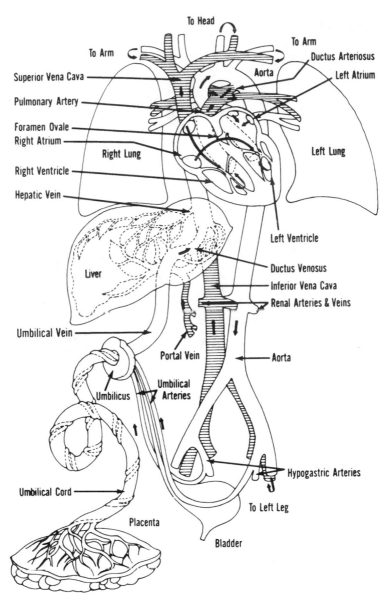

FIGURE 4-6. Schematic representation of fetal blood circulation. In the fetus, the placenta is the organ of oxygenation and gas exchange. Fetal circulation is often described in two parallel circuits which interact in the right atrium. In one circuit, blood from the placenta flows into the fetus through the umbilical vein. About one half of this blood enters the fetus's liver and the other half flows directly into the inferior vena cava. In the inferior vena cava, the well-oxygenated blood mixes with less well-oxygenated blood

(continued)

FIGURE 4–6. *(continued)*

returning from the fetus's gastrointestinal tract, lower extremities, and liver. This mixture enters the right atrium where more than half of it flows through the foramen ovale, an opening which closes shortly after birth, into the left atrium. Blood in the left atrium flows into the left ventricle where it is pumped into the ascending aorta to perfuse the heart and brain.

In a second circuit, blood from the fetus's head and upper extremities enters the right atrium via the superior vena cava. This poorly oxygenated blood mixes with blood from the inferior vena cava which did not flow through the foramen ovale. Blood in the right atrium is now a mixture of blood from the superior vena cava (returning head and upper extremity circulation) and blood from the inferior vena cava (umbilical vein and returning gastrointestinal tract, lower extremity and liver circulation). This mixture flows into the right ventricle where it is pumped into the pulmonary artery. Although a small amount of blood circulates into the fluid-filled fetal lungs, the majority is shunted through the ductus arteriosus (a second fetal circulatory opening which closes shortly after birth) into the descending aorta. The blood in this circulatory pattern is less well-oxygenated than the blood in the ascending aortic circulation; it perfuses the trunk and lower extremities and returns, via the umbilical arteries to the placenta for re-oxygenation. The lungs receive only enough blood to support lung tissue development; most blood is shunted away from the lung through the ductus arteriosus. Following birth, the ductus must close to ensure adequate shunting of blood into the lungs. (Courtesy of Ross Laboratories, Clinical Education Aid.)

In a second circuit, blood from the fetus's head and upper extremities enters the right atrium via the superior vena cava. This poorly oxygenated blood mixes with blood from the inferior vena cava which did not flow through the foramen ovale. Blood in the right atrium is now a mixture of blood from the superior vena cava (returning head and upper extremity circulation) and blood from the inferior vena cava (umbilical vein and returning gastrointestinal tract, lower extremity and liver circulation). This mixture flows into the right ventricle where it is pumped into the pulmonary artery. Although a small amount of blood circulates into the fluid-filled fetal lungs, the majority is shunted through the ductus arteriosus (a second fetal circulatory opening which closes shortly after birth) into the descending aorta. The blood in this circulatory pattern is less well-oxygenated than the blood in the ascending aortic circulation; it perfuses the trunk and lower extremities and returns, via the umbilical arteries to the placenta for re-oxygenation.

At birth, circulation must rapidly convert from this fetal pattern to the extrauterine pattern. This is accomplished by the complex interactions of clamping the umbilical cord and expanding the lungs with air. The resulting changes in pulmonary vascular resistance and oxygen tension result in closure of the foramen ovale and constriction of the ductus arteriosus. Closure of these fetal circulatory pathways and decreased pulmonary artery pressure results in blood flow into the lungs.

DEVELOPMENT OF THE EARS, FACE, AND PALATE

For professionals interested in human communication, knowledge of prenatal development of the ears, face, and palate is especially important. Major congenital anomalies such as aural atresia or cleft lip and palate typically result in speech and language delays that affect the infant's overall development.

The major features of the ears, face, and palate emerge and differentiate primarily during the fourth through eighth week of development (the embryonic period). Formation of the external structures of the head and neck depend largely on development of the branchial structures; development of the face, including the eyes, nose, lip, mouth, and palate, require contributions from both branchial and other embryonic structures.

The Branchial Structures

Most congenital malformations of the head and neck arise from abnormalities of the branchial structures. The branchial structures include: (a) the branchial arches, numbered one through four in a cranial-to-caudal sequence; (b) the pharyngeal pouches, outpocketings of the primitive foregut (pharynx) which arise internally and balloon out between the branchial arches; (c) the branchial grooves which separate the branchial arches externally; and (d) the branchial membranes which develop from the approximation of pharyngeal pouch and branchial groove epithelia. Figure 4–7 is a schematic representation of an embryo at 5 weeks development showing the relationship between branchial arches, pharyngeal pouches, branchial grooves, and branchial membranes.

Branchial Arches

The branchial arches emerge early in the embryonic period during the fourth week following fertilization. They appear as surface ele-

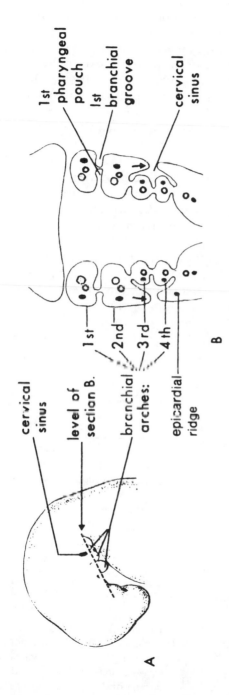

FIGURE 4-7. (A) Lateral view of the head and neck region of an embryo about 32 days showing the branchial arches and cervical sinus. **(B)** Diagrammatic horizontal section through the embryo illustrating growth of the second arch over the third and fourth arches. [From *The Developing Human Clinically Oriented Embryology*, Fifth Edition (p. 190), by Moore, K. L. and Persaud, T. V. N. (1993). Philadelphia, PA: W. B. Saunders Company. Copyright 1993 by W. B. Saunders Company. Reprinted with permission.]

vations on the head/neck area of the embryo lateral to the developing pharynx. The first and second branchial arches appear at about day 24, and the four most apparent arches are visible by about day 28. The branchial arches are composed of mesenchyme derived from embryonic mesoderm, covered externally with ectoderm and lined internally with endoderm. All three tissue layers are important in transformation of the branchial arches into their ultimate structures.

The branchial arches include arteries, cartilage, muscle, and nerve tissues. These components develop into structures associated with the head, neck, face, and/or ear. For example, the cartilage of the first branchial arch (Meckel's cartilage) contributes to formation of two middle ear ossicles, the malleus and the incus. Similarly, the cartilage of the second arch (Reichert's cartilage) evolves into the stapes. Table 4–2 summarizes the structures derived from branchial arch components.

The first branchial arch (mandibular) is especially important in head and face development. Derivatives from this structure include the mandible (lower jaw), maxilla (upper jaw), the zygomatic bone (cheekbone), and squamous portion of the temporal bone.

The second branchial arch (hyoid) contributes to development of the hyoid bone (suspension for the larynx). The third branchial

Table 4–2. Structures derived from components of the branchial arches.

Arch	Nerve	Muscles	Bone and Cartilage
Mandibular (First)	Trigeminal (Vth cranial)	Tensor tympani Tensor veli palatini Muscles of mastication	Malleus Incus
Hyoid (Second)	Facial (VIIth cranial)	Stapedius Stylohyoid Muscles of expression	Stapes Styloid process Upper part of hyoid bone
Third	Glossopharyngeal (IXth cranial)	Stylopharyngeus	Portions of hyoid bone
Fourth	Superior laryngeal branch of the vagus (Xth cranial)	Cricothyroid Levator veli palatini Muscles of the larynx and pharynx	Cartilages: Thyroid Aryteniod Cricoid Corniculate Cuneiform

arch also contributes to development of the hyoid bone. The fourth branchial arch contributes to formation of the larynx.

Pharyngeal Pouches

The pharyngeal pouches are outpocketings of the primitive foregut or pharynx. The pharynx will evolve into the digestive tract of the fetus; the pharyngeal pouches will contribute to structures important in head, face, and ear development.

Four functional pharyngeal pouches balloon out internally into the space between the branchial arches (e.g., the first pharyngeal pouch occupies the space between the first and second branchial arch). The first pharyngeal pouch evolves into the tubo-tympanic recess including the middle ear cavity, the mastoid antrum, and the eustachian tube. The second, third, and fourth pharyngeal pouches contribute to development of the lymphoid system, the parathyroid, and thymus gland.

Branchial Grooves

The four pharyngeal pouches separate the branchial arches internally; the four branchial grooves separate the branchial arches externally. Of these, only the first branchial groove persists into a permanent structure. The first branchial groove involutes into the external auditory meatus.

Swelling of mesenchymal tissue (auricular hillocks) on the first and second branchial arch around the first branchial groove evolve into the external ear. Auricular hillocks are clearly apparent on embryos of 5 to 6 weeks of development. The other three branchial grooves transform during embryonic development into a sinus which becomes obliterated as the neck develops.

Branchial Membranes

The branchial membranes appear where the branchial grooves approximate the pharyngeal pouches. Approximation of the ectoderm of the grooves with the endoderm of the pouches induces formation of mesenchyme. Only the mesenchyme of the first groove/pouch persists into an adult structure; it becomes the middle layer of the tympanic membrane (TM).

Development of the Ear

Formation and evolution of the branchial arch apparatus during the fourth through eighth weeks are signal events in development of the external and middle ear. As described above, these structures are important for development of the auricle, the external auditory meatus, the tympanic membrane, the middle ear cavity and eustachian tube, and the ossicles. The inner ear develops simultaneously with the external and middle ear but arises from different embryonic tissue. It is often normal in the presence of congenital malformation of the external and/or middle ear.

External Ear

Development of the external ear is initiated by formation of the branchial arches during the fourth week. Of the four identifiable arches, the first (mandibular) and second (hyoid) arches are critical to development of the external ear.

The auricle develops from swellings that arise around the first branchial arch during the fifth week. These irregular enlargements, auricular hillocks, grow and fuse into a recognizable external ear by about the eighth week. Scanning electron microscopic examination of human embryos has confirmed the contributions of each hillock to the structures of the auricle. In general, the auricular hillocks associated with the first branchial arch contribute to formation of the tragus; auricular hillocks associated with the second branchial arch contribute to formation of all other structures of the external ear. Figure 4–8 shows evolution of the auricular hillocks into the auricle from about the fourth week of development to birth.

The external auditory meatus (EAM) develops from the first branchial groove beginning at about the fourth to fifth week. The ectoderm-lined groove deepens towards the endoderm-lined first pharyngeal pouch; approximation of these two tissue layers induces formation of a third tissue layer, mesoderm. Eventually, the tympanic membrane arises from tissue derived from the ectoderm of the first branchial arch (outer, radial fiber layer), mesoderm (middle, fibrous layer) intermediate to the first branchial groove and the first pharyngeal pouch, and endoderm of the first pharyngeal pouch (inner, circular layer). Through the twentieth week of development, the EAM is occluded by a solid tissue plug, the meatal plug. The EAM opens during the twenty-first week with disintegration of the meatal plug.

Middle Ear

The middle ear cavity and eustachian tube develop from the endoderm-lined first pharyngeal pouch (the internal separation of the

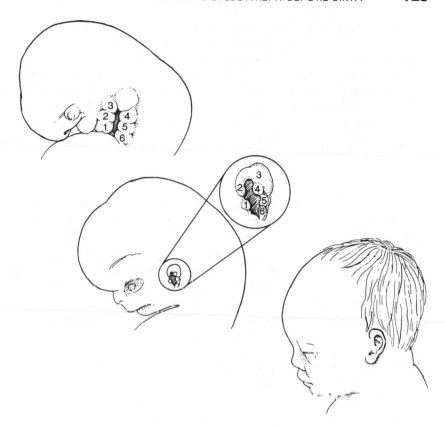

FIGURES 4–8. Evolution of the auricular hillocks into the external ear from about the fourth week of development to birth.

first and second branchial arches). As this pouch expands, it gradually encompasses the developing middle ear ossicles and their attachments. Development of the tympanic cavity begins at about five weeks and is virtually complete by the 30th week. The mastoid antrum arises from expansion of the middle ear cavity during late fetal development.

Cartilaginous derivatives of the first and second branchial arch contribute to development of the middle ear ossicles. Meckel's cartilage, associated with the first arch, gives rise to the head and neck of the malleus and the body and short arm of the incus. Riechert's cartilage, associated with the second arch, contributes to the manubrium of the malleus, the long arm of the incus, and the head, neck, and crura of the stapes.

The branchial arches contain primitive blood vessels termed aortic arch arteries. The stapes develops around the artery associated with the second branchial arch, the stapedial artery. The distinctive stirrup-like appearance of the stapes results from embryonic molding of the ossicle around this artery.

The malleus, incus, and stapes begin to ossify about the fourth month of development. These are the first bones to attain adult size in the human body; early in the sixth month growth of the ossicles is complete. The auricle, EAM, and middle ear space will continue to growth during the first decade of life.

Inner Ear

The inner ear sensory structures are derived from ectodermal tissue thickenings on the lateral surface of the head. These structures, the otic placodes, become apparent about the fourth week. Shortly thereafter, each otic placode invaginates to form an otic pit. The edges of the otic pit approximate and eventually fuse to form an otic vesicle (otocyst). The otic vesicle pinches off from the surface ectoderm and migrates internally.

Figure 4–9 shows development of the membranous labyrinth from the otocyst during weeks 5 through 8. During this period, the otocyst rapidly differentiates into the vestibular and cochlear portion of the membranous labyrinth. Initially, the otocyst lengthens more rapidly than it widens to form two pouches, a large, triangular pouch that will evolve into the vestibular membranous labyrinth and a slender, flattened pouch that will evolve into the cochlear membranous labyrinth. By the sixth week, the cochlear pouch begins to coil. One and one-half coils are apparent by the eighth week; by 9 weeks, the full two and one-half coils of the cochlea are complete. The membranous cochlea continues to growth through 16 weeks when the length of the cochlear duct approximates the adult length of 33–37 millimeters. Mesenchyme surrounding the otic vesicle forms the cartilaginous otic capsule. This capsule eventually ossifies to form the bony labyrinth.

From the seventh through the twentieth week, the sensory structures of the inner ear are developing from cells within the membranous labyrinth. As the membranous labyrinth attains its ultimate structure, six sensory structures develop and differentiate, the three ampullae of the semicircular canals, the maculae of the saccule and utricle, and the organ of Corti. By about the eleventh or twelfth week, incompletely differentiated hair cells are apparent. Inner hair cells can be identified throughout the cochlear duct, but outer hair cells are observed only in the basal half of the cochlea. Differentiated hair cells are visible by the sixteenth week, and by 17 weeks, the full number of adult hair cells

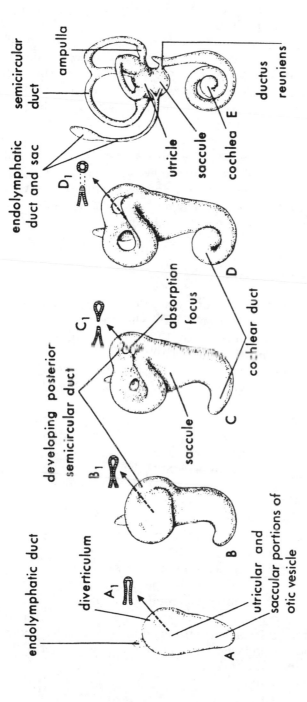

FIGURE 4-9. Diagrams showing development of the membranous labyrinth of the inner ear. **(A to E)** Lateral views showing successive stages in the development of the otic vesicles into the membranous labyrinth from the fifth to eighth weeks. (From *The Developing Human: Clinically Oriented Embryology*, Fifth Edition (p. 435), by Moore, K. L. and Persaud, T. V. N. (1993). Philadelphia, PA: W. B. Saunders Company. Copyright 1993 by W. B. Saunders Company. Reprinted with permission.)

is apparent in the cochlea of the developing fetus. Supporting cells in the organ of Corti (Deiter's cells, Hensen's cells) develop in parallel with the sensory structures.

Innervation of the cochlea progresses from the seventh through about the twentieth week. During the period, ganglion cells from the spiral ganglion start to grow toward the membranous labyrinth. Shortly after coiling of the cochlea is complete (ninth week), nerve fibers enter the developing sensory epithelium. Synaptic endings for both afferent and efferent nerve fibers form when the hair cells begin differentiating in the eleventh week. By 20 weeks, mature synaptic patterns are achieved on the inner hair cells; synaptic patterns on the outer hair cells continue to evolve. The fetus acquires rudimentary functional hearing around the twentieth week. By about 34 weeks, the cochlea has achieved its final size and structure, and growth and development are complete.

Development of the Face

The face includes the mouth, chin, jaws, lips, nose, cheeks, eyes, and forehead. The mouth evolves from a slight depression in the surface ectoderm of the embryo early in the fourth week of development. This depression, the stomodeum, is separated from the primitive pharynx by a membrane which ruptures on about day 24 and permits communication between the primitive digestive system and the amniotic cavity.

The other structures of the face arise from prominences or swellings surrounding the stomodeum. Five prominences are apparent early in the fourth week; facial development occurs primarily during the fourth through eighth week. The five prominence are the single, midline, frontonasal prominence and the paired maxillary and mandibular prominences.

The single frontonasal prominence surrounds the forebrain and accommodates the optic vesicles. These structures are projections from the forebrain which will evolve into the eyes. The frontal portion of the frontonasal prominence will become the forehead and the portion intermediary to the frontal portion and the stomodeum will contribute to development of the nose.

The maxillary and mandibular prominences arise from the first branchial arches. These structures contribute to development of the upper and lower jaws, the upper and lower cheeks, the upper and lower lips, and the chin.

Development of the Palate

The palate begins development during the fifth week and completes the process during the twelfth week. The critical period of palatal development encompasses the sixth through ninth week of development. Figure 4–10 shows development and fusion of the structures of the palate.

The palate arises from two structures, the primary palate, a wedge-shaped mass of mesenchyme formed midline between the two maxillary prominences (segments of the first branchial arches). The primary palate contributes to formation of a small portion of the hard palate.

The secondary palate evolves into both the hard and soft palate. It arises from lateral mesenchymal projections from the internal segments of the maxillary prominences. These projections elongate on each side of midline and fuse to form the complete palate.

Developmental Anomalies of the Ears, Face, and Palate

Not unexpectedly, developmental anomalies of the first branchial arch result in a complex range of anomalies affecting the external and middle ear, face, and palate. Although developing simultaneously with the external and middle ear, the inner ear is unaffected because it originates from different embryonic tissue.

First arch syndrome (for *first branchial arch*) describes a constellation of defects including aural atresia, microtia, and developmental anomalies of the middle ear ossicles, mandible, maxilla, eyes, and palate. It is believed to result from disruption in normal cell migration patterns during the fourth week of development. Mandibulofacial dysostosis (Treacher Collins syndrome; see Chapter 3), inherited through autosomal dominant transmission, includes malar hypoplasia (underdevelopment of the zygomatic bone); abnormalities of the external, middle, and inner ear; and defects of the lower eyelids. Pierre Robin sequence, a constellation of abnormalities secondary to the primary defect of mandibular hypoplasia (small lower jaw) includes cleft palate and defects of the external ear. Both mandibulofacial dysostosis and Robin sequence represents disorders within the spectrum of first arch syndrome.

During the period from 4 through about 10 weeks of development, the embryo/fetus is especially vulnerable to anomalies of inner ear development. Exposure to teratogens, for example, the

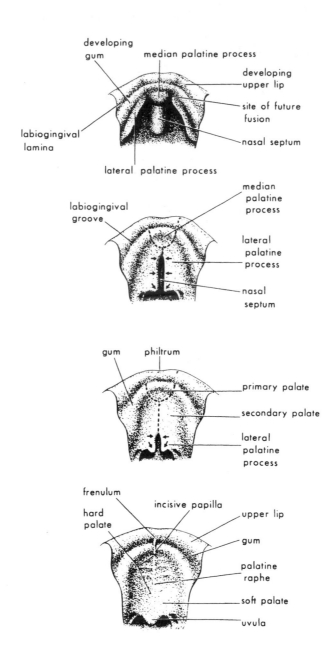

FIGURE 4–10. Drawings of the roof of the mouth from the sixth to twelfth weeks illustrating development of the palate. The broken lines indicate sites of fusion of the palatine processes. The arrows indicate medial and poste-

(continued)

FIGURE 4-10. *(continued)*
rior growth of the lateral palatine processes or palatal
shelves. (From *The Developing Human Clinically Oriented
Embryology*, Fifth Edition (p. 212), by Moore, K. L. and
Persaud, T. V. N. (1993). Philadelphia, PA: W. B.
Saunders Company. Copyright 1993 by W. B. Saunders
Company. Reprinted with permission.)

rubella virus, during this critical period may result in disruption of
the normal developmental sequence and congenital deafness.
Genetic effects are also capable of disrupting inner ear development
during this period; at least one form of congenital deafness of genetic origin, Mondini aplasia, originates from arrest in development of
the inner ear during about the seventh week to eighth week. This
disorder is characterized by one and one-half turns of the bony
cochlea rather than the normal two and one-half turns. Mondini
aplasia is also associated with several syndromal anomalies as well
as exposure to teratogens (e.g., cytomegalovirus). Regardless of the
etiology of the Mondini defect, its presence suggests developmental
effects during the seventh week to eighth week.

One of the most useful approaches for studying dysmorphology of the ear is evaluation of mutant mice strains. These animals
carry specific genes that cause congenital anomalies of the ear.
For example, there are mice whose congenital deafness has been
linked to developmental anomalies of the otic vesicle. Study of
these animals may uncover the phenomena that trigger disruption
of the normal developmental sequence and thus improve our
understanding of congenital sensorineural hearing loss.

Isolated cleft lip and/or palate are relatively common birth
defects. Cleft lip occurs in about 1 in 1,000 births; cleft palate
occurs in about 1 in 2,500 births. Cleft lip almost always refers to
fissure in the upper lip; cleft of the lower lip is exceedingly rare.
Cleft lip may be unilateral or bilateral; both unilateral and bilateral forms result when processes within the maxillary prominence
(derived from the first branchial arch) fail to fuse with medial
nasal prominences. Very rarely, median cleft lip results from dis-
turbance in embryonic development.

Cleft palate results from failure in fusion of either the primary
(intramaxillary mesenchyme) or the secondary (lateral maxillary
mesenchyme) palate, or both. A cleft palate may involve only the
uvula or both the hard and soft palate.

Cleft lip and/or palate typically results from multifactorial
inheritance (see Chapter 3). Both genetic and nongenetic effects
influence embryologic development of cleft lip and/or palate.

Single gene defects and chromosomal anomalies may also result in a cleft lip and/or palate. For example, infants with an extra copy of chromosome 13 (trisomy 13) commonly exhibit cleft lip and palate. Teratogenic agents are also implicated in cleft lip and palate. An association between anticonvulsant drugs and cleft lip and palate has been reported.

TERATOGENS AND THE DEVELOPING FETUS

In addition to disorders related to genetic and chromosomal factors, the developing fetus is vulnerable to injury from environmental factors such as infections, drugs, radiation, and mechanical compromise. Environmental agents that can damage a developing embryo or fetus are called teratogens. In general, teratogens result in malformations and anomalies of specific organ systems when the fetus is undergoing rapid differentiation (for most organ systems during the third through eighth week of development).

Three factors influence the possible teratogenicity of an agent: (a) critical period of human development, (b) concentration of the exposure or dosage, and (c) maternal/fetal and teratogen interaction.

Exposure of the embryo to teratogens during periods of rapid tissue and organ system differentiation typically results in major congenital anomaly of the organ system under development. Figure 4–11 illustrates the critical periods of human fetal development when exposure to teratogens results in either major congenital anomaly or minor abnormality and functional deficits. For humans, the critical period of development generally occurs between the third and eighth week for most organ systems, and extends through the 16th week for the central nervous system. During this period, all major sense and organ systems are undergoing rapid differentiation and development. Exposure to teratogens prior to the third week may result in early death and spontaneous abortion of the pre-embryo, but does not cause congenital anomalies because cell differentiation has not occurred. Prior to implantation (during week 2 following fertilization) the preembryonic cell mass is not susceptible to teratogens.

The dosage or concentration of the teratogen is a factor contributing to the development of congenital anomalies. Because of the complex interaction between the dosage or concentration of exposure and maternal and fetal reactions to that exposure, a specific dose threshold cannot be established for most teratogens. For this reason, pregnant women are advised to avoid *any* exposure to potentially teratogenic agents (e.g., eliminate consumption of alcohol and smoking prior to and during pregnancy).

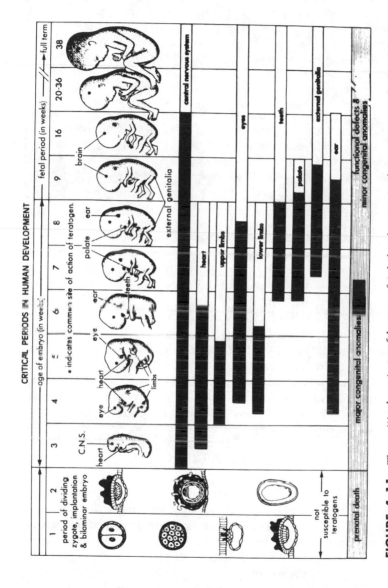

FIGURE 4-11. The critical periods of human fetal development when exposure to teratogens results in either major congenital anomaly or minor abnormality and functional deficits. (Adapted from *Before We Are Born*, Third Edition by K. L. Moore, 1989, p. 118. Philadelphia, PA: W. B. Saunders Company. Copyright by W. B. Saunders Company. Reprinted with permission.)

The sedative, thalidomide, has become the most notorious teratogen in history. From 1957 to 1962, an "epidemic" of congenital limb deformities occurred in many countries throughout Europe. The deformities ranged from amelia (absence of limbs) including babies born without either upper or lower limbs through intermediate forms of deformity (meromelia; rudimentary, nonfunctional limbs). The thalidomide tragedy highlights the relationship between the time of exposure to the teratogen and presence and type of congenital defect. For example, anomalies of the upper limbs are present in babies exposed on days 27 to 30 of development; anomalies of the lower limbs are present in babies exposed on days 30 to 33 of development. In addition, anomalies of the external ears develop if exposure occurs during days 21 to 27. It is estimated that more than 7,000 infants were affected by this potent teratogen. Because thalidomide was not approved by the United States Food and Drug Administration, less than two dozen cases were reported in the U.S.

Finally, animal studies have shown that there are genetic differences in response to teratogens. In humans, a similar response is suspected because not all embryos who are exposed to a specific teratogen develop major congenital anomalies. It appears, therefore, that the genetic characteristics of the embryo influence whether a teratogen will affect its development.

The teratogenic agents most familiar to audiologists and speech-language pathologists include infectious diseases such as rubella, cytomegalovirus, toxoplasmosis, and syphilis, and drugs such as alcohol, cocaine, thalidomide, nicotine and other agents in cigarette smoke, and retinoic acid (vitamin A). Environmental chemicals such as organic mercury and lead are also potent teratogens.

SUMMARY

The process of prenatal development is an exquisite succession of coordinated, programmed events. At any given instance in this development, critical mechanisms are ensuing which, if interrupted or altered, may result in death of the developing embryo or fetus or severe congenital abnormality. Because congenital anomalies are a major factor in neonatal morbidity and mortality, professionals who provide services to very young infants and their families should develop a basic understanding of the elegant process of human development before birth.

SUGGESTED READINGS

Moore, K. L., & Persaud, T. V. N. (1993). *The developing human clinically oriented embryology* (5th Edition.) Philadelphia: W. B. Saunders Company. *A comprehensive overview of human embryology.*

Gorlin, R. J., Toriello, H. V., & Cohen, M. M. (1995). *Hereditary hearing loss and its syndromes.* New York: Oxford University Press. *The definitive, current text detailing hereditary hearing loss.*

CHAPTER 5

Care of Premature and Critically Ill Newborns: The Neonatal Intensive Care Unit

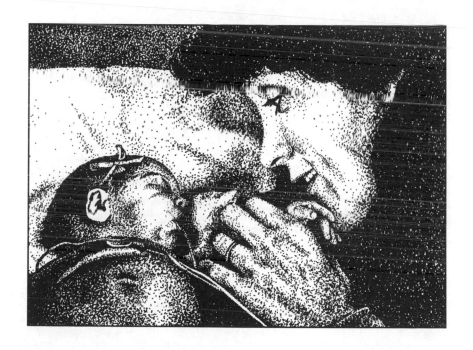

A daunting array of complex medical technology and sophisticated treatment is currently available to care for premature and critically ill newborns. The neonatal intensive care unit (NICU) contains medicine's most advanced technology including machines to monitor, infuse, view, stimulate, warm, and breathe for these fragile babies. Since the introduction of NICU care in the United States in the mid-1960s, newborn mortality rate has dropped significantly, and infants as small as 1,000 grams (approximately 2 pounds, 4 ounces) now routinely survive.

Babies have not always been considered candidates for medical care. Hospital care for children and routine health care for newborn infants are largely 19th and 20th century phenomena. From earliest times through the 19th century, infant survival was related more to chance and luck than medical intervention and treatment. Today, of course, infant survival is the routinely expected outcome of pregnancy, even for high-risk babies. For these vulnerable infants, the high-technology milieu of the NICU is a lifesaving necessity.

A BRIEF HISTORY OF WESTERN MEDICAL CARE FOR INFANTS

Antecedents

Although the foundations of traditional Western medicine originate with the ancient Greeks, medical care for infants was not practiced in Greek or Roman civilization. By custom, infants who were unacceptable by reason of deformity, gender, legitimacy, or economics were exposed and abandoned outside the city gates. Physicians recommended that infants who were weak or imperfect were not worth rearing and should be deserted to die.

Practices of childbirth had the greatest influence on infant medical care from the Middle Ages through the late 18th century. Birthing was a home event attended by a midwife with little or no medical background or experience. Neither mother nor infant received medical care for morbidity associated with labor and delivery. As medical practice advanced, physicians had more to offer laboring women but lacked experience in childbirth and delivery. To develop physician experience and to apply medical practice to labor and delivery, maternity hospitals were opened in Europe, and later in the United States. Through these institutions, physicians had an opportunity to observe medical problems of newborn infants and the concept of administering medical care to sick newborns developed. Infectious diseases of infants were described and, when possible, treatments introduced. Initially, infants were treated through the nursing mother or wet nurse, but eventually, infants received direct medical care. Prevention of infant disease through practice of antiseptic techniques during or immediately after delivery also developed during the late 19th century.

The Infant Welfare Movement

A variety of social and political forces emerged to stimulate the Infant Welfare Movement in Western Europe in the 1870s. Western European countries, and especially France, experienced an appalling infant mortality rate coupled with a declining birth rate. By 1870, the birth rate in France scarcely exceeded the death rate. To reverse the trend to depopulation, the French government encouraged increase in the birth rate and prompted efforts to improve the infant mortality rate. Attempts to increase the birth rate failed, but efforts to improve infant mortality rates succeeded. Two French obstetricians, Etienne Tarnier, and his student and successor, Pierre Budin, developed the technology and systems to provide vigorous medical care to premature and sick newborns. These two physicians were largely responsible for improving infant health care in France and for influencing Western medical tradition to consider newborn infants as patients rather than by-products of the birth process.

While practicing at the *Maternité Hôpital* in Paris in 1880, Tarnier introduced a closed infant incubator modeled after a device used to raise chickens for the Paris Zoo. Thermoregulation was accomplished by heat transfer from a water tank to the air surrounding the infant in a closed cabinet. Tarnier's incubator could house two or three "weaklings" (premature infants) comfortably. Although Tarnier did not develop the first incubator to be used with human infants, he was among the first to apply incubator care on a widespread basis. Babies from throughout Paris were taken to the *Pavilion les Debiles* at the *Maternité* for care and treatment.

Budin succeeded Tarnier as director of the *Pavilion* in 1895. Budin observed and cared for infants who were previously destined to die due to lack of knowledgeable and adequate care. Often considered the father of neonatal medicine, Budin described three fundamental principles in caring for sick and premature newborns: (a) their temperature and their chilling, (b) their feeding, and (c) the diseases to which they are prone. The first newborn medical record was developed in Budin's unit, and newborns officially became patients in their own right.

Incubator Baby Sideshows

Tarnier's technology and Budin's medical expertise spawned a peculiar sideshow attraction, the baby incubator shows. In 1896, live premature babies were displayed at the World Exhibition in Berlin to demonstrate incubator technology. The exhibit was an instant success. Premature babies received specialized technology and nursing care; the public received an amazing show. A German physician, Martin Couney, organized incubator exhibits with live babies throughout the continent. By summer 1898, Couney was in the United States exhibiting incubators with live babies at the Trans-Mississippi Exposition in Omaha. Couney settled in this country and continued to exhibit babies in incubators through the 1930s at exhibitions, worlds fairs, and annual shows at Coney Island. By the 1940s, public interest in incubator baby shows diminished, and Couney closed his Coney Island shows. Although the ethics of Couney's live baby shows remain questionable, it is sobering to consider that many infants survived because of the care that they received in these exhibits.

Newborn Care in the United States

Along with incubator baby sideshows, the Infant Welfare Movement emigrated to the United States in the early 20th century. Although hospitals for children had been established in this country as early as 1854, these institutions were not specifically dedicated to treating newborns and very young infants. It was not until 1922 that a special unit for premature infants opened at the Sarah Morris Hospital in Chicago. Chicago was one of the first cities to initiate a systematic program to save premature infants which included mandatory reporting of premature births to the Board of Health and transporting premature infants to special hospital care units. The first premature infant station in New York City opened in 1944.

In concert with establishment of special medical care units for children and infants, physicians also responded to the unique needs of children in the late 19th century. In 1880, the American Medical Association (AMA) established a Section on Diseases of Children; in 1888, the American Pediatric Society (APS) was founded. Despite these efforts, it would be more than 20 years before physicians could maintain a practice devoted exclusively to the care of children, and 50 years before this specialty was recognized with board-certification status. In the early part of the 20th century, pediatricians developed practices tending to the artificial feeding (i.e., formula feeding) of infants and treating diseases of childhood. By the 1930s, pediatricians began to provide systematic evaluation and management of sick newborns. Normative data about physical and physiological characteristics of newborn infants appeared, and recognition of congenital diseases and disorders improved. By the late 1940s, hospital birthing became routine, newborn nurseries were standard features of metropolitan hospitals, and pediatricians commonly controlled care of newborn infants.

Following the second world war, American society developed a renewed interest in children and the family. The baby boom began. New medical technologies emerged, benefitting both mothers and infants, and survival of premature and other sick infants was an expected medical outcome. By the mid-1950s, newborn infants were routinely assessed by the rating scale introduced by Virginia Apgar, an obstetric anesthesiologist (see Chapter 6). The scale permitted development of systematic guidelines for resuscitation of newborn infants and provided a reference point for newborn research.

Newborn Intensive Care

Despite rapid technological advances throughout the 1950s, infant mortality rates in the United States were poorer than those reported by other Western industrialized nations. Factors contributing to this relatively poor standing included the cultural diversity of our population, geographic dispersion of population centers, and lack of access to systematic health care for all Americans. In addition, neither expensive, sophisticated technology nor

---

Standard terms are used to describe the weight and age of newborns. These are also used to indicate the potential risk for these newborns. These terms are *low birth weight* and *preterm*.

Low birth weight (LBW) = under 5 lb, 8 oz, or 2,500 gm

Very low birth weight (VLBW) = under 3 lb, 5 oz, or 1,500 gm

Extremely low birth weight (ELBW) = under 2 lb, 3 oz, or 1,000 gm

Preterm birth = birth after fewer than 37 weeks of gestation

Very preterm birth = birth after fewer than 32 weeks of gestation

From *The Future of Children*, a publication of the Center for the Future of Children, The David and Lucile Packard Foundation (1995).

experienced personnel were available in all communities where premature and sick babies might be born. To address this issue, the medical community promoted the concept of "regionalization" of perinatal care. Under this model, a cooperative network of care providers is identified in a specific geographic region who (a) identify high-risk pregnancies, (b) refer pregnant women and newborn infants into high-technology labor-delivery and perinatal treatment centers, and (c) monitor outcomes of these interventions relative to the neonatal morbidity and mortality. Essentially, in an identified geographic region, a single tertiary perinatal program is connected by telephone "hot line" and ground- and air-transport facility to multiple hospitals throughout the region where labor and delivery occur. Women who are identified as high-risk, or who enter in premature labor, are transported to the perinatal center for delivery and care of their newborn. Infants who experience difficulty after birth are also transported to the perinatal center. As the infant improves, he or she may be transported back to the home community for less intensive inpatient care. This approach provides adequate medical care for most women and infants, avoids costly duplication of technology and personnel, and permits assessment of statistical outcomes against national and international standards.

There is little doubt that introduction of regionalized perinatal care improved neonatal mortality rates. Reports from programs in both rural and urban regions of the United States revealed reduction in fetal and newborn mortality, no increase in infant mortality (e.g., the improved neonatal mortality rate was not an artifact of postponing neonatal death), and reduction in obstetric and newborn morbidity.

The 1980s brought challenges to the concept of regionalized perinatal care. Largely in response to market forces and competition, centers that had previously provided only routine, well-baby care (level I nursery) or intermediary care (level II nursery) expanded services to include care to premature and critically ill newborns (level III nursery). Despite proliferation of higher levels of perinatal care, however, infant mortality rates did not significantly improve during this era. Infant mortality rates in the United States continue to exceed those of Western European countries and Japan. In addition, infant mortality rates for ethnic and racial minorities in the United States exceed those of caucasians by one and one-half to two times. Minority women are less likely to receive adequate prenatal care, and more likely to bear premature or low birthweight infants than caucasian women. Sophisticated perinatal care centers cannot substitute for adequate prenatal care.

THE NURSERY ENVIRONMENT

Within the past decade, audiologists and speech-language pathologists have expanded their professional practices to provide services to infants and their families in the nursery environment. Unfortunately, most training programs do not prepare these clinicians with an understanding of the organization, philosophy, personnel, technology, and care encountered in these units.

Organization

As recommended by the American Academy of Pediatrics and the American College of Obstetricians and Gynecologists (1992) perinatal care, that is, care around the time of birth, is organized into three levels depending on the complexity of services needed by the mother and her infant. Perinatal care programs are often coordinated jointly by medical and nursing directors for obstetrics and pediatric services. Most community hospitals offer level I perinatal services; higher levels of services, levels II and III, may be available only in larger institutions or institutions affiliated with teaching facilities.

Level I Perinatal Care

Level I care represents routine postdelivery care of the mother and infant. Mothers and babies in this setting require no unusual medical or nursing services. In hospitals with level I nurseries, babies with an uneventful prenatal and birth experience receive complete physical assessment and initial observation, care, and management. On discharge, usually within 24 hours of birth, parents assume responsibility for ongoing observation, care, and management of their babies. Services not necessary for routine care of an infant must be coordinated within the very short length-of-stay in the level I nursery.

In most institutions, parents have the option of "rooming-in" or nursery infant care. Infants who "room-in" receive care in the same hospital room where the mother is receiving postpartum care; infants who receive nursery care are housed in the nursery except for feedings and other care delivered in the mother's room. The nursery is typically an open room with unobstructed line-of-sight of babies in plexiglass-sided bassinets. Hearing testing in this environment is often complicated by excessive noise levels.

Level II Perinatal Care

Level II care is provided to mothers and infants who are at risk for complications due to premature delivery, small size/low birthweight, unusual conditions of labor or delivery, or other medical events. Infants who receive level II care require monitoring for development of complications associated with their underlying conditions. In these units, babies receive more interventions and treatments than babies in a level I nursery. Infants who develop respiratory or other complications may receive continuing care in the level II nursery, or they may be transferred to a level III nursery depending on the severity of their illness. Length-of-stay in a level II nursery ranges from 24 hours for infants who are under observation to several weeks for babies receiving uncomplicated treatment for prematurity or other conditions.

Babies who receive level II care are housed in nursery units that permit optimum observation and care of these higher risk infants. Level II nurseries access more technology than level I nurseries and include capability for isolation of infants with potentially infectious conditions. Cardiopulmonary monitoring and other electronic technology are common in level II nurseries and may affect hearing testing. Similar to level I nurseries, excessive noise is frequently encountered in this environment.

Level III Perinatal Care

Level III care is provided to mothers and infants at high risk for morbidity and mortality due to conditions of pregnancy, labor, or delivery. This care was originally organized on a regional basis; that is, one site in a geographic region was designated to provide level III perinatal care. Connected to regional level I and level II programs by telephone and transport services, the regional level III program provides rapid access to mothers laboring prematurely and to unstable newborns who required complex medical care. Medical and nursing personnel in level III settings are highly specialized in maternal and neonatal diseases and their complications. These professionals are trained to provide emergency medical care to every patient they receive.

Level III nurseries are typically designated as newborn intensive care units (NICU). In these units, services are highly individualized to the unique needs of the newborn's complex medical condition. Nursing staff-to-infant ratios may exceed one-to-one in the case of unstable infants with complicated medical conditions. Physicians who specialize in newborn intensive care medicine, neonatalogists are present 24 hours a day to admit incoming transports, and respond to medical emergencies of patients under care. Length-of-stay in level III nurseries may range from 24 hours or less for infants who need initial assessment and observation only to many months for babies with severe complications from their underlying condition or its treatment.

The physical environment of the level III nursery is intense with electronic equipment surrounding each bassinet and bassinets in close proximity to facilitate nursing care. Several professionals may surround a single infant, and monitors and other audible alarms are frequently activated. The level III nursery is one of the most challenging environments for accurate hearing testing.

Table 5-1 compares function and type of patients served at the three levels of perinatal care. The table shows that each level of care adds services to those already provided by the previous level of care. For example, a level II nursery should provide all services accessible in a level I nursery as well as ability to treat infants with birthweights less than 2,500 grams or with gestational ages of 32 weeks and greater. Infants with these conditions who develop complications may require higher levels of services in the level III NICU.

Table 5-1. Characteristics of level I, II, and III perinatal care.

LEVEL I
Management and care of uncomplicated patients
Normal pregnancy, labor, delivery
Identify at-risk patients and prepare for transport
Emergency management/stabilization of unexpected complications
Prepare patients for transport

LEVEL II
Provide all services of a level I facility
Management and care of selected high-risk patients
  (e.g., premature infants > 32 weeks)
Identify high-risk patients requiring care beyond level II
  capability (e.g., premature infants < 32 weeks)
Initiate and receive transport

LEVEL III
Provide all services of a level II facility
Management and care of all high-risk patients
Long-term care of high-risk infants
Coordination of transport services
Outcome evaluation of regional services

Quaternary Care

Most recently, a fourth level of medical care has been defined. The term, *quaternary care*, is used to refer to care required of patients who receive organ transplants. Newborn infants who receive organ transplants receive this highly technical support for weeks or months following transplantation. In general, quaternary care for newborn infants in available in only a few highly specialized medical centers.

Philosophy of Care in the NICU

NICUs are intensive care units. The basic premise of these units is to rescue newborns from life-threatening medical emergencies in the face of uncertain medical or developmental outcomes. The considerable resources of the NICU are directed at managing medical crises and perilous events in the earliest days and weeks of life.

Care in the NICU is complicated by unavoidable uncertainty. Prognoses for very low birthweight babies or infants with severe congenital disorders are often unknown and unpredictably affected by the very treatment necessary to sustain life. Until a situation is deemed final and hopeless, no effort may be spared in sustaining life.

As in any intensive care situation, there is no precrisis opportunity for parents and professionals to develop a comfortable working relationship. When the moment of crisis arrives, parents and professionals are thrown together in effort to save an infant's life. Despite these less-than-ideal circumstances, NICU staff adhere to a philosophy of informing parents of potential treatment options, respecting parent treatment decisions, and involving parents in the infant's care.

Although neonatalogists and other NICU professionals have been criticized for attempting medical rescue of marginally viable infants, there appears to be a deep public commitment in this country to expensive and expansive medical care of newborns. Public initiatives to lower infant mortality rates have targeted infants who require expensive NICU care, very low birthweight babies. With regularity, the popular media highlights the story of some "miracle" baby—a baby with the lowest birthweight ever recorded—who has survived because of the heroic efforts of the NICU physicians and nurses.

NICU Personnel

Core professionals who provide service in a NICU are neonatalogists and neonatal nurse specialists. Medical and health care consultants who also provide essential services in the unit include cardiologists, pediatric surgeons, neurologists, geneticists, radiologists, and other medical specialists, and radiology technicians, respiratory therapists, social workers, and other health care specialists.

Neonatalogists

Neonatology began as a subspecialty of pediatrics in the early 1970s. Physicians who specialize in neonatology are pediatricians with advanced training in fetal development, physiology, genetics, neurodevelopment, and prematurity. They are board certified by the American Academy of Pediatrics as both pediatricians and neonatalogists. In a level III nursery, neonatalogists are in-house 24 hours a day, 7 days a week. Because of the demands and stress associated with this intensive care environment, neonatalogists often rotate through the unit on a monthly basis.

Neonatalogists are intensivists who typically do not provide care to infants beyond the hospital period. If infants require long-term hospitalization for chronic medical problems, they may receive care in a level II nursery staffed by neonatalogists. At discharge, care of NICU or level II graduates with ongoing medical problems is typically transferred to pediatricians with special expertise in chronic medical and developmental problems. A professional priority for neonatalogists is preservation of life rather than management of developmental consequences of prematurity, significant birth defects, or trauma.

Neonatal Nurse Specialists

Neonatal nurse specialty training evolved simultaneously with the development of the NICU. These specialists are nurses with post baccalaureate training in neonatal nursing practices and care. Neonatal nurse specialists are credentialed by the National Association of Neonatal Nurses.

Neonatal nurse specialists assume a complex role of providing nursing care to infants, complementing medical and physician services, and supporting parent and family interaction and understanding. They continuously observe each infant's condition, administer prescribed medications and tests, perform monitoring procedures, counsel parents, and provide information to physicians and other consultants. To most parents, their infant's primary nurse is a vital communication link to the physicians and specialists and an essential support in understanding the complex treatments. In contrast to neonatalogists who rotate out of the nursery on a regular schedule, neonatal nurse specialists are assigned to the NICU on a continuous basis. They frequently provide continuity in care and communication among physicians, parents, and consultants.

Other Specialists

The complex care provided in the NICU cannot occur without the support of a host of other medical specialists. These consultants assess specific aspects of an infant's medical condition such as cardiac function or neurologic status through appropriate laboratory, radiographic, or physiologic techniques. Their findings and recommendations are communicated to the neonatalogist for incorporation into the infant's overall care plan.

Other health care specialists who provide services in the NICU include pharmacists, respiratory therapists, occupational and physical therapists, nutritionists, and developmental specialists. These individuals frequently assess an infant's status in a specific modality and administer and monitor results of prescribed treatments.

Care provided by any specialist in the NICU is dependent on technology. In many cases, sustaining life requires instruments to warm, monitor, view, and often breathe for the baby. Neonatal intensive care is possible only through this advanced technology.

Technology in the NICU

The history of the NICU is intimately related to technological achievements in respiratory and other biomedical instrumentation. The development and use of the neonatal positive pressure respirator in the 1970s provided one of the earliest breakthroughs in the management of premature infants and infants with respiratory distress syndrome. It has been followed by a host of complicated technology specific to monitoring and treating premature and critically ill newborns.

Cardiorespiratory Monitors

To detect potentially damaging episodes of bradycardia (slow heart rate) and apnea (periodic cessation of breathing), babies in the NICU are continuously monitored for heart rate and respiration.

Figure 5–1 shows a cardiorespiratory (CR) monitor commonly used in the NICU. CR monitors are passive devices; they monitor but do not alter the infant's state. Infants are monitored by electrodes attached on either side of the chest (active electrodes) and

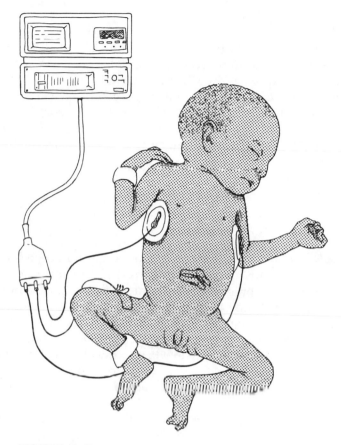

FIGURE 5–1. A cardiorespiratory (CR) monitor commonly used in the NICU. Electrodes are attached on either side of the infant's chest (active electrodes) and abdomen or leg (ground). The active electrodes detect the electrophysiologic signal that stimulates cardiac muscle contraction (heart beat) and chest expansion (respiration). These signals are displayed on the monitor oscilloscope and an electronic counter.

abdomen or leg (ground). The active electrodes detect the electrophysiologic signal that stimulates cardiac muscle contraction (heart beat) and chest expansion (respiration). These signals are displayed on the monitor oscilloscope and an electronic counter. Nursing staff set the limits of the acceptable range for heart rate and respiration for individual babies. Any deviation from this range for periods of 15 seconds or longer results in an audible alarm.

Pulse Oximetry

Pulse oximetry permits noninvasive monitoring of heart rate and blood-oxygen saturation level. The monitor consists of a light-emitting probe attached to a distal extremity (typically a finger or toe) which measures the arterial hemoglobin oxygen saturation. Oxygen saturation is calculated from the light absorption characteristics of the blood flow as it passes through the skin beneath the probe. If oxygen saturation drops below a preset limit, an audible alarm triggers. Pulse oximetry was an important development in infant monitoring because it permitted continuous noninvasive measurement of oxygen saturation.

Ventilators

Neonatal ventilators are one of the most important technologies in the nursery (Figure 5–2). Premature infants, and some term infants, may suffer progressive respiratory failure from a number of underlying conditions. The purpose of the ventilator is to maintain lung inflation and to deliver a measured flow of oxygen to the baby.

Figure 5–2 shows a schematic diagram of a neonatal ventilator. Oxygen from a compression tank or wall delivery system is mixed with room air to achieve the required concentration of oxygen. The respirator pump delivers the air and oxygen mixture at a prescribed rate and pressure through a nebulizer and heater system which adds moisture and warms the mixture. An inflow tube delivers the moist, warm oxygen to the infant through a pressure monitoring device which monitors the inflow to the infant. Oxygen may be delivered through an endotracheal tube, a polyethylene tube fed through the infant's mouth into the trachea and ending below the level of the vocal folds, or through nasal cannula. For infants with specific medical conditions, a continuous airway pressure may be maintained to prevent collapse of the alveoli and re-inflation of the lungs with each breath.

Extracorporeal Membrane Oxygenation (ECMO)

Extracorporeal membrane oxygenation (ECMO) is a variant of cardiopulmonary bypass first developed in the 1950s for open heart surgery. By these procedures, blood is removed from the patient and pumped through an oxygenator prior to return to the patient. These systems permit tissue preservation during surgery in which normal heart and lung function is stopped. In the 1980s, this concept was applied to neonatal medicine in the form of ECMO. The

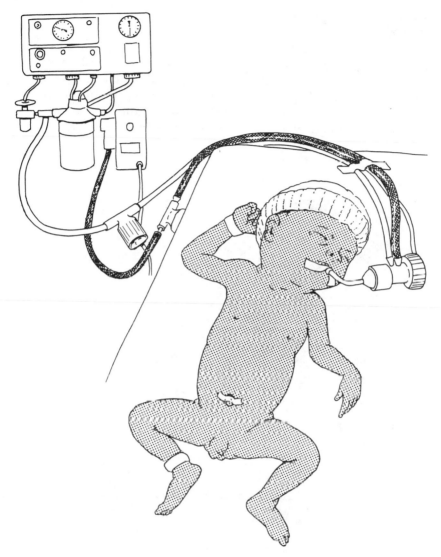

FIGURE 5–2. Schematic diagram of a neonatal ventilator. Oxygen from a compression tank or wall delivery system is mixed with room air to achieve the required concentration of oxygen. The respirator pumps the air and oxygen mixture at a prescribed rate and pressure through a nebulizer and heater system which adds moisture and warms the mixture. Moist, warm oxygen is delivered to the infant through a pressure monitoring device which monitors the inflow to the infant. Oxygen may be delivered through an endotracheal tube, a polyethylene tube fed through the infant's mouth into the trachea and ending below the level of the vocal folds, or through nasal cannula.

essential difference between surgical cardiopulmonary bypass and ECMO is length of time on the bypass machine. In the case of surgery, patients are on bypass for hours; in the case of ECMO, infants are on bypass for periods extending up to several days.

Figure 5–3 shows an ECMO array. A catheter in the infant's right atrium drains deoxygenated blood into a pressure-sensitive reservoir which is connected to the ECMO pump. A servocontrol mechanism, coupled with the pressure-sensitive reservoir, detects

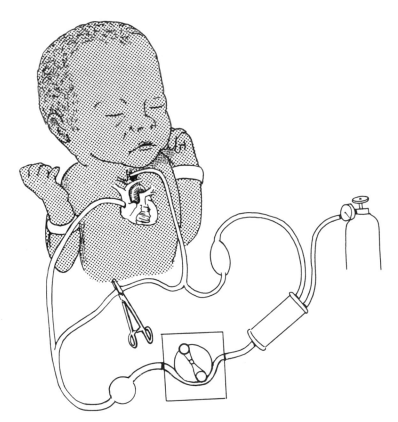

FIGURE 5–3. An ECMO array. A catheter in the infant's right atrium drains deoxygenated blood into a pressure-sensitive reservoir which is connected to the ECMO pump. A servocontrol mechanism, coupled with the pressure-sensitive reservoir, detects blood outflow from/inflow to the infant, and maintains a constant infant blood volume. Deoxygenated blood in the reservoir is pumped through a membrane lung for oxygenation prior to return through a heat exchanger back to the infant. Oxygenated blood is returned through the infant's aortic arch.

blood outflow from and inflow to the infant, and maintains a constant infant blood volume. Deoxygenated blood in the reservoir is pumped through a membrane lung for oxygenation prior to return through a heat exchanger back to the infant. Oxygenated blood is returned through the infant's aortic arch.

Although use of ECMO has become widespread, few well-controlled clinical trials have been reported. Morbidity and mortality associated with ECMO range from 13% to 33% depending on underlying disease process. Long-term adverse effects include intracranial bleeding and neurodevelopmental delays.

ECMO is an expensive, labor-intensive procedure. More recently, investigators have reported use of inhaled nitric oxide (NO_2) as a noninvasive, effective alternative to ECMO for some infants. NO_2 causes capillary dilation in lung alveoli which permits effective oxygenation in infants with specific lung disease.

Intravenous Infusion Pumps

In premature or sick infants, nutrition, fluids, and medication may have to be supplied directly into the bloodstream to avoid stressing the immature digestive tract. This is accomplished by insertion of an intravenous (IV) line into a superficial (small, peripheral) or central (larger, major) vein. An infusion pump attached to the IV line regulates the amount of nutrition, fluids, and medications that are delivered to the baby.

Figure 5–4 demonstrates an infusion pump/IV line in a premature infant. The IV fluid, usually a glucose/sterile water solution, is hung on a stand attached to the infusion pump. The fluid is gravity-fed into the pump through a calibrated burette. The pump controls rate of fluid dispersement through the IV line. A variety of junctures or membrane-capped joins are interspersed in the line to permit administration of medications. Flow through the line can be manually interrupted by stopcock valve.

An IV line may be inserted into a small, superficial vein of the arm, leg, or scalp, or into a larger central vein of the arm, leg, scalp, or neck. If the line is inserted into a central vein, a catheter is threaded into the vein into close proximity of the heart. A central IV line permits delivery of higher concentrations nutrients and medications than a superficial IV line. It is also less likely to infiltrate, or slip outside the vein, than a superficial line.

Gavage Feeding

One of the factors important to survival of premature infants is appropriate nutrition. Infants less than approximately 34 to 36

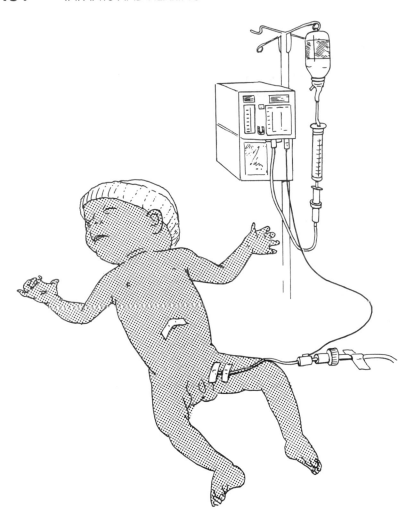

FIGURE 5–4. An infusion pump/IV line in a premature infant. The IV fluid, usually a glucose/sterile water solution, is hung on a stand attached to the infusion pump. The fluid is gravity-fed into the pump through a calibrated burette. The pump controls rate of fluid dispersement through the IV line.

weeks gestation do not exhibit neurologically mature swallow, gag, or cough reflex. These babies may not be able to coordinate sucking, swallowing, and breathing in the correct sequence and are at risk for aspiration of formula or breast milk into the lungs. In addition, babies on ventilators may aspirate if fed by mouth.

If an infant cannot be fed orally, he or she will receive nutrition via gavage feeding. Figure 5–5 shows an infant receiving gavage feeding. Feeding is accomplished by positioning a flexible polyethylene tube through the infant's nose or mouth directly into his or her stomach. A syringe containing a specified amount of breast milk or formula is connected to the tubing. By elevating the syringe above the baby, breast milk or formula flows through the tube into the baby's stomach by gravity. Rate of flow can be con-

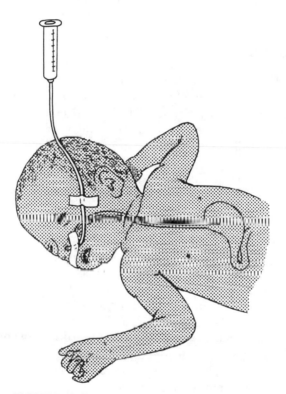

FIGURE 5–5. An infant receiving gavage feeding. Feeding is accomplished by positioning a flexible polyethylene tube through the infant's nose or mouth directly into his or her stomach. A syringe containing a specified amount of breast milk or formula is connected to the tubing. By elevating the syringe above the baby, breast milk or formula flows through the tube into the baby's stomach by gravity. Rate of flow can be controlled by raising or lowering the syringe.

trolled by raising or lowering the syringe. During feeding, the infant may be offered a pacifier to stimulate nonnutritive sucking, calm the infant, and promote earlier nipple feeding. Gavage feeding may be scheduled on an intermittent or continuous basis depending on the infant's tolerance for feeding.

Infants who cannot be fed orally or by gavage methods due to esophageal anomalies, or who require long-term tube feeding due to significant neurologic compromise, will receive gastrostomy placement, surgical insertion of a feeding tube through the abdominal wall directly into the stomach. These infants may require tube feeding for months or even years.

Bilirubin Lights

Mild hyperbilirubinemia is a condition in almost all newborn infants. Bilirubin, described more fully in Chapter 6, is a toxic by-product of the normal process of red blood cell breakdown. It is normally detoxified in the liver. In the first week of life, however, the liver is not fully effective in conjugating, or detoxifying, bilirubin. Increasing bilirubin levels in the blood lead to hyperbilirubinemia and jaundice. For most infants, the condition is transient and does not require any intervention. For premature infants, or infants with birth trauma or infection, potentially damaging levels of bilirubin may develop. For cases of hyperbilirubinemia that approach but do not exceed the bilirubin level associated with central nervous system damage, infants may receive phototherapy. Under this treatment, infants are exposed to a specific wavelength of light under special lights. These bililights alter the molecular structure of bilirubin which improves liver detoxification and natural excretion. An infant may receive bililight treatment for periods ranging from a few days to more than a week. Effective phototherapy prevents the need for exchange transfusion that occurs when hyperbilirubinemia reaches levels associated with central nervous system damage.

Other Technology in the NICU

In addition to monitors, ventilators, pumps and feeding devices, and phototherapy lights, sophisticated diagnostic technologies are readily available in the NICU. Radiology technicians use portable ultrasound, and conventional x-ray equipment to image the infant's head and body; electroencephalographic (EEG) technicians use portable EEG and evoked potential equipment to measure brain electrical activity; audiologists use evoked potential and otoacoustic emission technology to screen and evaluate peripheral hearing sensitivity. The infant may be transported to the radiology department for computerized imaging, and samples of blood and body fluids may be sent for laboratory analysis. Probably no other group of hospitalized patients receives as much technological support as infants in the NICU.

CONTROVERSIES IN NEWBORN INTENSIVE CARE

Without question, high technology NICU care has resulted in improved infant mortality rates. This care is not without controversy, however. Three primary issues emerge. First, does increased morbidity in some survivors of NICU care create an undue burden for families and society? Infants who require high-technology care may suffer permanent disability either from the underlying condition or care for that condition. Although statistics from most follow-up studies of infant outcome are encouraging, some infants do suffer severe disabilities.

Second, does the outcome of treatment justify its cost? Neonatal intensive care is extremely costly. Parents may find a maximum health insurance benefit of $1,000,000 quickly eroded by care and treatment of a critically ill newborn. Although individual investigators have analyzed cost of these programs by various formulae, and society has tacitly agreed to pay the costs, there are no universally agreed on guidelines to define the limits of care.

Finally, is it moral to provide care that may marginally prolong life but at the cost of unknown, and possibly inestimable suffering? Ethical dilemmas are not uncommon in the NICU, and the impact of these quandaries on caregivers and families is frequently profound. Because newborn intensive care makes it possible to rescue infants with underlying conditions of significant morbidity, it is often unclear how aggressively to extend treatment. In addition, it is possible for an infant to survive despite attempts to limit treatment. The Child Abuse Amendments of 1984 ("Baby Doe regulations"), promulgated by the federal government, attempted to address some of the issues surrounding treatment decisions affecting infants. Professional and societal consensus about the limits of care have not yet been achieved, however. As technology advances, health care costs increase, and health care dollars decrease, ethical dilemmas and debate in the NICU will become more complex and intense.

The newborn intensive care unit is one of the frontiers of medicine. Because of the sophisticated and highly technical care available in this environment, infants who previously would have perished from congenital disability, birth trauma, prematurity, or disease now survive, and most survive with very favorable outcomes. Audiologists and speech-language pathologists who provide services in the nursery should become familiar with their role and responsibility to the infants and their families, and to the other professionals in the NICU.

The birth of Baby Doe in 1982 provided the impetus for federal government involvement in the care of newborns with disabilities. Baby Doe was an infant with Down syndrome and a tracheoesophageal defect that was surgically correctable; without correction, the baby would die within a short period of time. After conferring with their physician, the parents decided not to permit surgery because of the baby's Down syndrome. The hospital brought action to overturn the parents' decision but the court as well as the Indiana Supreme Court ruled in favor of the parents' right-to-decide. Baby Doe died 6 days after birth. In response to the widespread publicity and public debate generated by the Baby Doe case, President Ronald Reagen requested development of federal regulations to address medical or surgical treatment of infants with disabilities. Ultimately, Congress passed the Child Abuse Amendments of 1984 which prohibit withholding of medically indicated treatment from infants and specifically proscribe discrimination in medical or surgical treatment on the basis of disability.

SUGGESTED READINGS

Guillemin, G. H., and Holmstrom, L. L. (1986). *Mixed Blessings: Intensive Care for Newborns*. New York: Oxford University Press. *A view of medical decision-making in the neonatal intensive care unit within the social context.*

Harrison, H. (1983). *The Premature Baby Book*. New York: St. Martin Press. *A parent's guide to coping with premature birth. This richly illustrated text includes basic medical information, and the most frequently encountered conditions and their treatment. Parents' experiences and reactions are woven throughout the text.*

CHAPTER 6

Disorders Affecting Newborns and Infants

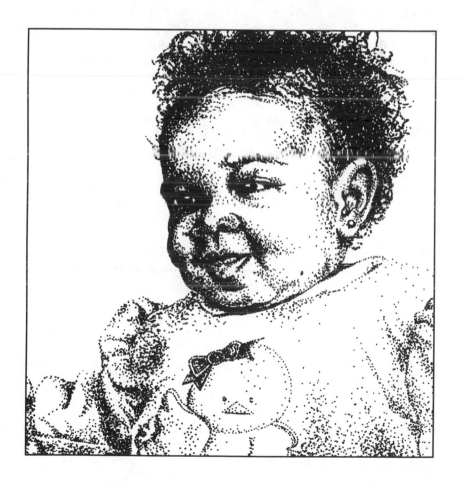

*T*he medical problems of babies in the neonatal intensive care unit (NICU) are often described by abbreviations resembling alphabet soup—NEC, BPD, RDS, MAS, SGA, VLBW, HMD, IVH, VSD, TOF, ASD, to name a few. To the audiologist or speech-language pathologist entering the NICU for the first time, this vocabulary is perplexing and unenlightening. These acronyms represent serious medical complications affecting the infant's respiratory, circulatory, central nervous, or other critical systems. Genetic defects, prematurity, birth trauma, or congenital malformations often result in serious or even life-threatening conditions.

ASSESSMENT OF NEWBORN INFANTS

All newborn infants receive multiple examinations shortly after birth. Typically, the first assessment is completed in the delivery room within moments of birth. During the initial hours of life, the infant receives a complete physical examination. In some instances, formal assessment of estimated gestational age is also made based on specific physical and neuromuscular characteristics.

Apgar Score

At birth, babies are rapidly assessed to detect obvious abnormalities and to determine the need for resuscitation. In 1953, Dr. Virginia Apgar, an anesthesiologist, developed a tool for evaluating an infant's condition in the delivery room. Evaluation is completed at 1 minute and again at 5 minutes, based on five standardized observations (heart rate, respiratory effort, reflex irritability, muscle tone, and color). A rating of 0 to 2 is assigned to each observation based on the scale summarized in Table 6–1. Maximum Apgar score attainable is 10.

The 1-minute evaluation provides a rapid method of determining the baby's initial adaptation to extrauterine life. As soon as delivery is complete (baby is completely delivered and umbilical cord is clamped), a timer is started so that the baby can be evaluated at precisely 1 minute. Infants with Apgar scores of seven or higher require only routine care and observation. Apgar scores between three and six indicate moderate cardio-respiratory depression. These babies will require some form of resuscitation and close observation for at least 24 hours. Infants with Apgar scores below three are severely depressed and will require ventilatory assistance and intensive care.

Table 6-1. The scoring system for initial assessment of newborn infants developed by Dr. Virginia Apgar (1953). The baby is assessed at 1 minute following birth to determine need for resuscitative efforts and again at 5 minutes following birth to evaluate response to resuscitative efforts.

	Score		
Observation	**0**	**1**	**2**
Heart rate	Absent	Slow (below 100)	Over 100
Respiratory effort	Absent; apnea	Slow, irregular, shallow, gasping	Sustained cry, regular respirations
Reflex irritability	No response	Grimace, frown	Sneeze, cry, active avoidance
Muscle Tone	Limp, flaccid	Some flexion of extremities	Active motion, good tone
Color	Cyanotic, pale	Body pink and extremities pale	Completely pink

Virginia Apgar, M.D., is considered one of the pioneers in neonatal assessment. The Apgar Score, a simple procedure to assess infants within minutes of birth, is used in modern hospitals throughout the world.

Although initially trained as a surgeon, Dr. Apgar became an obstetric anesthesiologist, one of the first women to practice this specialty. She reportedly developed the Apgar Score in 1949 in response to a lament from a medical student of the need for a standardized method to assess newborns. Apgar replied, "That's easy! You do it this way." She picked up the nearest piece of paper and jotted down the famous five-point criteria which became known as the Apgar Score. The Apgar Score was first published in 1953; for more than four decades it has provided the foundation of initial assessment of the newborn.

Virginia Apgar was a gifted medical school professor. She also enjoyed a distinguished career with the March of Dimes where she directed research into the causes, prevention, and treatment of birth defects. Dr. Apgar, who lived from 1909 to 1974, was recognized on a 20-cent definitive stamp issued by the U.S. Postal Service in October, 1994.

The 5-minute Apgar score permits re-evaluation of the infant's condition and assessment of the baby's response to resuscitative measures. Infants who score seven or less at five minutes are typically re-evaluated at 10 minutes.

Nursery-Based Physical Examination

Several hours following birth, the baby receives a complete physical examination by a nurse, pediatrician, or other health care practitioner. This examination permits assessment of the baby's adaptation to the stress of birth and extrauterine life and detection of any subtle abnormalities. The examination includes assessment of the baby's general appearance, vital signs, and measurements; detailed physical assessment (thorough examination of head, face and neck, chest, abdomen, genitalia, and upper and lower extremities); and assessment of neuromuscular integrity including neonatal reflexes.

Estimating Gestational Age

Both birthweight and gestational age are important determinants of the baby's general condition. Although gestational age can be estimated from the mother's last menstrual period, this calculation is often inaccurate and unreliable. Because certain physical and neuromuscular characteristics emerge in a predictable sequence during fetal development, these characteristics form the basis for an objective estimate of gestational age. Physical characteristics useful for estimating gestational age include skin appearance, presence of lanugo (fine hair present on the fetus which largely disappears by 40 weeks gestation), cartilage development in the ear, and appearance of the genitalia. Neuromuscular characteristics include resting posture and flexion and extension of the extremities. These features yield an estimate of gestational age which can be compared to birthweight to determine if the infant is small-for-gestational age (SGA), appropriate-for-gestational age (AGA), or large-for-gestational age (LGA).

DISORDERS AFFECTING PREMATURE AND NEWBORN INFANTS

Approximately 10% of newborns are at risk for medical problems and developmental disability. Although the risk status of some infants may be known prenatally, most infants at risk are detected either at birth, as reflected in low Apgar scores, or during the complete physical examination within a few hours of birth. Many of these babies receive initial care in the NICU.

Hearing loss is much more prevalent in infants who receive care in an NICU than in newborns who receive care in the normal newborn nursery. On the average, babies who receive care in an NICU exhibit hearing impairment 20 times more frequently than infants who receive care in a well-baby nursery (Simmons, 1980). Although the cause of hearing impairment among the normal newborn population remains largely unknown, hearing loss in infants in the NICU is often secondary to an identifiable disorder or treatment for that disorder.

Disorders of the Respiratory System

Babies are most often admitted to the NICU due to pulmonary immaturity and respiratory illness. The pulmonary and circulatory systems work in tandem to produce adequate oxygenation; both systems are involved when newborn infants develop respiratory dysfunction. Chapter 4 provides an overview of the development of the respiratory system and function of the fetal and extrauterine cardiorespiratory systems.

Respiratory Distress Syndrome (RDS)/ Hyaline Membrane Disease (HMD)

The terms respiratory distress syndrome (RDS) and hyaline membrane disease (HMD) are used interchangeably to describe the most common case of respiratory disease in premature infants.

Pathophysiology. As described in Chapter 4, a complex, coordinated cardiorespiratory response must occur at birth to change from a placenta-based to a lung-based gas exchange (oxygenation) system. Upon first breath, all infants must inflate their lungs and shunt blood flow into the lungs. Surfactant, a surface-tension reducing component produced in specific lung tissue, is essential to maintain lung expansion. Because the major period of differentiation of the lung cells that produce surfactant is between 24 and 34 weeks development, premature infants are especially vulnerable to RDS. Surfactant allows some air to remain in the lungs upon exhalation and thus prevents collapse of the alveoli. Subsequent breaths will require less effort than the first. In infants with inadequate surfactant production, all air will be expelled upon exhalation and the alveoli will collapse. Subsequent breaths will require as much effort as the first. During the early hours of life, the infant will become progressively fatigued with the effort of breathing. Over time, the baby will be unable to reinflate completely all alveoli with each breath. Oxygen/carbon dioxide gas exchange decreases. The infant works harder to obtain progressively less oxygen. Carbon dioxide in the bloodstream increases, and respiratory acidemia (shift in blood pH to an abnormally acid range) further impedes respiration. As the disease progresses, collapsed alveoli stick together (atelectasis), pulmonary cell death accelerates, and sloughed cells combine with fluid leaking from the capillaries to form thick hyaline membranes. These membranes further impede gas exchange in the lungs.

Treatment.   When premature birth is imminent, a mother may receive corticosteroids to accelerate lung maturation in the fetus. If birth can be delayed for days or even hours, severity of RDS may be lessened. After birth, treatment for RDS includes maintaining expanded lung volume, delivering oxygen through mechanical ventilation, and instilling a surfactant replacement. To sustain lung expansion, ventilators that supply continuous positive pressure are typically used (continuous positive airway pressure, CPAP, or positive end-expiratory pressure, PEEP). Artificial surfactant, usually extracted from bovine or sheep lung, is instilled through the ventilator. Infants are maintained on ventilatory support until they produce sufficient surfactant to sustain lung expansion and adequate gas exchange.

Complications of Disease or Treatment.   Infants with RDS may develop complications of the visual, respiratory, and central nervous systems. One of the first complications recognized in the treatment of premature infants with respiratory distress was retrolental fibroplasia or retinopathy of prematurity. ROP is a disorder of the retina which may result in blindness in premature infants. Although the pathophysiology of ROP is not completely understood, the association between prematurity, oxygen administration, and blindness was identified as early as the 1950s. ROP results in blindness in approximately 5% to 11% of infants with birthweights less 1500 grams.

Injury to the respiratory system is not uncommon. Delicate lung tissue may be injured by pressure created by mechanical ventilation and by oxygen toxicity. A cycle of injury-healing-reinjury of immature lung tissue results in chronic lung disease. Infants with chronic lung disease often require supplemental oxy-

Retinopathy of prematurity (ROP) is a disorder of premature infants in which scarring behind the lens leads to blindness. First described in 1942 as retrolental fibroplasia, ROP is one of the leading causes of childhood blindness. Prior to the development of high-oxygen concentration incubators in the mid-1940s, ROP was rarely observed. An epidemic of ROP developed during the mid- to late-1940s, however, and by 1953, approximately 10,000 children had been blinded by ROP. For more than a decade, various mechanisms underlying the development of ROP were proposed and debated. Although the precise etiology of ROP in premature infants is complex and not completely understood, an association between supplemental oxygen and ROP was demonstrated in the 1950s. Following this report, supplemental oxygen therapy for premature infants was curtailed and the number of cases of ROP fell dramatically until the early 1960s. At that time, clinicians recognized that, although oxygen curtailment reduced ROP in premature infants, increased infant deaths and neurologic damage in surviving premature infants were the result of oxygen deprivation. By the early 1980s, the number of infants with serious loss of vision due to ROP again increased, probably related to improved survival of very low birthweight infants. The ROP dilemma reveals the complex problems underlying care in the neonatal intensive care unit. Treatment needed to save lives may result in survival with lifelong disability.

gen during the early years of life. Other respiratory complications include pneumothorax, or air leakage from the lungs into surrounding chest cavity. Pneumothorax is a life-threatening complication because pressure within the chest cavity compromises lung excursion and cardiac output. Without emergency surgical relief of pressure, the infant will not survive.

The most serious central nervous system (CNS) complication is intracranial hemorrhage, or periventricular or intraventricular hemorrhage (P/IVH). P/IVH is classified by the severity of the bleed which can range from mild to severe. Infants with severe P/IVH typically exhibit serious neurodevelopmental delay.

Because infants with RDS receive treatment by invasive procedures such as intubation and suctioning, they are at increased risk of developing infection. Infants who become septic (generalized infection) are typically treated with antibiotics with potentially ototoxic properties.

Persistent Pulmonary Hypertension of the Newborn (PPHN)

PPHN results from complex cardiopulmonary dysfunction shortly after birth. It is diagnosed in infants who maintain a fetal pattern of blood circulation instead of converting to an extrauterine pattern of circulation. For this reason, PPHN is also termed persistent fetal circulation, or PFC. The critical differences between fetal and extrauterine circulation are described in Chapter 4.

Pathophysiology.   As outlined in Chapter 4, blood circulation in the fetus is markedly different than blood circulation after birth. In infants with PPHN, pulmonary vascular resistance remains high (pulmonary hypertension) after birth and blood does not shunt into the lungs. PPHN is diagnosed in infants who exhibit pulmonary hypertension, shunting of blood through the fetal cardiovascular channels (foramen ovale, ductus arteriosus, or both) away from the lungs, and a structurally normal heart. The syndrome may be without a known cause (idiopathic), or it may be secondary to other disorders such as RDS, congenital diaphragmatic hernia, sepsis, or meconium aspiration syndrome (MAS). Infants with PPHN experience inadequate oxygenation leading to diminished cardiac output and further decreased oxygenation. PPHN is a disorder of near-term or term infants.

Treatment.   Maintaining adequate oxygenation is the primary goal in caring for infants with PPHN. Treatment is directed at decreasing pulmonary resistance through mechanical ventilation and infusion of vasodilators. Within the past decade, extracorporeal membrane oxygenation (ECMO) was introduced as a treatment for PPHN. This treatment involves shunting the blood to an oxygenation circuit outside the body (extracorporeal). Babies are typically maintained on ECMO for durations less than 72 hours. More recently, an experimental protocol utilizing inhaled nitric oxide has been investigated at several institutions. This treatment may reduce morbidity associated with mechanical ventilation and ECMO.

Complications of Disease or Treatment.   Mortality from PPHN is high. Prior to ECMO, mortality rates as high as 80% were reported in infants with PPHN. Mortality rates in infants treated by ECMO range from 13% to 33%. For infants who survive, complications include those associated with mechanical ventilation such as chronic lung disease and pneumothorax. Infants treated with ECMO may also develop P/IVH, cerebral and generalized edema, and uncontrollable bleeding resulting in death. Because of the risk of P/IVH in infants treated with ECMO, premature infants who are already at risk for P/IVH typically are not candidates for ECMO therapy.

Meconium Aspiration Syndrome (MAS)

MAS is compromise of respiratory function secondary to obstruction of the respiratory tract and lung tissue by meconium, a blackish-green substance produced in the intestinal tract of fetuses.

Pathophysiology. Meconium is normally passed shortly after birth and represents the newborn infant's first bowel movement. Fetuses who experience hypoxia in utero may pass meconium prior to birth because decreased oxygen causes the anal sphincter to relax. With on going hypoxia, the fetus may perform gasping respiratory movements which suction meconium-stained amniotic fluid into the nose, mouth, and oropharynx. MAS results when deeply inspired meconium obstructs the respiratory tract and compromises gas-exchange in the lungs following birth. Because greatest quantities of meconium are produced in fetuses age 34 weeks and older, MAS is a disorder of term or near-term infants.

Treatment. To prevent MAS, the infant with meconium-stained amniotic fluid must be suctioned before first breath. Upon delivery of the infant's head, and before delivery of the body, the attending physician suctions the infant's nose, mouth, and oropharynx. Immediately after birth, the infant may be intubated, and meconium suctioned from below the vocal folds.

Despite aggressive suctioning, some infants will develop MAS. The principle pathology in MAS is mild to severe hypoxemia. These babies may require supplemental oxygen by hood, or more vigorous treatment with mechanical ventilation.

Complications of Disease or Treatment. PPHN is a frequent complication of MAS. Infants who require mechanical ventilation are susceptible to mechanical injury to the lung and oxygen toxicity resulting in chronic lung disease.

Bronchopulmonary Dysplasia (BPD)

In the late 1960s, investigators described chronic radiographic changes in lungs of infants who survived RDS/HMD. BPD is an iatrogenic disease, that is, it is an adverse condition resulting from medical treatment.

Pathophysiology.   The pulmonary changes observed in BPD reflect the cycle of injury/healing/reinjury of delicate lung tissue in infants who receive supplemental oxygen and/or mechanical ventilation. Infants with BPD exhibit decreased lung compliance, increased pulmonary resistance, and pulmonary edema.

Treatment.   Because BPD affects oxygen/carbon dioxide exchange in the lungs, infants with this disorder often require mechanical ventilation and supplemental oxygen for weeks or even months after birth.

Complications of the Disease or Treatment.   Infants with BPD are at risk for respiratory infections, emphysema, and pulmonary hypertension. To manage the complications associated with BPD, infants may receive diuretics and antibiotics with ototoxic properties.

Effects on Hearing of Respiratory Systems Disorders

Several important studies document an association between respiratory system disorders in premature and term newborns and sensorineural hearing loss.

In 1986, Nield, Schrier, Ramos, Platzker, and Warburton reported that 11 infants with RDS who demonstrated normal auditory brainstem responses (ABR) on discharge from the NICU were found to have sensorineural hearing loss at follow-up. All infants required prolonged mechanical ventilation and sustained chronic lung damage. All of the infants received treatment with gentamicin (an aminogylcoside antibiotic), and 10 of the 11 infants also received furosemide (a loop diuretic). Other frequent clinical complications included abnormal CNS findings during the NICU stay (10 infants), acidosis on initial blood gas (8 infants), and persistent fetal circulation (persistent pulmonary hypertension of the newborn, PPHN) in the 7 infants greater than 1,500 grams birthweight. Although the etiology of hearing loss in these 11 infants cannot be specifically identified, RDS and its treatment appear to place an infant at risk for hearing loss.

In 1985, Sell, Gaines, Gluckman, and Williams were among the first to report long-term neurodevelopmental outcome of infants with PPHN. In this investigation, more than 50% of infants demonstrated sensorineural hearing loss at follow-up. Naulty, Weiss, and Herer (1986) and Hendricks-Munoz and Walton (1988) documented increased risk for hearing loss in infants with PPHN and also reported risk for progressive loss in these babies.

In 1991, Walton and Hendricks-Munoz reported on follow-up of 51 infants with PPHN. Nineteen of the 51 infants (37%) were diagnosed with sensorineural hearing loss; 16 with bilateral and 3 with unilateral loss. Five infants demonstrated progressive losses with hearing worsening an average of 55 dB at 2000 to 4000 Hz. In general, the hearing loss was downward sloping and ranged from mild to severe.

In addition to sensorineural hearing loss, infants with PPHN who are treated with ECMO may demonstrate abnormal auditory brainstem responses (ABR) with prolonged interpeak latencies. Schumacher, Spak, and Kileny (1990) reported abnormally prolonged wave I to V interpeak latencies in 10 of 23 infants treated by ECMO. On follow-up at age 4 to 12 months, six infants demonstrated additional neurologic abnormalities. The authors speculate that prolonged wave I to V interpeak latencies in this population prognosticate future neurologic abnormalities.

Conservative management of infants with PPHN may reduce prevalence of neurologic abnormalities and sensorineural hearing loss. Marron et al. (1992) evaluated neurologic status, hearing loss, and intelligence in 27 children who were diagnosed with severe PPHN at birth and received conservative medical management (treated without paralysis or hyperventilation). Children were tested between 10 months and 6 years of age; children who were younger than 1 year of age at the initial hearing test were retested after they reached 2 years of age. The average intelligence quotient in the 27 children was within the normal range. Four children demonstrated severe neurologic abnormalities, three of them had been severely asphyxiated at birth. An additional five children demonstrated mild neurologic abnormalities. No children were diagnosed with sensorineural hearing loss.

Disorders of the Cardiovascular System

Congenital heart disease (CHD) is among the most common birth defects affecting as many as 1 in 100 newborns. Some conditions are benign and require no intervention; other conditions are life-threatening and require immediate surgical treatment. In some centers, complex surgical procedures, including heart transplantation, are performed on newborn infants.

Figure 6–1 shows a schematic diagram of a normal adult heart including the major arteries, veins, and valves associated with normal heart anatomy and physiology. The heart is a double pump. The right side of the heart receives blood returning from

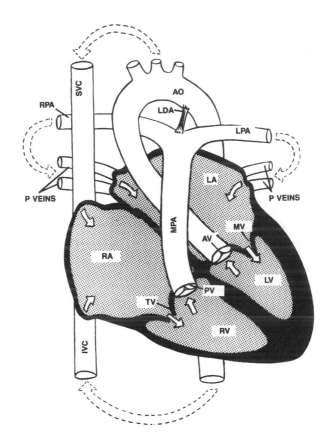

The normal heart.

AO	Aorta	MV	Mitral valve
AV	Aortic valve	PV	Pulmonary valve
IVC	Inferior vena cava	P VEIN	Pulmonary vein
LA	Left atrium	RA	Right atrium
LDA	Ligamentum ductus arteriosus	RPA	Right pulmonary artery
LPA	Left pulmonary artery	RV	Right ventricle
LV	Left ventricle	SVC	Superior vena cava
MPA	Main pulmonary artery	TV	Tricuspid valve

FIGURE 6–1. Schematic diagram of a normal adult heart including the major arteries, veins, and valves associated with normal heart anatomy and physiology. The heart is a double pump. The right side of the heart receives blood returning from the head and body via the superior and inferior vena cavae into the right atrium. This poorly oxygenated blood enters the right ventricle through the tricuspid valve. From the right ventricle, it is pumped through the main, right, and left pulmonary arteries into the lungs. The left atrium receives the now well-oxygenated blood from the lungs through the pulmonary veins. This blood enters the left ventricle through the mitral valve. From the left ventricle, it is pumped through the aortic valve into the aorta for distribution to all parts of the body. (Courtesy of Ross Laboratories, Clinical Education Aid.)

the head and body via the superior and inferior vena cavae into the right atrium. This poorly oxygenated blood enters the right ventricle through the tricuspid valve. From the right ventricle, it is pumped through the main, right, and left pulmonary arteries into the lungs. The left atrium receives the now well-oxygenated blood from the lungs through the pulmonary veins. This blood enters the left ventricle through the mitral valve. From the left ventricle, it is pumped through the aortic valve into the aorta for distribution to all parts of the body.

The heart develops during the first 7 weeks following fertilization. During this critical period, major CHD can arise from genetic and chromosomal abnormalities, infection, exposure to teratogens, or maternal metabolic or nutritional factors. Approximately 85% to 90% of congenital heart disease is assumed to result from an interaction of genetic and environmental factors (multifactorial; see Chapter 3); 10% to 12% is associated with specific chromosomal anomalies (e.g., trisomy 18, trisomy 21); 1% to 2% is identified with known environmental factors (e.g., congenital rubella syndrome, maternal alcohol consumption).

Newborns with severe CHD may exhibit cyanosis, respiratory distress, and/or congestive heart failure and decreased cardiac output. Cyanosis is a characteristic bluish discoloration of the skin, nail beds, and mucous membranes which results from generalized poor oxygenation. Respiratory distress may occur because of the CHD or as a result of primary pulmonary disease and CHD. Congestive heart failure is a clinical syndrome signaling inability of the heart to meet the metabolic needs of the body. Signs of congestive heart failure include enlarged heart, increased heart rate, generalized malaise, fluid retention and edema, and failure to thrive and feeding problems.

CHDs often encountered in the NICU include ventricular septal defect, atrial septal defect, patent ductus arteriosus, coarctation of the aorta, tetralogy of Fallot, and hypoplastic left heart syndrome.

Ventricular Septal Defect (VSD)

VSD is an opening or defect in the wall separating the right and left ventricles. It is the most common congenital heart malformation. VSD is shown in Figure 6–2.

Pathophysiology. A VSD can occur anywhere in the membranous or muscular septum separating the ventricles. VSD may occur in isolation or in combination with other congenital heart

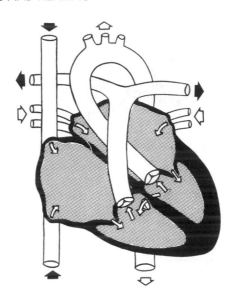

Ventricular septal defect.

An abnormal opening exists between the right and left ventricles. Ventricular septal defects can occur anywhere in the ventricular septum, but most commonly involve its membranous portion. Occasionally, more than one defect is present. Because the pressure is higher in the left ventricle than in the right and the systemic vascular resistance is greater than the pulmonary vascular resistance, blood shunts from left to right through the defect. Size of the defect is more important than its location. The clinical and laboratory features, treatment, and natural history vary with the size of the defect. The defects are classified as small and large.

FIGURE 6–2. Ventricular septal defect, an abnormal opening between the right and left ventricles of the heart. (Courtesy of Ross Laboratories, Clinical Education Aid.)

malformations. Infants with VSD demonstrate abnormal movement of blood between the left and right ventricles (left-to-right shunting).

Treatment. Approximately 50% to 75% of small VSDs close without surgical intervention. Larger VSDs require surgical intervention to repair the defect.

Complications of Disease or Treatment.   Mortality from VSD is less than 5%. Mortality is highest in premature newborns and in infants with multiple heart defects.

Atrial Septal Defect (ASD)

Similar to a VSD, an ASD is an opening or defect in the septum between the right and left atria. Figure 6–3 shows an ASD.

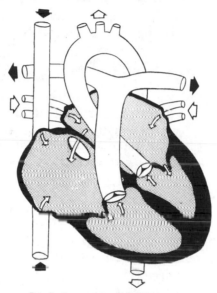

Atrial septal defect.

A hole in the atrial septum permits blood to flow between the atria. Before birth, blood flows from the right to the left atrium through the foramen ovale. This trapdoor-like opening in the septum normally closes after birth when left-atrial pressure exceeds right-atrial pressure. The foramen ovale then gradually undergoes anatomic fusion in infancy. However, if the foramen ovale retains its patency instead of becoming anatomically fused and is subsequently subjected to tension, it may gap open, permitting a right-to-left shunt. Likewise, if the left atrium dilates because of a large blood flow, the foramen ovale may be stretched, permitting a left-to-right shunt.

FIGURE 6–3.   Atrial septal defect, an abnormal opening between the right and left atria of the heart. (Courtesy of Ross Laboratories, Clinical Education Aid.)

Pathophysiology.   An ASD results in exchange of blood between the right and left atria. Because the right atrium is more compliant than the left atrium, left-to-right shunting also occurs in ASD.

Treatment.   ASDs spontaneously close in approximately 40% of children by age 5 years. Management of ASD includes prevention of congestive heart failure and surgical correction, if necessary, at age 2 to 5 years.

Complications of Disease or Treatment.   Mortality rate of surgery for ASDs is less than 1%. Mortality is highest for premature newborns who develop congestive heart failure.

Patent Ductus Arteriosus (PDA)

The ductus arteriosus is a normal pathway in the fetal circulatory system between the pulmonary artery and the descending aorta. Figure 6–4 shows a patent ductus arteriosus (PDA). At birth, the ductus constricts and completely closes within hours or days. Failure of the ductus to close results in PDA.

Pathophysiology.   The ductus arteriosus permits blood in the fetal pattern of circulation to shunt from the right ventricle through the pulmonary artery into the descending aorta, effectively bypassing the lungs. This pathway closes shortly after birth in response to increased arterial oxygen concentration and other metabolic factors. In preterm infants, the ductus does not respond to increased oxygen concentration as readily as in term infants and the ductus remains patent. PDA causes blood to shunt from the aorta into the pulmonary artery (left-to-right) and may result in enlargement of the heart and congestive heart failure.

Treatment.   Infants with PDA may be asymptomatic and require only close monitoring for evidence of progressive cardiac disease. Infants with evidence of congestive heart failure may receive medical or surgical management. Medical management involves inducing the PDA to close through intravenous medication in infants less than 7 days of age. Surgical closure is required for infants who fail to close with medical management. A newer method of closure involves placement of a small occluding device during cardiac catheterization.

Complications of Disease or Treatment.   The mortality rate following treatment for PDA is low, less than 2% in preterm infants

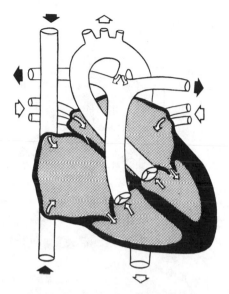

Patent ductus arteriosus.

Vascular communication persists that short-circuits the pulmonary vascular bed and directs blood from the pulmonary artery to the aorta during fetal life. Functional closure of the ductus normally occurs soon after birth. If the ductus remains patent after birth, the direction of flow through the ductus is the opposite of that in the fetus, passing instead from the aorta into the pulmonary artery.

FIGURE 6–4. Patent ductus arteriosus, the abnormal persistence of a fetal vascular communication after birth. (Courtesy of Ross Laboratories, Clinical Education Aid.)

and less than 1% in term infants. Mortality rate is highest in very small preterm babies. For infants without other significant conditions, the prognosis is excellent.

Coarctation of the Aorta (COA)

Coarctation is a narrowing or localized constriction of the aorta that most commonly occurs in the vicinity of the ductus arteriosus. The constriction may occur in isolation or in combination with other cardiac defects such as PDA, VSD, and an abnormal aortic valve. COA is shown in Figure 6–5.

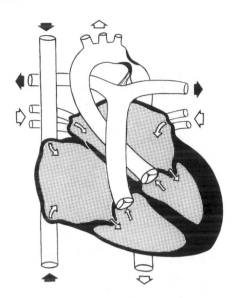

Coarctation of the aorta.

It consists of a narrowed aortic lumen, usually at the entrance of the ductus arteriosus. A long, narrowed area (hypoplastic segment) may be located proximally to the coarctation and co-exists with additional intracardiac defects. A bicuspid aortic valve coexists in at least half of patients. The constricted segment of the aorta obstructs blood flow, causing a difference in pressure across the segment. The elevation of pressure that occurs proximally increases left-ventricular systolic pressure, which is accom-panied by hypertrophy and, in symptomatic infants, dilation.

FIGURE 6–5. Coarctation of the aorta, a narrow-ing of the aorta in the region of the ductus arte-riosus. (Courtesy of Ross Laboratories, Clinical Education Aid.)

Pathophysiology. Because COA causes obstruction to blood flow, pressure is elevated in the portion of the aorta between the heart and the obstruction. This leads to increased pressure in the left ventricle and ventricular hypertrophy. In severe cases, babies exhibit symptoms of cyanosis, congestive heart failure and low cardiac output.

Treatment. Surgical correction or interventional cardiac catheterization to reduce the obstruction may be required for

COA. Interventional cardiac catheterization involves threading a balloon catheter through an artery to the site of the COA. Inflation of the balloon expands the constriction and permits normal blood flow through the previously constricted site. Intervention is required if medical management fails to prevent congestive heart failure.

Complications of Disease or Treatment.   If surgical repair of COA must be attempted in early infancy because of unmanageable congestive heart failure, mortality rates exceeding 30% have been reported. Newborns who receive cardiac catheretization may require recatheretization or surgical correction if the COA reoccurs.

Tetralogy of Fallot (TOF)

TOF is a complex cardiac disorder characterized by four anomalies: (a) a large VSD, (b) pulmonary artery stenosis or other obstruction to blood flow out of the right ventricle, (c) an enlarged aorta, and (d) hypertrophied right ventricle. TOF is shown in Figure 6–6.

Pathophysiology.   Large VSD and obstruction of blood outflow from the right ventricle decrease blood flow to the lungs. Cyanosis develops from poor generalized oxygenation.

Treatment.   Surgical repair of TOF is not typically recommended in the neonatal period. Surgery is usually delayed until the infant is age 6 months or older to permit growth of the pulmonary arteries. Surgical treatment includes repair of the VSD and reduction in the right ventricular outflow obstruction.

Complications of Disease or Treatment.   Mortality rate from TOF varies with the severity of the disorder and its effect on circulation. Mortality rate is 5% to 10% in the first 2 postoperative years for uncomplicated TOFs and higher for infants with more severe anomalies.

Hypoplastic Left Heart Syndrome (HLHS)

HLHS is a constellation of cardiac defects including severe coarctation of the aorta, stenosis or atresia of the aortic and mitral valve, and a small left atrium and ventricle.

Pathophysiology.   In infants with HLHS, blood outflow from the left ventricle, the main pump supplying blood to the head and

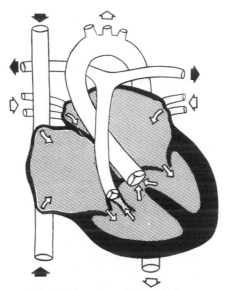

Tetralogy of Fallot.

Four conditions are present: pulmonary stenosis, ventricular septal defect, overriding aorta,
and hypertrophy of the right ventricle. The
obstruction can be located in the outflow area
(infundibulum) of the right ventricle or at the pulmonary valve or valve ring. Or the pulmonary
arteries may be reduced in caliber. A combination of these obstructions is usually present.
The ventricular defect is usually large, causing
equalization of pressure between the ventricles. Because of the obstruction to blood flow
from the right ventricle into the pulmonary
artery, unsaturated blood flows through the ventricular septal defect into the aorta.

FIGURE 6–6. Tetralogy of Fallot, a complex of
congenital heart defects. (Courtesy of Ross
Laboratories, Clinical Education Aid.)

body, is severely restricted or eliminated altogether. In the presence of a PDA, blood shunts from the pulmonary artery into the
aorta, bypassing the lungs. Infants with HLHS rapidly develop
metabolic acidosis and circulatory shock.

Treatment.   HLHS is usually considered a lethal lesion. A multistage surgical procedure, the Norwood procedure, is performed
in some centers but mortality rates remain high. Infants with

HLHS may be candidates for heart transplantation if they can survive until a suitable donor is identified.

Complications of Disease or Treatment. Without surgery, mortality from HLHS is 100% within days or weeks of birth. Mortality rates of 75% are reported with the first stage of the Norwood procedure and 50% with the second stage. Heart transplantation may provide the only chance for survival.

Effects on Hearing of CHD

Although there is no reported association between hearing impairment and isolated CHD, hearing loss is often present in infants with CHD and other congenital anomalies. Several syndromes have been identified which include cardiac and auditory dysfunction. CHARGE association includes a characteristic constellation of disorders: coloboma (defect in the retina); heart defects including TOF, PDA, VSD, ASD, or other heart anomalies; choanal atresia (obstruction of the bony passage of the nose); growth deficiency; mental retardation; external ear anomalies; and hearing loss. Hearing impairment is frequently moderate to severe and includes conductive and sensorineural components, both of which may be progressive (Thelin, Mitchell, Hefner, and Davenport, 1986).

Jervell and Lange-Nielsen syndrome affects a small percentage of individuals with congenital deafness. Although individuals with this disorder have no structural abnormality of the heart, they exhibit electrocardiac abnormalities with associated fainting spells which may result in sudden unexplained death in childhood. Because there are no other distinguishing characteristics of Jervell and Lange-Nielsen syndrome, it is often misdiagnosed and improperly treated. Further information about this syndrome is presented in Chapter 3.

Among chromosomal disorders, CHD and hearing loss are frequent findings in infants with trisomies. Approximately 40% of babies with Down syndrome, for example, will experience some form of congenital heart anomaly, typically VSD, PDA, or ASD. Hearing loss is very common in infants with Down syndrome. CHD also frequently occurs in infants with trisomy 13 and trisomy 18. Most babies with trisomy 13 and trisomy 18 also exhibit sensorineural and/or conductive hearing loss. More than 95% of infants with trisomy 13 and trisomy 18 die in early infancy.

CHD is a frequent finding in infants with congenital rubella syndrome (CRS). Fortunately, a successful vaccination program has virtually eliminated rubella in the United States although CRS may frequently be encountered in countries where a widespread vaccination program is not available.

Medical management of CHD may include use of ototoxic medications (loop diuretics and/or aminoglycoside antibiotics). Loop diuretics may be used to reduce stress on the heart associated with fluid overload; aminoglycoside antibiotics may be given at the first sign of infection. Hearing impairment is significantly associated with combined loop diuretic and aminoglycoside therapy in premature and low birthweight infants. Salamy, Eldredge, and Tooley (1989), for example, reported that, in very low birthweight infants, sensorineural hearing loss was statistically associated with greater amounts of furosemide administration for longer durations and in combination with aminoglycoside antibiotics. It is important to consider the effects of both the infant's underlying condition and the treatment for that condition as potential etiologies in sensorineural hearing loss.

Disorders of the Central Nervous System (CNS)

The CNS is vulnerable to genetic and teratogenic disorders, as well as to iatrogenic effects secondary to treatment for respiratory, cardiovascular, infectious, and metabolic dysfunction. The CNS is one of the first major organ systems to initiate development in the embryo, and functional development continues through the early years of childhood. Because the brain controls all other organ systems and is responsible for all learning, CNS disorders and their related neurologic effects are among the most feared complications of prematurity and neonatal disease.

Anencephaly

Anencephaly is lack of development of the brain and cranium. Anencephalic infants have no normal brain tissue above the brainstem. This neural tube defect occurs in approximately 1 in 1,000 births.

Pathophysiology.   Anencephaly is a neural tube defect that occurs when the neural tube fails to close in the cranial area. It arises from genetic, environmental, or genetic-environmental interactions before day 24 or 25 of development (see Chapter 4). The neural tube closes at the cranial end of the embryo at about day 24 to 25 after fertilization; the disruption resulting in anencephaly must occur prior to this time.

Treatment. Anencephaly is incompatible with independent life. Many infants with anencephaly are stillborn and those who are born alive die shortly after birth. Recently, two ethical issues have arisen in medical treatment of infants with anencephaly. In the first, the suitability of maintaining an infant with anencephaly on life support to permit use of her normally developed organs for transplantation created substantial ethical debate. In the second, parental demands to maintain life through artificial means in an infant with anencephaly generated an equally perplexing ethical dilemma.

Spina Bifida

Spina bifida is a neural tube defect of the spinal cord and vertebrae. Spina bifida refers to defects in the caudal region of the neural tube with the majority of defects in the lumbar region of the spine. The most common form of spina bifida occurs in about 1 in 500 births.

Pathophysiology. Fusion of the neural tube occurs from the middle to both the cranial and caudal ends of the developing embryo (see Chapter 4). Closure in the lumbar region, the last area of fusion, occurs at about day 26 or 27. Figure 6–7 shows the normal relationship of the spinal cord within the vertebral column, and the two principal forms of spina bifida, meningocele and meningomyelocele. The normal spinal cord (A) is enclosed in the bony segments of the spine, the vertebra. In infants with meningocele (B), an outpocketing of meninges (tissue covering of the brain and spinal cord) and cerebrospinal fluid (CSF) extrudes into a sac outside the spinal column; the spinal cord and its associated nerve roots are in their normal anatomical position. In infants with meningomyelocele (C), the most common form of spina bifida, an outpocketing of meninges, CSF, spinal cord, and nerve roots extrudes into a sac outside the spinal column. A third form of spina bifida, myeloschisis, is a defect in which a portion of the spinal cord is exposed with no covering. In severe cases, the entire length of the spinal cord is exposed; the infant may also be anencephalic.

Treatment. Prompt surgical closure of the defect is the treatment of choice for most infants with spina bifida. Surgical closure typically is performed within the first 24 hours of life with severe defects requiring multiple, staged procedures.

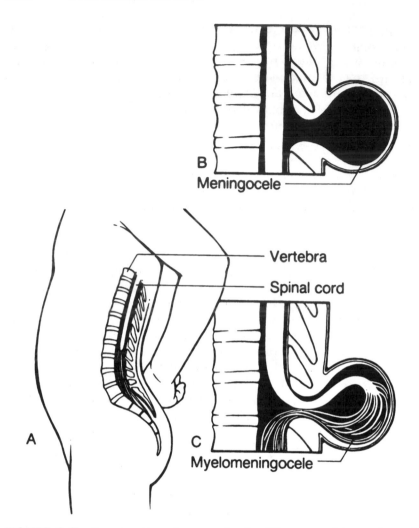

FIGURE 6-7. Cross section of a normal spine (A) compared to meningocele (B) and myelomeningocele (C). (From *Maternal and Neonatal Nursing—Family-Centered Care*, Third Edition, by K. A. May and L. R. Mahlmuster, 1994, p. 1059. Baltimore, MD: J. B. Lippincott Publishing Company. Copyright 1994 by J. B. Lippincott Publishing Company. Reprinted with permission.)

Complications of Disease or Treatment. With surgical intervention, more than 90% of infants with meningomyelocele without other life-threatening complications survive the neonatal period. Disability associated with spina bifida may range from minor malformations with no clinical significance to major anomalies with resulting para- or quadriplegia and bladder and bowel dysfunction. Some infants with spina bifida exhibit additional neural anomalies involving the medulla, fourth ventricle, and lower cerebellum. This defect, Arnold-Chiari malformation, may result in abnormal auditory brainstem response (ABR) studies on the basis of neural conduction abnormality.

Intracranial Hemorrhage

Spontaneous, uncontrolled bleeding in the brain or within the skull is termed intracranial hemorrhage. In newborns, the most common sites of intracranial bleeds are into the ventricles (intraventricular hemorrhage, IVH) or in the area around the ventricles (periventricular hemorrhage, PVH).

Pathophysiology. P/IVH is primarily a condition of premature infants and represents the most common and serious neurologic disorder of preterm babies. It is estimated that intracranial hemorrhage occurs in as many as 25% of infants weighing less than 1,500 grams, or babies born at 32 weeks or younger. Premature and low birthweight infants are at risk for intracranial bleeding because of complex anatomical and physiologic processes occurring in this stage of fetal development.

P/IVHs are categorized on the basis of location and severity of the bleed. Four categories of bleeds are recognized, grade I through grade IV. Grade I hemorrhage represents the least severe bleed. In grade I hemorrhage, bleeding is limited to the subependymal germinal matrix, an area which is transitionally present in the fetus but disappears by term. Grade IV is the most severe bleed. In a grade IV hemorrhage, bleeding occurs into the subependymal germinal matrix, lateral ventricles, and brain tissue. The ventricles dilate and blood spreads throughout the ventricular system. Neurologic outcome of infants with intracranial bleeds appears correlated with severity of the bleed; infants with grade I or II bleed have a better prognosis for normal outcome than infants with grade IV bleeds.

Treatment. There is no direct medical or surgical intervention for infants with P/IVH. Infants receive supportive management and ongoing assessment to detect ventricular dilation and hydrocephalus. Progressive hydrocephalus secondary to P/IVH may require shunt placement.

Complications of Disease or Treatment. Complications from P/IVH are related to the underlying cause of the bleed and its severity. Very sick or premature newborns with severe intracranial bleeding have more pronounced neurologic or developmental sequelae than healthier infants with a milder degree of bleeding. The most common complication of P/IVH is posthemorrhagic hydrocephalus.

Hydrocephalus

Hydrocephalus is alteration in circulation or production of CSF and results in head enlargement. It may be congenital, occurring in 3 to 4 in 1,000 live births, or acquired shortly after birth.

Pathophysiology. Hydrocephalus develops in infants before birth due to obstruction either within the ventricular system (aqueductal stenosis resulting in noncommunicating hydrocephalus) or external to the ventricles (communicating hydrocephalus). Figure 6–8 shows the brain/CSF relationship in an infant with hydrocephalus. As shown in the figure, if left untreated, infants with hydrocephalus will develop significant enlargement of the ventricles and corresponding compression of the cortex. Eventually, skull size will enlarge.

Treatment. Treatment for hydrocephalus includes identification of the underlying cause and relief of CSF pressure. Infants

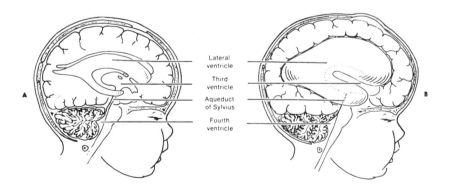

Lateral ventricle

Third ventricle

Aqueduct of Sylvius

Fourth ventricle

FIGURE 6–8. Hydrocephalus, a block in the flow of CSF. Patent cerebrospinal fluid circulation (A); enlarged lateral and third ventricle caused by obstruction of CSF circulation—stenosis of the aqueduct of Sylvius. (From *Whaley and Wong's Essentials of Pediatric Nursing*, Fourth Edition, by D. L. Wong, 1993, p. 976. St. Louis, MO: Mosby Publishing Company. Copyright 1993 by Mosby Publishing Company. Reprinted with permission.)

with uncomplicated hydrocephalus that spontaneously arrests may not require surgery to drain excess CSF. The most common surgical treatment for hydrocephalus in infants, the ventriculoperitoneal (VP) shunt, is shown in Figure 6–9. One end of a radiopaque catheter is placed in the lateral ventricle and the other end into the peritoneal cavity. A one-way valve, palpable under the skin near the ear, allows CSF to flow out of the ventricles into the peritoneal cavity. A VP shunt requires multiple revisions during childhood to account for growth.

Complications of Disease or Treatment. The prognosis of infants with hydrocephalus depends on the underlying cause of the disease. Infants with hydrocephalus secondary to congenital malformations, grade III or IV P/IVH, or meningitis are at highest risk for developmental and neurological complications. In contrast, infants with an isolated defect of the ventricular aqueduct and infants whose hydrocephalus arrests spontaneously have a good prognosis.

Hypoxic Encephalopathy

Hypoxic encephalopathy is injury to the brain secondary to both decreased oxygenation of the blood and decreased blood flow to the brain.

Pathophysiology. In the absence of adequate oxygenation, the entire cortex of the brain may become edematous (swollen with excess fluids). Further damage to the developing brain then results from compression of the cortex against the skull. Permanent cerebral injury can occur. In premature infants, hypoxic encephalopathy is often associated with intracranial bleeds; in term infants is often associated with perinatal asphyxia. It is estimated that moderate to severe postasphyxial encephalopathy is seen in 1 in 1,000 births.

Treatment. There is no direct treatment for hypoxic encephalopathy. Close monitoring for ventricular dilation and development of hydrocephalus is important to detect other neuropathologic changes.

Complications of Disease or Treatment. Prognosis for normal recovery and development depends on the extent and severity of the hypoxic injury. Sequelae of hypoxic encephalopathy may include mental retardation, microcephaly, cortical blindness, and cerebral palsy.

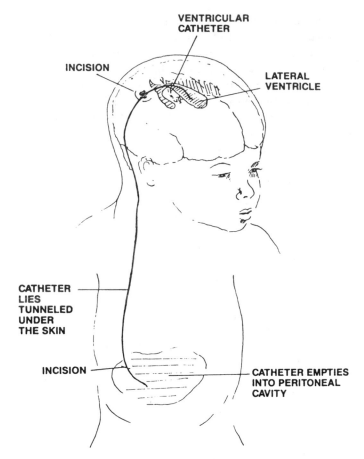

FIGURE 6–9. A ventriculo-peritoneal (VP) shunt. A catheter is inserted under the scalp into the lateral ventricle; it is connected to a long tubing that empties into the peritoneal (abdominal) cavity. (From *Shunts*, by the American Brain Tumor Association, 1994. Des Plaines, IL. Copyright 1994 by the American Brain Tumor Association. Reprinted with permission.)

Neonatal Seizures

Seizures are excessive, synchronous, electrical discharges within the brain. The behavioral manifestations of seizures are inappropriate, involuntary, and uncontrolled movement or muscle contraction and brief absence (lack of awareness) or brief or sustained loss of consciousness.

Pathophysiology. Seizures are not a disease but rather a clinical manifestation of an underlying pathologic process. Seizures in newborn infants are associated with primary CNS disorders, asphyxia, systemic diseases, and metabolic effects. Most neonatal seizures are acute; seizure activity disappears within the first few weeks after birth. Seizures occur in less than 1% of all newborns but in as many as 25% of unstable premature infants.

The exact mechanism underlying neonatal seizures is un-known. Seizures in newborns are different than seizures in older children and adults due to immaturity of brain organization. Newborns do not sustain generalized seizures but rather demonstrate more subtle signs of seizure activity. Because clinical manifestations may be subtle, seizures can be difficult to diagnosis in newborn babies.

Treatment. Phenobarbital or other antiepileptic drugs are used to control acute seizures in newborns. Long-term management involves identification and treatment of the underlying pathologic process.

Complications of Disease or Treatment. Because neonatal seizures typically indicate insult to the vulnerable developing brain, long-term neurologic or developmental effects from the condition precipitating the seizures are not uncommon. Infants with seizures secondary to birth asphyxia, grade III or IV P/IVH, CNS malformation, and some viral and bacterial infections have the poorest prognosis for normal recovery.

Effects on Hearing of CNS Dysfunction

Any primary disorder that results in hypoxia may affect an infant's hearing and neurologic status. Neurologic dysfunction per se does not result in hearing impairment but may substantially affect central auditory processing, speech, and language development. Infants with neurologic dysfunction in the newborn period should be monitored closely for neurodevelopmental effects.

Congenital Infections

The impressive, damaging effects of congenital infections on the developing fetus were first described more than 50 years ago. In 1941, N. McAllister Gregg, an ophthalmologist in Australia, recognized the association between congenital cataracts in infants and maternal rubella. His pioneering observation initiated investigation into the potential teratogenicity of fetal exposure to maternal infection.

Although the fetus develops within the normally protected environment of the womb, specific microbes can cross the placental membranes and infect the fetus. Infections acquired transplacentally during the first trimester of pregnancy are especially damaging. Because organ systems are undergoing rapid differentiation and growth, infection during this period results in major congenital anomalies and multisystem disease.

Congenital Rubella Syndrome (CRS)

Rubella, also called German measles, is a viral infection that results in a mild flu-like illness. Rubella was first isolated in 1962 in monkey kidney and human amnion cell cultures. The rubella virus has a world-wide distribution; prior to the introduction of the rubella vaccine, epidemics generally occurred in spring and early summer months in countries with temperate climates.

Pathophysiology. Transmission of rubella virus occurs from close contact with infected individuals. Characteristic features of primary rubella infection in adults are rash, malaise, swollen lymph nodes, and joint pain. As many as 10% of cases may be asymptomatic. For this reason, primary rubella infection in a pregnant woman may be undetected. If a primary maternal infection occurs during the first trimester of pregnancy and the virus crosses the placenta, the fetus may develop generalized infection and multi-organ system disease. Spontaneous abortion occurs in as many as 20% of cases when maternal rubella occurs in the first 8 weeks of pregnancy. In fetuses exposed during the first trimester who survive, the reported incidence of congenital anomalies ranges up to 54%; the incidence of congenital anomalies in fetuses exposed between 13 and 16 weeks gestation is approximately 17%. For fetuses exposed after 16 weeks gestation, risk of congenital anomaly is low. The only abnormalities reported in infants infected after the first trimester are deafness and retinopathy.

Infants who are born infected characteristically exhibit lethargy, petechiae (small subdermal hemorrhages; "blueberry muffin" rash), intrauterine growth retardation (IUGR), and enlarged liver and spleen (hepatosplenomegaly). Cultures for rubella virus may remain positive in infants up to age 1 year, and rubella virus has been recovered from intracellular tissue of children with congenital infections up to age 3 years. Congenital rubella infection is a chronic disease and may result in progressive disability.

Treatment. Prevention of maternal infection is the most effective treatment for CRS. In the United States, CRS has been virtually eliminated as a major cause of birth defects because of successful vaccination programs initiated in the late 1960s and early 1970s.

Complications of Disease or Treatment. The characteristic features of CRS are cardiac defects, congenital cataracts, and deafness, and other features include mental retardation, glaucoma, and microphthalmia. During the last large-scale rubella epidemic in the United States in 1964, an estimated 10,000 to 20,000 infants were born with hearing loss secondary to CRS.

Cytomegalovirus (CMV)

CMV is a member of the herpes family of viruses which includes herpes simplex, Epstein-Barr, and varicella (chickenpox) virus. CMV is endemic throughout the world. Like other herpes viruses, exposure to CMV results in a primary infection which then becomes dormant for extended periods of time. Reinfection results in recurrence of CMV. It is the most common viral infection in the human fetus. The incidence of congenital CMV infection is reported to range from 0.3% to 3% of live births. If 1% of all babies born in the United States are infected, then as many as 40,000 infants with congenital CMV infection are born in this country each year (Raynor, 1993).

Pathophysiology. CMV is not highly contagious. Transmission occurs through direct contact with infected secretions (urine, blood, semen, vaginal secretions, breast milk, and other bodily fluids). Because CMV is ubiquitous, most people acquire CMV infection at some time in their lives. Although adults with both primary and recurrent CMV infections are usually asymptomatic, some individuals may experience a mild flu-like illness. Primary CMV infection in a pregnant woman results in congenital CMV infection in the infant in about 30% to 40% of cases. Much less frequently, recurrent infection in the mother results in congenital infection in the fetus. Unlike rubella, infection by CMV in any stage of gestation may result in damage to the fetus.

As many as 90% to 95% of infants with congenital CMV infection are asymptomatic at birth. Although most of these infants develop normally with no developmental deficits attributable to their infection, about 5% to 10% of these normal newborns will be identified with sensorineural hearing impairment which is often progressive.

Approximately 10% of infants infected from primary maternal disease are symptomatic at birth. These babies demonstrate characteristics similar to those seen in CRS including IUGR, microcephaly, congenital cataracts, hepatosplenomegaly, and petechiae.

Treatment.   There is no treatment for congenital CMV. Although congenital infection can be detected at birth through urine, saliva, or blood cultures, screening for congenital CMV infection is not routinely performed.

Complications from Disease or Treatment.   Figure 6–10 compares outcome of congenital CMV infection in infants infected from primary (panel A) versus recurrent (panel B) maternal infection. Primary maternal disease is more devastating; congenital CMV infection occurs in 30% to 40% of infants born to mothers with primary disease. Approximately 15% of these infants will by symptomatic at birth; of these, as many as 30% will die. Ninety percent of survivors will exhibit neurodevelopmental deficits including deafness, microcephaly, mental retardation, cerebral palsy, and chorioretinitis. The remaining 85% to 90% of infants with congenital CMV acquired during primary maternal disease will be asymptomatic at birth, but as many as 15% of these infants will develop neurodevelopmental deficits.

Infants born to mothers with recurrent disease (Figure 6–10, panel B) are much less likely to be infected. Only about 1% of recurrent maternal disease results in congenital CMV infection, and 10% or less of infected infants demonstrate neurodevelopmental sequelae.

Studies have shown that congenital CMV may result in progressive hearing loss in infants; recent research suggests that the hearing impairment may first appear after the newborn period. Identification of hearing loss in asymptomatic infected infants may be delayed because these babies will not be recognized as at risk for progressive hearing loss.

Toxoplasmosis

Toxoplasma gondii is a single-celled protozoan parasite that is widespread in domestic and wild animals (e.g., dogs, cats, rabbits). *Toxoplasma gondii* infections are found world-wide, but are less common in cold climates, hot and arid regions, and at high altitudes.

Pathophysiology.   Human infection by *toxoplasma gondii* occurs following ingestion of toxoplasma cysts in undercooked meat or contaminated raw vegetables or through close contact with domestic animals harboring the infection (typically cats). Cat feces carry oocysts which may contaminate cat box filler, soil, or garden vegetables, and infection may spread through contact with these materials. Most infections are asymptomatic or result in a

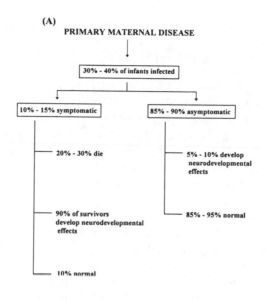

(A)
PRIMARY MATERNAL DISEASE

30% - 40% of infants infected

10% - 15% symptomatic

85% - 90% asymptomatic

20% - 30% die

5% - 10% develop neurodevelopmental effects

90% of survivors develop neurodevelopmental effects

85% - 95% normal

10% normal

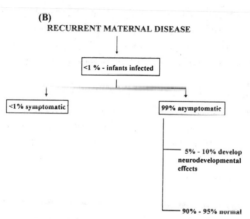

(B)
RECURRENT MATERNAL DISEASE

<1 % - infants infected

<1% symptomatic

99% asymptomatic

5% - 10% develop neurodevelopmental effects

90% - 95% normal

FIGURE 6–10. Comparison of the outcome of congenital cytomegalovirus (CMV) infection related to (A) primary vs. (B) recurrent maternal disease. Primary maternal disease is more devastating; congenital CMV infection occurs in 30% to 40% of infants born to mothers with primary disease. Approximately 15% of these infants will by symptomatic at birth; of these, as many as 30% will die. Ninety percent of survivors will exhibit neurodevelopmental deficits including deafness, microcephaly, mental retardation, and chorioretinitis. The remaining 85% to 90% of infants with congenital CMV acquired during primary maternal disease will be asymptomatic at birth, but as many as 15% of these infants will develop neurodevelopmental deficits. Infants born to mothers with recurrent disease (panel B) are much less likely be be infected. Only about 1% of recurrent maternal disease results in congenital CMV infection, and 10% or less of infected infants demonstrate neurodevelopmental sequelae.

mild, nonspecific illness characterized by malaise, lethargy, and enlarged lymph nodes.

Toxoplasma infection crosses the placenta and infects the fetus in about 40% to 50% of untreated maternal infections. Manifestation of toxoplasmosis at birth range from infants who are infected but asymptomatic (approximately 80% to 90% of cases) to infants with severe disease. If untreated, asymptomatic infants will develop retinal disease in about 85% of cases. In fact, visual disease is the most important sequelae of congenital toxoplasmosis (Stagno et al., 1977; Stein and Boyer, 1994). Late development of hearing impairment and mental retardation have also been reported.

Clinical features of severe congenital toxoplasmosis at birth include hydrocephalus, infection of retinal tissue, cerebral calcification, and other organ system disease.

Treatment. Unlike rubella or CMV, acute maternal toxoplasmosis infection can be treated to prevent the parasite from infecting the fetus. Infected infants also receive direct treatment for congenital toxoplasmosis. Infants are treated with antiparasitic medications and vitamin supplements. Treatment appears effective in reducing morbidity associated with congenital toxoplasmosis infection.

Complications of Disease or Treatment. Neurodevelopmental sequelae of untreated congenital toxoplasmosis include mental retardation, microcephaly, microphthalmia, and hearing loss. The most common disorder is visual defects and blindness.

Syphilis

Syphilis is a sexually transmitted disease caused by the bacterium *Treponema pallidum*. It is estimated that 1 in 10,000 live-born infants in the United States is infected with congenital syphilis. Although the incidence of syphilis steadily declined through the 1970s, syphilis is on the increase with more reported cases of the disease now than in the previous two decades.

Pathophysiology. *Treponema pallidum* is a frail organism that does not survive long outside a host organism. It is transmitted through sexual intercourse when the lesions of the infected individual come into intimate contact with minute breaks in the epithelial surfaces of his or her partner. There are several stages of syphilis infection. During the first and second stages (early syphilis), viable organisms are present and the individual can transmit the disease through sexual contact. During the third, or latent, stage (late syphilis), the individual no longer transmits the disease through sexual contact although the infection can be transmitted to the fetus.

The first stage of syphilis is characterized by development of a primary lesion, or chancre, at the site of inoculation of the bacteria. This occurs approximately 3 weeks after exposure and may be undetected, especially in women. These lesions heal spontaneously within 2 months, and are followed by a secondary stage of generalized illness characterized by sore throat, low-grade fever, malaise, headache, enlarged lymph nodes, and rash. During this stage, there is a multiplication and spread of treponemas throughout the body. The secondary stage of early syphilis is followed by the development of latent syphilis. This third stage may persist for years or even for life. In early latent syphilis, relapses of mucocutaneous lesions may occur. Recurrent lesions do not appear in late latent syphilis and the individual is generally asymptomatic. Approximately 30% to 40% of individuals with latent syphilis will develop late complications including neurosyphilis and/or cardiovascular syphilis.

An infected mother in either the early or late stage of syphilis may transmit the infection to her fetus. In early, untreated syphilis, transmission to the fetus occurs in 80% to 90% of cases. Approximately 25% to 30% of infected fetuses die in utero, 25% to 30% die postnatally, and 40% of survivors develop late symptomatic syphilis. Transmission can occur in any stage of pregnancy; untreated maternal infection in the first two trimesters leads to significant fetal morbidity but maternal infection in the third trimester does not always result in fetal infection.

Treatment.   Treatment of primary syphilis with penicillin during pregnancy is highly effective in preventing infection of the fetus. Penicillin is also an effective treatment for congenital syphilis.

Complications of Disease or Treatment.   Approximately 60% of infants with congenital syphilis are asymptomatic at birth. Congenital syphilis is defined as early or late depending on whether clinical signs are present before or after the second year of life. In early congenital syphilis, the infant develops rhinitis (snuffles) and treponemas are present in the discharge. Shortly thereafter, a rash develops that especially affects the palms, soles, perianal and perioral regions. Skin on the palms and soles is vulnerable to sloughing.

Late congenital syphilis manifests after age 2 years with a variety of lesions affecting the bones, connective tissue, and central nervous system. Progressive sensorineural hearing loss is a common finding in late congenital syphilis.

Human Immunodeficiency Virus (HIV)

In 1981, the first cases of acquired immunodeficiency syndrome (AIDS) were recognized. HIV is a retrovirus that is now known to cause AIDS. HIV replicates in the host's immune system, thereby diminishing the host's immune response.

HIV first developed in the sub-Saharan Africa where spread of the virus began in the 1970s. By the late 1970s the virus had spread to western Europe and the United States. HIV was introduced to Asia and the Pacific rim countries in the 1980s. HIV is rapidly increasing among women of childbearing age and children. In the United States, it is estimated that more than 22,000 infants and children are HIV-positive. At the present time, there is no treatment for AIDS and death results from opportunistically acquired infections. AIDS is among the 10 leading causes of death for children ages 1 to 4 years.

Pathophysiology.   HIV is transmitted through sexual intercourse, infected blood products, infected breast milk, or transplacentally. Typically, no symptoms are present at initial infection although some individuals demonstrate a mild flu-like illness. Most infected individuals remain asymptomatic for years after infection. An individual who is HIV positive develops AIDS when he or she exhibits signs of generalized constitutional disease, opportunistic infections, neurologic disease, secondary cancers, and other systemic effects. AIDS is the end stage of a complex disease process.

The risk of transmission of the HIV from an infected mother to her fetus is estimated to range from 10% to 40%. Factors affecting the risk of transmission are largely unknown, but the virus load in the mother is thought to contribute to risk. Early treatment of the infected pregnant woman with antiviral drugs has been shown to reduce transmission of HIV to the fetus. Because the virus can be transmitted both transplacentally and through breast milk, it is important to know a mother's HIV status to prevent transmission to the infant from breastfeeding and to provide appropriate follow-up and care to the infant with congenital infection.

The spectrum of embryopathologic effects of HIV is not entirely known. Early reports of growth retardation, premature birth, low birthweight, and dysmorphic features in infants with prenatally acquired HIV have not been universally substantiated. In about

80% of cases, diagnosis is apparent by age 3 years and one half of these children will demonstrate clinical symptoms by age 1 year. Approximately 75% of children die within 2 years of diagnosis of AIDS; survival time is shortest for infants diagnosed before 1 year of age.

Treatment.   Treatment for HIV infection includes prophylaxis against other infections and use of antiviral drugs. Because no effective treatment is available to eliminate HIV infection, treatment is directed to avoiding other life-threatening infections (e.g., meningitis, measles, pertussis) and postponing development of AIDS.

Complications of Disease or Treatment.   Individuals do not die of AIDS per se but rather from the opportunistic infections and disease. CNS complications include neurodevelopmental delay, ataxia, and acquired microcephaly. Hearing loss may develop secondary to meningitis or use of ototoxic antibiotics.

Effects on Hearing of Congenital Infections

Congenital infections are an important cause of hearing impairment in infants. Previously, rubella was considered the single most important cause of nongenetic, congenital hearing loss. In the United States, rubella has been virtually eliminated through successful vaccination programs. In countries without a widespread vaccination program, CRS remains an important cause of deafness. Health care services in the former Soviet Union declined in the late 1980s, for example, and CRS emerged as an important cause of childhood disabilities in Russia and other former Soviet bloc countries.

CMV is now considered a leading cause of nongenetic, congenital, and progressive hearing impairment in infants and young children (Strauss, 1985). Based on the annual birth rate and the estimated number of babies born with congenital CMV infection, McCollister et al. (1996) project that more than 6,000 children born in the United States each year experience sensorineural hearing impairment as a consequence of congenital CMV infection.

In children with symptomatic congenital CMV infection, bilateral temporal bone anomalies have been reported. Bauman et al. (1994) reported features of bilateral Mondini dysplasia in a child with symptomatic congenital cytomegalovirus and severe, bilateral sensorineural hearing loss. Follow-up evaluation of other children with congenital CMV also revealed radiographic evidence of temporal bone abnormalities.

Primary maternal CMV infection is associated with more severe neurodevelopmental effects than recurrent maternal infection. Fowler et al. (1992) compared neurodevelopmental outcomes in CMV-infected infants born to mothers who acquired primary CMV infection during pregnancy with outcomes in CMV-infected infants born to mothers with recurrent infection. Only babies in the primary-infection group were symptomatic at birth (18%). After almost 5 years of follow-up, neurodevelopmental effects were observed in 25% of the primary-infection group and 8% of the recurrent-infection group. Sensorineural hearing impairment was present in 15% of the primary-infection group and 5% of the recurrent-infection group.

Most infants with congenital CMV infection are asymptomatic at birth. Because newborn nurseries do not routinely screen for congenital CMV, most children with asymptomatic congenital CMV infection are undetected. Appearing as apparently healthy newborns, hearing impairment in these infants will be undetected if newborn hearing screening is limited to infants with known risk criteria. Hicks et al. (1993), for example, assessed the ability of risk criteria-based newborn hearing screening to identify infants with hearing loss resulting from congenital CMV infection. In their study of more than 12,000 newborn infants, 167 (1.3%) were identified with congenital CMV infection by routine urine cultures. Of these, 14 (10.4%) had sensorineural hearing loss. Risk criteria-based screening of the 12,000 infants resulted in hearing screens on 2,036 babies; of these, only 34 of the infants with congenital CMV infection were screened and only 2 of the 14 infants with sensorineural hearing loss were detected. These authors concluded that newborn hearing screening based on the presence of risk criteria will fail to identify the majority of infants with sensorineural hearing loss secondary to congenital CMV infection.

Congenital CMV infection frequently results in progressive hearing loss. Dahle et al. (1979) provided one of the first reports on congenital CMV infection and progressive sensorineural hearing loss in children. More recently, Williamson, Demmler, Percy, and Catlin (1992) reported that hearing loss continued to worsen in children with asymptomatic congenital CMV infection through age 5 years. In the same report, the authors documented development of unilateral sensorineural hearing loss during the first year of life in an infant with asymptomatic congenital CMV and normal hearing at birth. Any child identified with congenital CMV infection should receive regular audiologic follow-up to detect development and progression of hearing impairment regardless of hearing status at birth.

In children with inadequately treated congenital toxoplasmosis infection, visual deficits are the most common neurodevelopmental effect (Stagno et al., 1977). Hearing impairment has been reported in as many as 14% to 26% of cases. Recent reports from a national collaborative study (Stein and Boyer, 1994) indicate that auditory, visual, and central nervous system sequelae of toxoplasmosis can be virtually eliminated with long-term (i.e., 1 year) treatment with antiparasitic drugs. In that study, none of 57 treated children developed sensorineural hearing loss.

Hearing impairment from congenital syphilis typically is not present at birth (Gleich, Urbina, and Pincus, 1994). Prompt antibiotic treatment of the mother to prevent infection of the fetus or treatment of the infant with congenital infection eliminates the risk of later development of syphilitic hearing loss.

Infants with congenital HIV infection are at risk for acquiring hearing loss secondary to either opportunistic infections, such as meningitis and otitis media, or ototoxic antibiotic treatment for these infections. At the present time, there is limited information on the long-term consequences of HIV infection on hearing function in children.

Any infant with congenital infection should receive audiologic assessment during the newborn period and routinely thereafter to identify late onset or progressive sensorineural hearing loss. Congenital infections have been identified as a risk factor on every registry published by the Joint Committee on Infant Hearing since 1972. In the future, widespread screening of infants for congenital CMV infection may improve both identification of infected infants with hearing impairment and infants at risk for acquired/progressive hearing loss.

Perinatally and Postnatally Acquired Infections

At birth, the infant's immune system must respond to the challenges of extrauterine life. Although many defense mechanisms are present, the newborn infant's immune system is not as effective as that of older infants, children, and adults. Newborn infants, and premature infants in particular, are at risk for acquiring infection in the perinatal and neonatal period (birth through 28 days of age).

Mothers with active birth canal infections may transmit disease to their infants during the birth process. Whenever possible, infants of infected mothers are delivered by caesarian section to prevent exposure of the infant to these diseases. In addition, premature infants are at increased risk for acquiring generalized infections due to immature immune system development.

Herpes Simplex Virus (HSV)

HSV is a member of a large family of herpes viruses that infect both invertebrates and vertebrates. Two types of HSVs infect humans. HSV-I is often acquired during childhood and is isolated from the mouth, nose, and oropharynx (cold sores). HSV-II is usually acquired in adolescence or adulthood from sexual transmission and is isolated from the genital mucosa (genital herpes). Each type of HSV may infect either or both sites, however. Like other herpes viruses, HSV-I and HSV-II cause latent infections that may reactivate or recur at periodic intervals.

Pathophysiology.   HSV is transmitted by direct contact with an infected individual. Transmission to the fetus occurs most commonly during the birth process in a mother with an active primary infection. Transmission from an active recurrent infection is much less common. Transplacental HSV infection is rare and the effects range from no abnormality to multisystem congenital anomalies including skin lesions, microcephaly, microphthalmia, spasticity, and mental retardation. Unfortunately, perinatally acquired infection can also result in devastating consequences to the infant. The spectrum of disease in these infants can range from localized skin lesions to disseminated infection involving the liver, lungs, and central nervous system.

Treatment.   Caesarian section delivery is recommended for mothers with active primary genital HSV infection. Mothers with active recurrent infections are less likely to transmit HSV to their infants despite vaginal delivery. Any infant who is exposed at delivery is closely monitored and early antiviral therapy is initiated if symptoms develop.

Complications of Disease or Treatment.   Infants with herpes infection may demonstrate symptoms ranging from localized skin lesions to generalized infection involving the lungs, liver, and central nervous system. Generalized infection and disseminated disease have a high mortality and morbidity. Neurologic and sensory system complications include microcephaly, encephalitis, chorioretinitis, and sensorineural hearing loss. The CNS is involved in 70% to 90% of infected infants.

Bacterial Sepsis

Bacterial infections are the most common infections in the newborn period and result from exposure to common microorganisms.

Older children and adults typically are not affected because they have developed immunities to these ubiquitous bacteria. Postnatally acquired bacterial infections are often life-threatening in newborn and premature infants.

Pathophysiology.   Bacterial infections are observed in infants with significant obstetrical histories (premature rupture of membranes, premature onset of labor, or maternal fever). In general, the infant acquires the infection from the birth canal during delivery. Early-onset (e.g., within the first few days of life) bacterial infections can result in fulminant, multisystem illness with high mortality, especially in premature infants. Organisms commonly responsible for early onset bacterial infections are Group B streptococcus, *Escherichia coli,* and *Haemophilus influenzae.* Typically, the infant with early-onset bacterial infection presents with lethargy, irritability, poor feeding, abnormal heart rate, abnormal respiratory rate, and cyanosis. Without prompt treatment, the infant may develop increased oxygen requirement and PPHN. Early-onset disease may mimic respiratory distress syndrome. Late-onset (e.g., after the first week of life) bacterial disease results from exposure during delivery or after delivery from human contact or contaminated equipment. The most common presentation of late-onset disease is bacterial meningitis with septicemia (manifestation of systemic illness with infectious organisms present in the blood).

Treatment.   On first sign of sepsis, newborn infants are treated with broad-spectrum antibiotics (typically ampicillin with an aminoglycoside) until the specific organism is identified.

Complications of Disease or Treatment.   Overall mortality from bacterial infections has been reported as high as 20%, with greatest mortality occurring in small preterm infants. Mortality is greatest in early-onset disease. Complications in survivors include mental retardation, spastic quadriplegia, cortical blindness, deafness, hydrocephalus, and uncontrollable seizures. Early treatment is important for preventing or diminishing neurologic sequelae.

Effects on Hearing from Peri- or Postnatally Acquired Infection

There is limited information about hearing impairment in infants with herpes infection. Dahle and McCollister (1988) reported developmental and audiologic results in 20 children diagnosed with symptomatic neonatal herpes infection. Although many of the

20 children demonstrated developmental and sensory deficits secondary to the infection including psychomotor retardation (13 children), visual abnormalities (11 children), and CNS involvement (10 children), only two children had sensorineural hearing loss, one moderate-severe bilateral loss and one moderate-severe unilateral loss. The authors speculate that the lack of clear documentation and extensive literature citations about the effects of neonatal herpes on hearing may be related to the relatively high mortality and morbidity of this disease.

Hearing impairment in infants with peri- or postnatally acquired bacterial infections is most often secondary to meningitis. Extension of a vaccination for *Haemophilus influenzae type B* (HiB) to young infants in the early 1990s has significantly reduced the incidence of bacterial meningitis in infants more than 3 months of age (Bent and Beck, 1994; Stein and Boyer, 1994). In infants less than approximately 2 months of age, e. coli and streptococcus type B are the most common organisms resulting in bacterial meningitis. The incidence of hearing loss has been reported as 31% with Streptococcus pneumoniae meningitis, 10.5% with Neisseria meningitidis, and 6% with Hemophilus influenzae infections (Dodge et al., 1984). Limited data are available regarding the incidence of hearing loss following e. coli meningitis.

An important consideration in the treatment of sepsis and bacterial meningitis in newborns and young infants is the ototoxicity of aminoglycoside therapy. Simmons (1980b) reported that, although the incidence of sensorineural hearing impairment is much higher in infants cared for in intensive care nurseries relative to well-baby nurseries, aminoglycosides did not have an obvious effect on incidence of hearing loss. Finitizo-Hieber et al. (1979) evaluated the long-term effects of gentamicin and kanamycin use in newborn infants. They performed audiometric, vestibular, and psychometric evaluations in three groups of children: children treated with gentamicin, children treated with kanamycin, and matched control infants and children who received no aminoglycoside antibiotics in the neonatal period. The authors found no substantial sensorineural hearing loss or vestibular dysfunction that could be attributed to aminoglycoside therapy. In addition, there were no differences among the three groups on psychometric measures.

In 1985, Finitizo-Hieber, McCracken, and Brown published results of a controlled, prospective evaluation of hearing in infants who received either netilmicin or amikacin during the neonatal period. The authors compared auditory function in the treated infants with auditory function in a group of age- and gender-matched control subjects who did not receive aminogylcoside antibiotics. Bilateral sensorineural hearing loss was confirmed in three (2%) infants, one each in the netilmicin and amikacin treated groups and one control infant.

As described previously, aminoglycoside ototoxicity is exacerbated when used in combination with loop diuretics, specifically furosemide. Salamy, Eldredge, and Tooley (1989) reported a statistically significant association between sensorineural hearing loss and duration and dosage of furosemide and the combination of furosemide and aminoglycoside antibiotics. Aminoglycoside administration alone was not systematically related to hearing impairment in very low birthweight babies, however.

It appears that, with meticulous monitoring to assure safe levels, effective aminoglycoside therapy can be administered to newborns without adversely affecting hearing. The combination of aminoglycosides with loop diuretics, however, substantially enhances the potential ototoxicity of therapy.

Hematologic Disorders

Several important disorders of newborn and premature infants are related to production or breakdown of blood and its various components. The developing embryo is nourished only briefly by direct maternal blood supply. At about age 18 days, development of the fetus's own blood supply and circulatory system begins. Blood circulation is functional by the third to fifth week, and the developing embryo obtains nutrients through the interface of fetal and maternal circulations. Incompatibility of blood type between fetus and mother, natural temporary cessation of red blood cell production in newborn infants, and clotting problems can lead to newborn morbidity and mortality.

Hyperbilirubinemia (Jaundice)

Bilirubin is a by-product of red blood cell breakdown. When it exceeds a specific range in the circulating blood (hyperbilirubinemia), it becomes potentially toxic to the CNS. Hyperbilirubinemia results in a characteristic yellow pallor to the skin and whites of the eye known as jaundice. Nonsignificant jaundice occurs in almost all normal newborns; clinically significant jaundice is observed in many premature infants and infants with maternal-fetal blood group incompatibility, congenital or perinatally acquired infection, and birth trauma.

Pathophysiology. Red blood cells are formed in the bone marrow and make up approximately 50% of blood volume. These cells contain hemoglobin, the red substance of the blood that carries oxygen to and carbon dioxide from tissue and organ systems. Natural breakdown of red blood cells releases hemoglobin and one of its components, the yellow pigment bilirubin, into the blood stream. Bilirubin is a potentially toxic substance which binds with the protein albumin and is transported to the liver where it is detoxified, or conjugated. Conjugated bilirubin is harmless and is excreted through the intestines and kidneys.

The newborn infant's liver is not maximally efficient in conjugating bilirubin. For this reason, higher than normal levels of bilirubin can be measured in the blood. Infants whose bilirubin level exceed a specific range demonstrate clinically significant hyperbilirubinemia. Very high levels of bilirubin can damage the CNS and result in neurologic dysfunction. This condition, kernicterus, occurs when unconjugated bilirubin crosses the blood-brain barrier and stains specific structures in the CNS with the characteristic yellow pigment.

Treatment.   Specific wavelengths of light alter the molecular structure of bilirubin and facilitate its binding with albumin, transport to the liver, and conjugation. For infants with clinically significant hyperbilirubinemia in the lower range of toxicity, phototherapy is effective in decreasing unconjugated bilirubin in the bloodstream. Infants whose jaundice cannot be controlled by phototherapy receive exchange transfusion of red blood cells to eliminate unconjugated bilirubin from circulation. Multiple exchange transfusions may be required to control hyperbilirubinemia.

Complications of Disease or Treatment.   Despite phototherapy or even exchange transfusions, some infants may develop kernicterus from hyperbilirubinemia. Structures at greatest risk are the basal ganglion, nuclei in the brainstem and cerebellum, and hippocampus. Damage to these structures may result in athetoid cerebral palsy, mental retardation, and sensorincural and/or central deafness.

Anemia

Anemia is deficiency in red blood cells; it is clinically important because red blood cells are necessary for oxygen/carbon dioxide transport and exchange in all tissues in the body. Anemia is diagnosed when the hematocrit, a measure of the percentage of red blood cells in circulation, drops below 40%. The opposite of anemia, polycythemia, occurs when there is an abnormally high percentage of red blood cells in circulation. It is treated by replacing some of the infant's blood with a saline solution chemically similar to blood serum.

Pathophysiology. Newborns stop producing red blood cells in their bone marrow for 2 to 3 months after birth resulting in normal physiologic anemia at about 6 weeks of age. Anemia that is present at birth may indicate blood loss before or during birth, maternal-fetal blood group incompatibility, decreased red blood cell production, or congenital conditions that alter red blood cell function.

Treatment. Normal physiologic anemia is self-limiting and requires no treatment. Treatment for pathologic anemia includes transfusion with whole blood or concentrated red blood cells. Homozygous alpha thalassemia, a genetic condition that occurs occasionally in Asian infants and alters red blood cell function and oxygen transport, cannot be treated.

Complications of Disease or Treatment. Anemia may cause tissue hypoxia and acidosis. In infants with primary respiratory or cardiac disease who are already hypoxic, anemia further complicates resolution of poor oxygenation. Anemia secondary to maternal-fetal blood group incompatibility may lead to hyperbilirubinemia and kernicterus. Complications of exchange transfusions include metabolic dysfunction, clotting disorders, and infection.

Maternal-Fetal Blood Group Incompatibility

Human blood is categorized or typed by specific inherited properties into blood group (A, B, AB, and O) and Rh factor (Rh-negative or Rh-positive; Rh, for rhesus monkey, the animal used in blood factor experiments in the 1940s). The blood groups and Rh factors indicate the presence of specific proteins (antigens and antibodies) in the blood cells and serum. Blood groups and Rh factors cannot be mixed indiscriminately; specific reactions occur with some combinations that result in destruction of red blood cells and systemic disease. Incompatibility in either blood type or Rh factor between the mother and the developing fetus may result in morbidity and mortality to the fetus or newborn infant.

Pathophysiology. A mother whose blood group or Rh-factor is incompatible with her developing fetus will develop antibodies against the fetus's blood type/Rh factor. These antibodies will cross the placental barrier and attack the fetus's red blood cells which carry the sensitizing proteins. Consequences to the fetus/newborn infant vary depending on the nature of the incompatibility.

Treatment.   One serious form of maternal-fetal blood incompatibility involves a Rh-negative mother who is carrying a Rh-positive fetus. Because antibody formation is relatively slow on initial exposure, infants from a first pregnancy are not typically at risk for blood incompatibility reaction. Future pregnancies with Rh-positive fetuses will be affected, however, because the mother has been sensitized by initial exposure. Affected infants manifest erythroblastosis fetalis (production and circulation of immature red blood cells in an attempt to compensate for destruction of mature red blood cells) with severe anemia, rapidly rising unconjugated bilirubin concentration, and enlarged liver and spleen. Rh-negative mothers who have been sensitized by pregnancy with an Rh-positive baby are given a human gamma globulin (RhoGAM) after delivery to prevent antibody formation and erythroblastosis fetalis in subsequent pregnancies.

Complications of Disease or Treatment.   Prior to development of RhoGAM, fetus and infant mortality and morbidity from erythroblastosis fetalis was common. The most serious consequences were spontaneous abortion, stillbirth, or premature birth. Kernicterus resulted in CNS damage (cerebral palsy, mental retardation, sensorineural and central deafness) in survivors.

Effects on Hearing of Hematologic Disorders

Hematologic diseases are important considerations in sensorineural hearing impairment and central auditory dysfunction. Prior to the development of RhoGam, kernicterus resulting from Rh incompatibility led to substantial disability in affected infants. Evaluation of individuals affected by Rh incompatibility revealed both cochlear and central components to their auditory disorders (Goodhill, 1967; Matkin and Carhart, 1966).

More recently, investigators have evaluated auditory brainstem response (ABR) in jaundiced infants and infants receiving treatment with either exchange transfusion or phototherapy. In 1983, for example, Perlman et al. reported ABR results in 24 infants with hyperbilirubinemia and jaundice. These infants showed abnormal waveform morphology and significantly prolonged brainstem transmission compared to nonjaundiced infants who had similar gestational and postnatal ages. For the majority of jaundiced infants, the abnormal ABR results rapidly reversed as their hyperbilirubinemia resolved. Perlman et al. concluded that neonatal jaundice is associated with significant transient aberrations of ABR suggesting transient brainstem encephalopathy. Nwaesei, Van Aerde, Boyden, and Perlman (1984) confirmed the findings of Perlman et al. and observed that brainstem abnormalities, as reflected on aberrant ABRs, reversed after exchange transfusion. Nakamura et al. (1985) compared ABR responses in three groups of infants, two groups with hyperbilirubinemia of differing total bilirubin levels and one group without jaundice. These investigators described prolonged wave I in jaundiced infants and prolonged waves I and V in the jaundiced infants with the higher total bilirubin levels. Following exchange transfusion, the latencies of both waves I and V decreased within 24 to 96 hours after the procedure. Tan, Skurr, and Yip (1992) demonstrated improvement in latencies of wave V and interpeaks I-V and III-V in jaundiced infants receiving phototherapy. Deliac, Demarquez, Barberot, Sandler, and Paty (1990) followed jaundiced newborns who received exchange transfusions by ABR both prior to and for up to 12 months following exchange transfusion. These investigators again confirmed that hyperbilirubinemia results in prolonged ABR responses which improve with treatment. At 1 year following exchange transfusion, ABRs were normal in the affected infants. Hung (1989) demonstrated elevated ABR threshold in a group of infants with kernicterus as well as improvement in ABR central conduction in jaundiced infants who received either exchange transfusion or phototherapy.

It is important to recognize that hematologic disorders may result in neurotoxic effects that alter the ABR. Because these effects are transient in successfully treated infants, audiologists should carefully interpret tests of auditory function that may be compromised by these transient neurologic abnormalities. Although limited information is available about OAEs in jaundiced infants, abnormal ABRs in the face of normal OAEs would not be unexpected in these babies.

Feeding/Swallowing and Gastrointestinal Disorders

Almost a century ago, Budin, the father of neonatal medicine, observed that feeding was one of the most important factors in the survival of "weaklings," or premature infants. Difficulty in feeding, swallowing, or food tolerance is alarming and potentially fatal to the newborn infant. The digestive tract is a long, complex tube running through the body; an abnormality at any level can affect the infant's nutrition, growth, and survival.

Esophageal Atresia and Tracheoesophageal Fistula

Esophageal atresia (EA) results when the esophagus ends in a blind pouch; tracheoesophageal fistula (TEF) results when the trachea and esophagus fail to separate completely and are joined together are some juncture. Figure 6–11 shows examples of EA and TEF.

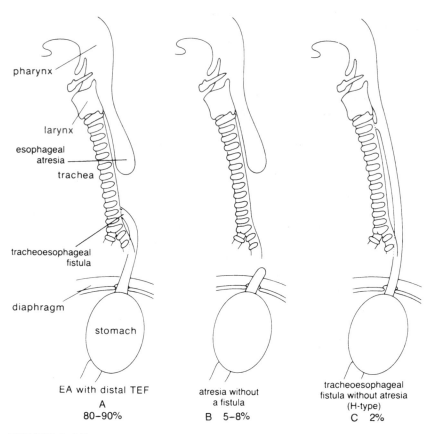

pharynx

larynx

esophageal atresia

trachea

tracheoesophageal fistula

diaphragm

stomach

EA with distal TEF
A
80–90%

atresia without
a fistula
B   5–8%

tracheoesophageal
fistula without atresia
(H-type)
C   2%

FIGURE 6–11. The three most common types of esophageal atresia and tracheoesophageal fistula. Esophageal atresia with a distal fistula comprises 80% to 90% of all cases (A); atresia without fistula accounts for 5% to 8% of cases (B); Isolated tracheoesophageal fistula without esophageal atresia (H-type defect) constitutes 1% to 2% of cases (C). (From *Family-Centered Nursing Care of Children*, Second Edition, by C. L. Betz, M. Hunsberger, and S. Wright, 1994, p. 1448. Baltimore, MD: W. B. Saunders Company. Copyright 1994 by W. B. Saunders Publishing Company. Reprinted with permission.)

Pathophysiology. Both EA and TEF are embryologic defects. EA probably arises from a spontaneous anomaly of the esophagus or a deviation of the foregut. TEF occurs when the trachea incompletely separates from the esophagus. Normally, the esophagus and trachea separate at about days 34 to 36 of development. EA occurs in approximately 1 in 3,000 to 1 in 4,500 births, and TEF is present in approximately 80–90% of these cases. Other congenital abnormalities are present in 30% to 70% of affected infants; congenital heart anomalies are the most common associated abnormalities. VATER association or VACTERL association may be identified in infants with a complex of vertebral anomalies, ventricular septal heart defects, EA and TEF, anal atresia, and limb abnormalities. The terms VATER and VACTERL are often used interchangeably.

Treatment. Definitive treatment for EA and TEF requires surgical connection (anastomosis) of the proximal and distal ends of the esophagus and elimination of the fistula. The surgical approach and technique depend on the location of the atresia and fistula, and the distance separating the two ends of the esophagus. During postoperative recovery, the infant is typically fed via gastrostomy tube for 5 to 10 days to facilitate healing.

Complications of Disease or Treatment. With early identification and intervention, survival rate for full-term infants exceeds 95%. Survival rate for premature infants or infants with other major, congenital anomalies is substantially less. Postoperative complications may include gastroesophageal reflux, stricture of the anastomosis, and recurrence of the fistula.

Gastroesophageal Reflux

Retrograde passage of acidic contents from the stomach into the esophagus is gastroesophageal reflux (GER). In adults, gastroesophageal reflux is commonly called "heartburn."

Pathophysiology. Normally, gastric contents are maintained in the stomach by several mechanisms including high pressure in the terminal section of the esophagus, a long segment of intrathoracic esophagus, and a sharp angle between the proximal stomach and esophagus. When any of these mechanisms is compromised, the infant is at risk for developing GER. Infants with congenital anomalies, especially TEF, are at greatest risk for GER.

Treatment. Medical treatment of GER includes thickening the infant's feeds, feeding more frequently and in smaller volume, and positioning the infant in a prone position after feedings. Several medications are available to decrease the acidity of the gastric contents and to speed gastric emptying.

Infants whose GER does not resolve with medical intervention require surgical invention. The most common surgical procedure is a Nissen fundoplication in which the proximal stomach (gastric fundus) is partially or completely wrapped around the distal esophagus at the gastroesophageal junction. A gastrostomy is often placed for feeding or relief of gastric pressure postoperatively.

Complications of Disease or Treatment. Chronic conditions associated with GER include vomiting, failure to thrive (FTT), aspiration pneumonia, and recurrent apneic spells. These infants often dramatically improve with surgery. Recurrence of GER postoperatively may necessitate a second, more difficult Nissen procedure.

Omphalocele and Gastroschisis

Omphalocele and gastroschisis are embryologic defects that result in extrusion of visceral organs outside the abdominal cavity. In these conditions, the infant is born with intestines extruding through the abdominal wall.

Pathophysiology. Omphalocele results when the intestines, which initially develop in the umbilical cord, fail to migrate completely into the abdomen during fetal development; intestines and other organs protrude through the abdominal wall into a transparent, moist sac. Gastroschisis is a full-thickness defect in the abdominal wall in which uncovered intestines protrude from the abdomen.

Treatment. Return of visceral organs to the abdominal cavity and closure of the abdominal wall defect are accomplished by either a single or multistaged surgical procedure.

Complications of Disease or Treatment. Injury to the bowel, respiratory compromise, and diminished venous return are complications of surgical intervention for omphalocele and gastroschisis. Intestinal function is typically diminished in the weeks immediately following surgery and the infant requires intravenous feeds (total parenteral nutrition).

Necrotizing Enterocolitis

Necrotizing enterocolitis (NEC) is a gastrointestinal disorder of premature infants. It is characterized by necrosis (tissue death) of the mucosal and submucosal layers of the bowel.

Pathophysiology. NEC is the result of complex interactions of bowel ischemia often secondary to asphyxia, RDS, or apnea, bacterial colonization of the intestine, and formula feeding. NEC is most commonly observed in premature infants, and infants less than 1,500 grams birthweight are at greatest risk of developing the disease. Infants with decreased oxygen intake develop a reflexive mechanism to protect the brain and heart from hypoxia by shunting blood away from the visceral and peripheral vasculature. This results in selective ischemia to the bowel. Bacteria colonize the intestines during the first few weeks of life. In infants with tissue compromise due to bowel ischemia and diminished immune system response due to prematurity, further bowel damage results from the toxins of these normally beneficial bacteria. Infant feeding formulas provide the fuel on which bacteria thrive. Infants who receive breast milk seldom develop NEC. If the full thickness of the intestinal wall is damaged, the infant's bowel perforates and releases gas and toxins into the peritoneal cavity.

Treatment. Medical management of NEC includes bowel rest with intravenous feeds, release of gas in the intestinal tract, and control of infection. Surgical management to resect necrotic bowel tissue and to create an ostomy (diversion of bowel emptying through the abdominal wall) is necessary in advanced cases or cases intractable to medical management. The overall mortality rate in infants who receive medical management is approximately 1 in 3 and 1 in 2 for infants who require surgical intervention.

Effects on Hearing of Feeding/Swallowing and Gastrointestinal Disorders

Infants with multiple congenital anomalies that include the gastrointestinal system should receive evaluation for genetic and/or syndromal abnormalities that might include hearing loss. For example, an infant with the complex of EA, TEF, vertebral anomalies, and cardiac disorder should receive hearing evaluation to rule out hearing impairment associated with VATER association. In isolation, infants with embryologic defects resulting in gastrointestinal disorders such as omphalocele or gastroschisis are not at increased risk for hearing loss. Infants with serious infections of the gastrointestinal tract such as NEC may receive ototoxic antibiotics to control sepsis and should receive hearing evaluation.

SUMMARY

As described in this chapter, a host of complex disorders affect newborns and young infants. These disorders may be relatively benign, and prompt treatment in the newborn period restores the infant to health with the potential for normal development. Conversely, many ominous conditions result in lifelong disease and disability.

Fortunately, techniques for early identification and treatment of infants at risk for these disorders are continually evolving. Diseases that previously affected scores of infants (e.g., congenital rubella syndrome, hemophilus type B meningitis, congenital toxoplasmosis) have been virtually eliminated by effective vaccination and/or treatment programs.

Significant advances in audiologic assessment of infants have resulted in better understanding of the etiology of hearing impairment in newborn infants and very young babies. Improved understanding of the etiology of hearing impairment in these babies hopefully will yield better methods to prevent and to treat these hearing disorders.

RECOMMENDED READINGS

Greenough, A., Osborne, J., and Sutherland, S. (Eds.). (1992). *Congenital, perinatal and neonatal infections.* New York: Churchill Livingstone.
A medical text describing major infections affecting newborns.
Kenner, C., Brueggemeyer, A., and Gunderson, L. P. (1993). *Comprehensive neonatal nursing: a physiologic perspective.* Philadelphia: W. B. Saunders Company.
An exhaustive description of the assessment and management of major organ system dysfunction in the newborn from a nursing perspective.
Merenstein, G. B. and Gardner, S. L. (Eds.). (1993). *Handbook of neonatal intensive care, third edition.* St. Louis: Mosby Year Book.
A comprehensive medical text with chapters covering major diagnostic categories. Additional chapters discuss the NICU environment, impact of NICU care on the infant and family and bioethics in the NICU.

SECTION III

Evaluation and Management

CHAPTER 7

Hearing Screening

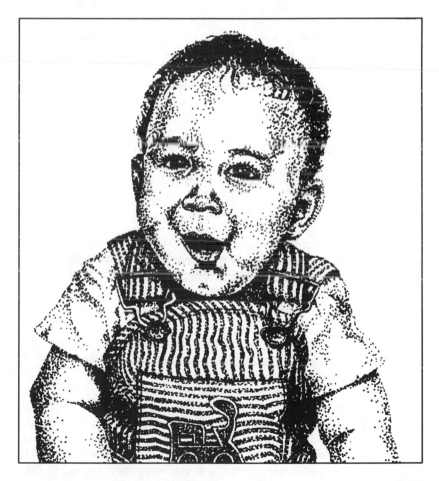

*H*earing impairment in infants is nearly impossible to detect during the routine clinical examination. Hearing loss is an invisible disability in newborns and young children. Yet, early detection is the key to successful treatment and management. The problem of early detection of hearing loss in newborns is a complex issue and each recommended solution brings forth both proponents and opponents. There is a paucity of longitudinal research data to provide verification of the efficacy of infant hearing screening. For example, Stein (1995) points out that the accepted conclusions regarding the average age of identification of hearing loss in infants is based on fewer than 10 published studies limited by retrospective analyses.

The answers to the pertinent questions have not yet been provided to the satisfaction of all the critics. The controversies about health screening are by no means limited to our special interest in the hearing of infants. But with crucial health and education concerns as important as the late detection of hearing loss in young children, to postpone action while we wait for definitive answers puts us in an untenable position, one with potentially devastating results for untold numbers of yet-to-be identified infants with hearing impairment.

Screening for health problems in the general population has been a generally accepted concept for many years. Feightner (1992) points out that, in the early years, health screening was based more on enthusiasm than science, but this has been largely corrected over the past two decades. During recent years, higher quality data have come from the improved design of research studies, which in turn has lead to better understanding of the necessary elements in mass screening programs. Acceptance of screening for health problems is best accomplished when supported by a solid data description of a screening procedure's performance. Of course, the success of a screening program rests on the effectiveness of the protocols used to identify those who are likely to have the target disorder and to pass over those who do not have the target disorder. Screening tests should accurately identify those who are predisposed to develop disease or who have the disease and are asymptomatic so that they can be effectively treated early to avoid more severe complications of the disorder.

Certainly the basic premise of screening, or early detection, of health problems makes good sense. Early identification offers the opportunity to initiate treatment and institute management procedures prior to the onset of symptoms which should result in long-term social and economic advantages. Treating a disability early should improve the prognosis for the patient while reducing suffering and hardship. The main goal of screening is to identify asymptomatic disease that can be managed medically, surgically, or through rehabilitation. But controversy persists over the role and value of health screening for a wide variety of medical conditions in the general population.

In every state in the United States, newborn infants are routinely screened for phenylketonuria and hypothyroidism, and many states choose to have mandatory screening for at least one of nine other disorders (Holtzman, 1991). The differences in states' policies on screening may be at least partially based on pressure from special interest groups. In the states where screening is not advocated for additional diseases, the reasons cited include uncertainty about the benefits and risks of the tests, competition for health dollars, and the absence of public pressure. The benefits of screening are of major importance in policy making, but in many situations clear guidelines for achieving the levels of optimal predictive accuracy are simply not available. The Colorado Committee for Advocacy of Universal Hearing Screening for Infants summarized available state screening statistics for various health problems as shown in Table 7–1.

As example of the opposition to screening, Lindner (1992) questions the rational for newborn-screening policies and suggests that they are driven by a "technological imperative." As new screening techniques and tests are developed, advocates institute the policy into health programs. Once a test is introduced into a program and infants are identified with the target disorder, there is a reluctance to discontinue the screening, because public pressure becomes an overriding issue and objective review is difficult.

The economic view is represented by Holtzman (1992) who states that the savings from screening depend primarily on how much the costs of medical care for children with detected disorders can be reduced. Further, there is a widely held position that screening should be supported only when the costs of not performing the screening test are greater than those of performing the test. Opponents to the economic viewpoint argue that the benefit to the patient should be considered in addition to the cost of the screening. Lindner (1992) responds that, when an effective test and therapeutic strategy are available, prenatal and neonatal screening are much more cost-effective than many highly publicized intervention procedures that absorb huge amounts of our health care dollars.

The very nature of screening brings special obligations for the professionals involved (Frankenberg and North, 1974). When a provider takes the intiative in discovering health problems in indi-

Table 7-1. Colorado Newborn Screening Programs based on 54,000 annual births.

	Sensorineural Hearing Loss	Hypothyroidism	Phenylketonuria (PKU)	Cystic Fibrosis	Hemoglobinopathies (HGB)
Frequency per 100,000 births	564 (376 Bilat)	25	25	50	13
# Positive - First Screen	3650	600	5	600	600
# Children Diagnosed	304 (203 Bilat)	15	4	27	7
Positive Predictive Value	8%	3%	80%	4%	1%
Average age of diagnosis if unscreened	30 months	3-12 months	3-12 months	42 months	3 - 36 months
Cost of Initial Screen Per Child	$25	$3	$3	$3	$3
Cost Per Confirmed Diag.	$ 4440	$10,800	$40,500	$10,800	$40,800
Effectiveness of Treatment	2+	3+	3+	1+	1+
Personal Cost of Delayed Diagnosis	Language delay; academic delays; psychosocial difficulties; cognitive delays	Lethargy; confusion; poor memory; myxedema coma; cretinism; pares thesias; myalgia.	Seizures; tremors; Gait disorders; sever, irreversible mental retardation.	Malnutrition	Bacterial sepsis (infancy); anemia and sickling crises and other complications.

Source: The Colorado Committee for Advocacy of Universal Newborn Hearing Screening (1996), Colorado Department of Health, Denver, CO.

viduals without complaints, the provider must be certain that identification of such problems will do more good than harm. Health screening may cause inconvenience and discomfort to children and their parents, but providers must be aware that anxiety also will be created about the meaning of positive or equivocal findings. To assure patients that knowing about the problem is better than not knowing about it, the following criteria must be met:

- Medical knowledge should be adequate to deal effectively with the problem identified.
- Sufficient numbers of skilled providers should be available to care for any problems that are discovered, and the providers should be linked to adequate laboratory, consultant, hospital, and other specialized health facilities as necessary.
- Financial resources should be adequate to pay for the necessary diagnosis and treatment of problems discovered.
- Services should be available to help the patient and family find and use the financial and medical support they need.

With the widespread discussion and concern for public health screening policies in today's changing health care atmosphere, it is important to note that the scientific evidence available for evaluation across different screening efforts varies considerably. Therefore, conclusions about health screening in general are difficult to apply to all of the disorders for which screening tests are available. A literal mountain of material has been written about screening. In the following sections, we attempt to clarify some basic principles and guidelines as they apply to hearing screening of infants.

SCREENING

Screening is an all-encompassing term which is defined as the preliminary acquisition of information for early detection of a condition. More specifically, screening is a process of applying certain rapid and simple tests and procedures to a generally large population to identify individuals with a high probablility of having the target condition from individuals who probably do not have the disorder. The concept of identifying disease before it is clinically apparent is an appealing public health consideration. Screening allows large numbers of persons to be evaluated for a disease or a condition with less commitment of time, cost, and inconvenience than with specific diagnostic tests.

Two important considerations are implicit in the above definitions: (1) *screening* is an issue of likelihood probabilities rather than a certainty of accuracy-the identification of persons who are likely to have the disorder from those who probably do not have the disorder. The results of screening procedures are never likely to be 100% accurate in separating normal from abnormal individuals and (2) *screening* must not be misconstrued into the totally separate issue of *diagnosis.*

Screening generally is applied to large groups of asymptomatic persons to identify those few persons who might have the undetected disorder. As a final descriptor of screening, it is the process that separates individuals with high and low probablity for a particular disease or disorder. Individuals identified with a "positive outcome" during the screening procedure must be considered only "at risk" for the problem until careful diagnostic testing can determine accurately the presence or absence of the disorder (Feightner, 1992).

The *validity* of a screening test is defined as the frequency with which the result of the test is confirmed by diagnostic evaluation. Validity may be considered the accuracy of the test in separating normal individuals from target individuals (i.e., the diseased from the nondiseased). Ideally, all individuals found positive on the screening test will indeed have the disease, and all of those with negative findings will be free of the disease. Unfortunately, this is seldom the case with hearing screening because diagnostic hearing tests are far more complex and more accurate in identification of mild or high-frequency hearing losses which are likely to be missed during the screening procedure.

The selection of a *screening cutting point* is the key to the performance characteristics of the screening test as described below. The *screening cutting point* is the value or level chosen to separate suspected positive individuals from suspected negative individuals. This has been a particularly difficult concept to apply in hearing screening because the cutting point for school-age populations is typically defined as a hearing level in decibels (i.e., 30 dB HL) for selected test frequencies (i.e., 500, 1000, 2000 Hz). With infant hearing screening techniques based on otoacoustic emissions and auditory brainstem response measurements, the screening cutting point is much more difficult to establish because of the complexity of the test results. To date, no thorough validity studies have been conducted as a function of screening cutting point for either infant screening technique. In fact, at this time, no recognized or agreed on screening cutting point exists for otoacoustic emission or auditory brainstem response screening in infants.

Performance Characteristics in Screening Tests

Prevalence and *incidence* are two important concepts that describe disease frequency within populations. Sometimes it is difficult to interpret screening data because the terms prevalence and incidence are often incorrectly used interchangeably even through they have two very different definitions:

- *Prevalence* is a census measure that expresses the presence of diseased patients per 100,000 persons in the general population at the time of the investigation.
- *Incidence* is the frequency of new outbreak of a disease condition in a population for a given time period.

An example of the relationship between the concepts of prevalence and incidence may be shown in the frequency of middle ear effusion found in infants and young children. The incidence may be high during the winter months when upper respiratory infection among children is common, whereas the prevalence rate may be low in the population of the southwestern states during the same time period. The operating characteristics of screening tests described below may vary as a function of both prevalence and incidence rates.

The model most frequently used to evaluate the performance characteristics of screening tests is known as the decision matrix analysis. In this model, analysis is focused on screening test outcomes and relates the results of screening to the actual presence or absence of the target disease which has been confirmed by follow-up testing. The results are traditionally presented in a 2 × 2 matrix as shown in Figure 7–1. The four components of the matrix table are the number of *true-positives* (those who turn out to actually have the target disease), *false-positives* (those identified in the screening who turn out not to have the target disease), *true-negatives* (those who are correctly identified as not having the target disease), and *false-negatives* (those who are not identified by the screening test, but in fact, turn out to actually have the target disorder). The "best" screening test results in the highest proportion of true-positives and the lowest false-negative rate (Jacobson and Jacobson, 1987).

The three terms used to describe the efficacy of a screening procedure are *sensitivity*, *specificity*, and positive and negative *predictive value.*

- The *sensitivity* of a test is its ability to correctly identify individuals who have the target disorder. If a test is described as hav-

	Impaired	Normal
Refer	A	B
Pass	C	D

FIGURE 7-1. A decision matrix demonstrating the computation of a test's operating characteristics. Sensitivity is the ratio of true positives (A) to the total number of impaired newborns (A + C). Specificity is the ratio of true negatives (D) to the total number of unimpaired newborns (B + D). False positives are represented by B, and false negatives are represented by C.

ing 80% sensitivity, it means that 8 out of 10 inividuals with the disease will be correctly detected. Sensitivity is the true-positive rate. In Figure 7–1 sensitivity is equal to (A/A + C) × 100.

- The *specificity* of a test reflects the number of individuals without the target condition that will be accurately identified. Specificity is the true-negative rate. In Figure 7–1 specificity is equal to (D/B + D) × 100.

- The *predictive value* of a test describes how accurately the test estimates disease or nondisease in a given population. The positive predicitive value is defined as the percentage of individuals who test positive and actually have the target disease. The negative predictive value represents the percentage of all negative results obtained from individuals who truly do not have the target disorder. Predictive value is dependent on sensitivity and specificity rates.

In general, the most effective screening tests have high sensitivity and high specificity rates. Sensitivity and specificity are regarded as fairly stable characteristics of a screening procedure, but their rates of accuracy can be manipulated by changing the pass and fail criteria (i.e., the screening cutting point).

Sensitivity and specificity share a reciprocal relationship: As sensitivity increases, specificity decreases, and as specificity increases, sensitivity decreases. This concept can be demonstrated for hearing screening by manipulating the pass-fail criterion based on a specific auditory threshold value. If the criterion level for passing the hearing screen is changed from 20 dB to 30 dB, more hearing-impaired persons will pass the screening test. Thus, the sensitivity for the screening test will increase (i.e., all the normal hearing persons will pass the test easily), but the specificity rate will decrease because more persons with hearing impairment will not be correctly identified by the screening test. If, on the other hand, the criterion level is made more stringent with a change from 20 dB to 10 dB, it will be more difficult for normal hearing persons to pass the screening, thereby creating a lower sensitivity rate, but fewer hearing-impaired persons will pass the screening test, thus increasing the specificity (false-negative) of the protocol.

It may be noted that the screening protocol criterion can be set to favor a specific test outcome. That is, if too many over-referrals are being generated by a screening protocol, altering the cutoff criterion will result in reduction of the apparent prevalence of the target disorder and fewer screening failures because more individuals will "pass" the screening test. A stringent pass criterion level will help assure that no individuals with the target condition will escape being correctly identified, but the cost of such a low criterion will be a high false-positive rate.

A practical demonstration of the importance of the precise criteria that are chosen to define screening outcomes is presented by Hyde, Riko, and Malizia (1990). These researchers reduced over-referral (false-positive rate) by altering ABR pass-fail criterion at the expense of increasing their false-negative rate. Decreasing the false-positive rate to 1%, for example, would result in an over-referral of less than 0.2% normal hearing infants for every baby identified as having a hearing loss.

However, when screening is being conducted for a low-prevalence condition, even a test with relatively high specificity may generate a large number of false-negative results. Individuals with the target disease who are missed by the screening test may not be aware that they have the disease until symptoms appear. Screening tests with high sensitivity are often responsible for a high number of false-positives identifications. These are individuals who are erroneously identified for further testing. This may create administative and economic problems in terms of the additional tests needed to correct this problem. High numbers of false-positive cases (over-referral) may overload the diagnostic capabilities available to the program, whereas an excessive number of false-negative cases (under-referral) undermines the purpose of the screening effort by missing the target patients. Any screening program can be tailored to meet the services available through manipulation of the screening cutting point or the algorithm used to determine referral from the screening test result.

These problems may be diminished by using a two-stage screening process, whereby a second low-cost screening test is applied before moving to additional diagnostic evaluations. Because of economic and time considerations, in the typical two-stage screening protocol, only individuals who fail the first screening test receive the second screening test. An example of this approach was described in Chapter 1, whereby the recommendation of the 1993 NIDCD Consensus Panel was for a two-stage protocol for universal infant screening based on first-stage otoacoustic emission screening for all infants followed by second-stage auditory brainstem response screening for infants who failed the initial screening. Obviously, the two-stage protocol is of value only in correcting the misidentification of the false-positive (over-referral) individuals. The false-negatives cases will be overlooked in the two-stage protocol until their disease becomes overtly symptomatic.

The problem in follow-up of false-negative persons is a difficult one. It is the most common fault in health screening programs. When only individuals who are detected as true-positives are followed and treated, sensitivity and specificity cannot be calculated; thus, the validity of the testing procedure cannot be accurately established. In reality, the only way to identify and follow-up the false-negative cases is to maintain contact with the entire population sample over an extended time period-a concept that is in direct opposition to the reasons for screening. However, true validation of any screening test must account for the diagnostic confirmation of all individuals screened.

Hearing Screening Applications in Infants

There are many unanswered questions regarding the various principles of screening when applied to newborn populations. Many of the issues in infant hearing screening have been debated for decades. Bess and Paradise (1994), in their outspoken criticism of universal screening for hearing impairment, argued that such an endeavor should not be undertaken without stronger justifications regarding practicality, effectiveness, cost, and harm-benefit ratio.

Answering these questions will require extensive research. In fact, the 1993 NIDCD Consensus Panel identified numerous areas they considered important for future studies . These topics included controlled trials of screening conducted by trained volunteers and qualified audiologists, the effectiveness of different screening techniques and protocols, evaluation of early intervention versus later intervention, careful investigation of the validity and reliability of the screening techniques, one- versus two-stage screening programs, and study of the cost-effectiveness of universal screening of infants for hearing impairment.

The 1994 Joint Committee also concluded their guidelines for screening with suggestions for areas in which additional research was needed. The Joint Committee recommended several research projects to facilitate establishing and maintaining infant hearing programs. Their recommendations included the need to develop a uniform state and national database with standardized screening protocols and cost-benefit analysis; the development of a tracking system to insure that newborns identified with or at risk for hearing loss have access to diagnostic evaluation, appropriate follow-up, and intervention services; the systematic evaluation of infant hearing screening techniques; ongoing studies of current indicators associated with hearing loss; and outcome studies to investigate the impact of early identification on the communication and education competencies achieved in life (Appendix F).

Before implementing a health screening program of any type, it is necessary to select testing procedures that meet standards of acceptability, simplicity, reliability, validity, reasonable cost, and appropriateness for the population to be tested. These factors are not necessarily independent of each other. For example, a test may be simple to administer, yet have poor validity. If the cost of follow-up testing on normals is considered important to the program, it may ultimately be less expensive to select a more complex and expensive test which has been determined to have strong validity to reduce the number of false-positive cases. The other, less favorable, approach is to apply some simple, less expensive screening procedure with questionable validity which may then require additional follow-up to substantiate the identification of target individuals.

Many authors have attempted to analyze the infant hearing screening issue by answering the following classic questions.

Is Hearing Loss in Infants Sufficiently Prevalent to Warrant Screening?

It is somewhat surprising that, after nearly four decades of debating the need and value of early identification of hearing loss, few data exist regarding the actual prevalence of childhood deafness in the general population. Most research reports are based on small samples of "inadequately collected and vaguely described data which lead to conclusions that are uncertain and inaccurate" (Mauk and Behrens, 1993, p. 2). Conclusions about the prevalence of congenital hearing loss have been questioned by Stein (1995) who points out that the frequently cited data are based on fewer than 10 published studies.

Published estimates of the prevalence of childhood deafness vary widely because the various projects and researchers defined significant hearing loss at different cutoff levels. Early studies used nonstandardized infant screening procedures to identify hearing loss and generally lacked confirming follow-up of the identified infants. Few, if any, studies reported verification that the "passed" infants actually had normal hearing. The contribution of these uncontrolled variables has resulted in the inability to generalize results of specialized sample studies to the population as a whole. Further, when mild or moderate hearing losses, as well as unilateral or conductive hearing losses are included in the statistical analysis, prevalence estimates are considerably higher than when only permanent, bilateral hearing loss is considered.

For many years, 1 deaf child per 1,000 live births was the accepted and quoted prevalence of hearing loss in children. However, this 1:1,000 estimate was based on the identification of newborns with congenital, profound, bilateral, sensorineural hearing loss of 80 dB HL or greater. This prevalence estimate was often questioned because it failed to include (1) the higher incidence of sensorineural hearing loss among infants with developmental disabilities and (2) well-babies with a lesser degree of sensorineural hearing loss. Considering that the prevalence rate for mild-to-moderate developmental disabilities in the general population is greater than the prevalence rate of profound disabilities, 3 infants with significant hearing impairment per 1,000 may be a more realistic (although still conservative) estimate of prevalence for the well-baby population. Adjusting the prevalence rate to account for infants at risk for developmental disability including hearing loss (30 to 50 of every 1,000 are hearing-impaired) and well-babies with moderate, severe, or profound sensorineural hearing loss yields a prevalence estimate of 6 babies with significant hearing loss for every 1,000 births (Hayes and Northern, 1994).

Bess and Paradise (1994) attempted to estimate the number of over-referrals if the NIDCD Consensus Panel recommendations were put into operation by screening all 4 million infants born in the United States each year (Table 7–2). Based on 1 infant with hearing impairment in every 1,000 live births, they calculated that 43,960 infants will be referred for comprehensive diagnostic evaluation; of these, 4,000 will be truly hearing impaired, and 39,960 will have normal hearing. In their calculations, almost 10 infants with normal hearing are referred for every baby who truly turns out to have a hearing loss. Northern and Hayes (1994) recalculated the Bess-Paradise estimate based on a more precise estimate of prevalence rates for childhood hearing loss. Table 7–3 shows that 62,572 infants from a universal screening sample of 4 million babies will be referred for comprehensive auditory evaluation of which 22,800 are truly hearing-impaired and 39,722 have normal hearing.

New technologies and comprehensive efforts at universal hearing screening for infants have produced better estimates of hearing loss prevalence than previously available. The Rhode Island Project, which is dedicated to universal hearing screening of infants, has reported a prevalence rate for all degrees of sensorineural hearing loss of 3.98/1,000 from a sample of 3,300 newborns and a rate of 2.61/1,000 from a larger sample of 7,000 babies. As reported by the Colorado State Program in unpublished statistics (1996), hospital-based programs screened 20,700 new-

Table 7–2. Bess-Paradise (1994) calculations to show 43,960 infants referred for complete auditory evaluation to identify 4,000 infants with hearing impairment. Calculations based on prevalence of 1:1000.

| | EOAE Screening | | | ABR Screening | |
	Impaired	Normal		Impaired	Normal
Refer	4,000	399,600	Refer	4,000	39,960
Pass	0	3,596,400	Pass	0	359,640

Source: Northern and Hayes (1994). Universal screening for infant hearing impairment. *Audiology Today, 6*(2), 11.

Table 7–3. Northern-Hayes (1994) re-calculation of Bess-Paradise (1994) paradigm from Table 7–2. The above paradigm is based on more precise prevalence rates for childhood hearing loss. Table 7–3 shows 65,572 referred for comprehensive auditory evaluation to identify 22,800 infants with hearing impairment. Calculations based on a prevalence estimate of 6:1,000.

| | **EOAE Screening** | | | **ABR Screening** | |
	Impaired	Normal		Impaired	Normal
Refer	22,800	397,720	Refer	22,800	39,772
Pass	0	3,579,480	Pass	0	357,948

Source: Northern and Hayes (1994). Universal screening for infant hearing impairment. *Audiology Today,* 6(2), 11.

borns to derive a prevalence rate of 4.58/1,000. In Utah, 1,900 infants were screened with a prevalence rate of 4.2/1,000 for sensorineural hearing loss in infants (Mahoney and Eichwald, 1987). However, it is difficult to compare these state programs because screening techniques and pass-fail criteria differ substantially.

Northern and Hayes (1994) developed a theoretical model to estimate the prevalence of sensorineural hearing loss in two populations: infants with no known risk factors and infants with high-risk factors for deafness. They based their calculations on the facts that approximately 10% of the 4,000,000 newborns born in the United States annually are at risk for developmental disability and at least 30 of every 1,000 at risk infants have been shown to have hearing loss. Calculations supporting this estimate of a prevalence ratio of 5.7/1,000 are shown in Table 7–4.

By comparison with other diseases that are routinely screened at birth, hearing loss has a much higher prevalence. In statistics reported for Rhode Island by Johnson et al. (1993), phenylketonuria (PKU), hypothryoidism, and sickle cell anemia have prevalence rates of 0.10/1,000, 0.25/1,000 and 0.20/1,000 respectively. Comparable statistics for the State of Colorado are shown in Table 7–1.

Table 7–4. Estimated number of infants with hearing impairment in two populations: infants with no known risk factors and infants at high-risk.

Category	Number Born Annually	Prevalence	Total Hearing-Impaired
No known risk	3,600,000	3:1000	10,800
At high-risk	400,000	30:10000	12,000
Total	4,000,000	5.7:1000	22,800

Source: Northern, J., and Hayes, D. (1994). Universal screening for infant hearing impairment. *Audiology Today, 6*(2), 11.

Are the Consequences of Hearing Loss in Infants Sufficiently Serious to Merit Screening?

The issue of early versus late treatment for hearing impairment seems clear: the future of a child born with signficant hearing impairment who is not identified and provided with appropriate intervention, has no way to acquire the fundamental language, social, and cognitive skills required for later schooling and success in society (Healthy People 2000, p. 460). Language is essential to learning; the earlier intervention begins for youngsters with hearing impairment, the more likely they are to develop communication skills on par with their normal hearing peers.

The cost of education for children with hearing impairment presents a viewpoint about the merits of hearing screening which can lead to earlier identification of hearing impairment. A detailed cost analysis done for the U.S. Department of Education concluded that every hearing-impaired child who is educated in a special self-contained classroom costs $6,306 more per year than hearing-impaired children who are mainstreamed into regular classrooms. Hearing-impaired children educated in state residential progams cost $32,397 per child per year more than children educated in regular classrooms (Johnson et al., 1993). These findings suggest that hearing-impaired children who enter school with better language and communication skills due to earlier identification are less likely to need extensive special education services.

The Educational Audiology Association (Von Almen et al., 1994) states that early identification is a bargain as educational costs increase significantly with the intensity of services required. Children with mild to moderate degrees of hearing impairment have the potential to be educated in regular classrooms with minimal special support. Deaf children can be educated in regular classes with the services of an educational-interpreter if they posses age-appropriate language skills. Table 7–5 compares regular classroom education and special education costs for Colorado children with hearing impairment. The EAA concludes that taxpayers can pay a little bit early in a child's life (i.e., cost of hearing screening and early intervention services) or pay more later due to the specialized eductional requirements for children with developmental delay due to late identification of their special needs.

A different point of view as answer to this question has been presented by the European community. For every child rehabilitated in Europe, it is estimated that the social expenses required during the adult years are reduced by at least $300,000.

Table 7–5. Regular education versus special education in terms of cost.[a]

Placement	Annual Cost	Excess Cost/Yr
Regular Education[a] (No special education services)	$4064.75	
Itinerant/Consultative (Usually up to 5 h/wk of special education services)	$5767.55	+702.80
Resource (Usually up to 20 h/wk of special education services)	$6397.55	+2332.80
Self-Contained (More than 20 h/wk of special education services)	$12,389.75	+8325.00
Preschool (Special education preschool 3 /day)	$8193.98	+2129.23
Residential (Placement at Colorado School for the Deaf and Blind)	$31,139.00	+27,074.25
Early Home Intervention Program[b] (In home family intervention- 90 min/wk)	$2600.00	

[a]Non special education student cost based on 1993 state average per pupil operating revenue

[b]Home Intervention Program-Colorado Department of Health, Handicapped Children's Program (Birth-2)

Source: From Executive Board of the Educationl Audiology Association (1994). Letters to the Editor, Pediatrics, 94(6), 957.

Do Screening Techniques Exist That Are Accurate, Efficient, and Cost-Effective for Identifying Hearing Loss in Infants?

Most infant screening programs at this time use either or both the auditory brainstem response (ABR) technique or otoacoustic emissions (OAE) measurement as the primary screening tool(s). Numerous research studies have confirmed sensitivity and specificity rates in excess of 96% for auditory evoked response screening on newborns (Hall, Kripal, and Hepp, 1987; Hyde et al., 1990; Jacobson, Jacobson, and Spahr, 1990). This high level of sensitivity and specificity is far more efficient and accurate than screening tests that are more commonly used such as mammography and Pap smears. Although less data are available concerning the operating characteristics of otoacoustic emissions used for screening the hearing of infants, preliminary data suggests that OAE screening sensitivity is high, but the procedure's specificity is lower than for ABR screening. Data reported from screening more than 3,700 infants in the Rhode Island Project with OAEs results in a test sensitivity of 100% and specificity of 82% (White, Vohr, and Behrens, 1993).

Are There Available Proven Treatments That Will Change the Outcome of Hearing Loss for Infants if Detected Earlier Rather Than Later?

The answer to this question is the essence of the importance of early intervention as discussed in detail in Chapter 10. Early intervention for infants with hearing loss is delivered in a family-centered approach and includes substantial family support and counseling by a multidisciplinary team; selection, evaluation, fitting, and monitoring of appropriate amplification; and auditory and language stimulation. For ethical reasons, it is not possible to implement a prospective study comparing early with late intervention in infants with hearing loss (Hayes, 1994).

Certainly, the predominance of evidence strongly favors a better prognosis for children with hearing impairment who are identified early and provided with appropriate early intervention. As one example, Markides (1986) reported a large longitudinal study in which children who were identified with sensorineural hearing loss and received amplificiation within the first 6 months of life showed far greater language development than children who did not receive amplification until later.

Are Services and Facilities Available for Diagnosis and Treatment for Infants Identified as Having Significant Hearing Loss?

This is considered by many critics to be an important liability in existing infant screening programs. We have repeatedly emphasized that an infant screening program serves no purpose if appropriate follow-up facilities for diagnosis, treatment, and management are not readily available. We agree that professionals who are trained in the management of infants with hearing impairment are not evenly distributed among rural and urban communities. Nonetheless, it is imperative for the persons responsible for the administration of an infant hearing screening program to insure that access to early intervention specialists will be available for infants identified with hearing loss and their families.

Because there may be wide variation in the needs of infants identified in the screening process, referral options must include audiologic, medical, surgical, educational, psychological, and other allied health and social service sources. Intervention services should be instituted as soon as possible following identification of an infant with hearing impairment. Home intervention and parent educational services are usually available in the local communities and often at no direct cost, or at least minimal cost, to families in need. Concern has been expressed concerning the availability, accessibility, and compliance of treatment of hearing loss in infants, especially in rural and impoverished communities. However, the same concerns may be expressed equally to all areas of health services. Access to services for infants and young children with hearing impairment has been enhanced as a result of federal and state legislative actions. Amendments to the federal Education of the Handicapped Act (P.L. 99-457) provided for statewide, comprehensive, coordianated multidisciplinary, interagency progams of early intervention services for all handicapped children and their families.

Cost of Infant Hearing Screening Commensurate with Benefits Derived for the Identified Individuals?

Accountability for outcomes, as well as the economics in hearing screening programs, is an important consideration. Infant hearing screening programs often are established and conducted on an emotional basis rather than on sound accounting principles (Finitzo, 1995). The determination of cost for infant hearing screening can be evaluated by several different techniques, again making comparison among studies difficult. Recently, however, several reports have been published which, although not conclusive, can begin to provide insight into the cost of infant hearing screening.

Turner (1992a) examined in theory every variable possible to estimate a cost of less than $7,000 per hearing-impaired infant from the intensive care nursery; in applying the same rational to the well-baby nursery, his estimate of cost jumped to $71,000 for each infant identified with hearing impairment. Based on actual costs of operating a universal newborn hearing screening program, the Rhode Island Infant Hearing Assessment Project calculated a cost of $26.05 per infant screened (Maxon, White, Behrens, and Vohr, 1995). Based on their prevalence data of 5.95/1,000, the screening of 4,253 infants over a 6-month period produced an estimated cost of $4,378 per infant identified with sensorineural hearing loss (Table 7–6). The reported cost of screening for each infant identified with phenylketonuria (PKU), hypothyroidism, or sickle cell anemia in Rhode Island is $40,960 (Johnson et al., 1993). Raffin and Matz (1994) estimate the cost of a national hearing screening program to be $233,320,000 for 1 year, or $58,330

Table 7–6. Actual costs of operating a unversal newborn screening program.[a]

Personnel	$60,654
Screening technicians (avg of 103 hrs/wk)	
Clerical (avg of 60 hrs/wk)	
Audiologist (avg of 18 hrs/wk)	
Coordinator (avg of 20 hrs/wk)	
Fringe benefits (28% of salaries)	$16,983
Supplies, telephone, postage	$12,006
Equipment[b]	$ 5,575
Hospital overhead (24% of salaries)	$14,557
Total Costs	$110,775

Cost per infant screened = $110,775/4253 = $26.05.

[a]These costs were calculated based on actual expenditures at Women and Infants Hospital of Rhode Island between July 1 and December 31, 1993.

[b]Equipment includes 3 EOAE unites, 1 ABR unit, 4 personal computers, 2 printers amortized over a 5-year period. Costs presented here are for 6 months only.

Source: White, K., and Maxon, A. (1995). Universal screening for infant hearing impairment: simple, beneficial, and presently justified. *International Journal of Pediatric Otorhinolaryngology, 32,* 205.

per child identified as hearing-impaired. They point out that this estimated price of a national program amounts to about 90 cents per United States resident.

Turner (1991, 1992a, 1992b) developed a series of three papers devoted to modeling the cost and performance of various early identification protocols for infant hearing screening. Turner refuted the historical approach to these problems, which generally was based on intuition and clinical experience, as unacceptable because of the lack of quantitative data and the inherent vulnerability to personal bias and undetected errors. He argued that, although the best approach to evaluating the cost and performance of various protocols for early identification of hearing loss in infants was to perform detailed cost-benefit analysis, he noted that this model was too difficult to be practical. Turner suggested that the most reasonable model of cost and performance analysis was based on a compromise of the above two methods. He used certain factors for which he could calculate cost with reasonable accuracy, as well as subjective analysis of factors for which it was not easily to determine actual costs. Turner carefully includes every aspect of the early identification program in his evaluation including the costs of the screening protocol, diagnostic evaluation, and patient follow-up. He reports that many factors influence the cost of early identification, but the greatest economic impact is related to two factors: (1) the false alarm rate (percentage of normal hearing infants in the nursery who are incorrectly called hearing impaired by the protocol) and (2) the success of the follow-up percentage. Obviously, with a higher follow-up success rate, more babies receive diagnostic testing, and diagnostic testing carries the highest expense burden of the protocol. This triad of excellent essays provides realistic considerations which may be used to develop and analyze early identification program protocols.

SUGGESTED READINGS

Goldbloom, R. and Lawrence, R. (Eds.). (1990). *Preventing Disease: Beyond the Rhetoric*. New York: Springer-Verlag Publishers.
    A comprehensive textbook which joins together public health officials and primary care physicians for an overview of the current state of knowledge regarding all areas of health screening and intervention.
Oleske, D. (Ed.). (1995). *Epidemiology and the Delivery of Health Care.* New York: Plenum Press.
    A general presentation of the concepts and considerations necessary for the provision of public health care and delivery of health services.

CHAPTER 8

The Hearing Evaluation
of Infants

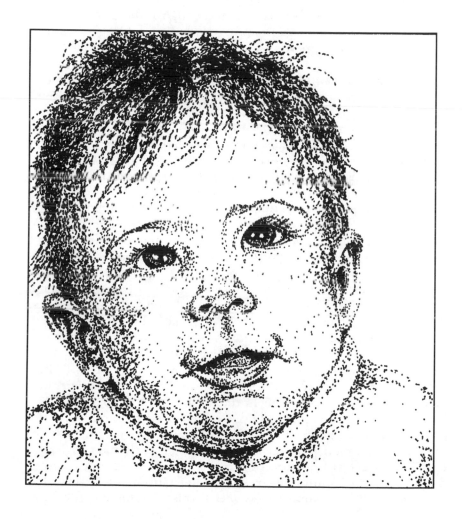

Assessment of hearing is the cornerstone of the field of audiol-ogy. The challenge of accurately determining the hearing sta-tus of an infant or young child is met through specialized training and extensive clinical experience. Behavioral assessment of pedi-atric patients is complicated by developmental and maturational limitations. However, establishing the precise degree and configu-ration of hearing loss in each ear is critical to the provision of medical treatment as well as individualized intervention services for children (ASHA, 1991). Although nonbehavioral electrophysio-logic measurements are useful and may be necessary in the evalu-ation of hearing in infants, the ultimate confirmation of hearing loss by behavioral audiometry is mandatory.

No single auditory test is precise enough to be a perfect and complete assessment tool. Defining the nature and degree of an infant's hearing loss inevitably requires the use of multiple tests and techniques that include threshold and suprathreshold mea-sures. Behavioral observation audiometry cannot yield precise predictions of hearing sensitivity in infants and young children, but may, in conjunction with a physiological test such as auditory brainstem response audiometry or otoacoustic emission measure-ment, provide useful information. In fact, Jerger and Hayes (1976) strongly recommended the use of the crosscheck principle in pedi-atric audiometry (i.e., using a physiologic test such as acoustic immittance or ABR, as confirmation of behavioral test results).

The basic pediatric hearing evaluation consists of a thorough developmental history followed by behavioral frequency-specific threshold tests, acoustic immittance measurements, and brain-stem auditory response (ABR) and otoacoustic emission (OAE) tests as necessary. The pediatric hearing test typically is an ongo-ing, age-specific activity because, as the infant grows older, more accurate hearing results can be expected. Pediatric audiologists depend on a test battery approach, with measurements obtained in sound field and under earphones, when possible, to complete the hearing evaluation of infants and young children.

Each infant or young child presents unique behavioral and developmental characteristics to the audiologist; the specific behavioral audiometry protocol utilized should be adaptable to dif-fering circumstances. Obviously, the approach to each pediatric audiology evaluation needs to be flexible within the confines of the individual situation. The pediatric audiologic evaluation includes careful behavioral observation assessment of unconditioned responses and conditioned response measurement by various techniques. It is beyond the scope of this chapter to provide a complete description of pediatric audiology procedures, therefore our discussion is limited to techniques appropriate to the evaluation of hearing in infants. A comprehensive description of pediatric audiology used with young children is available in Northern and Downs (1991).

The importance of establishing the precise type, degree, and configuration of hearing impairment for each ear should not preclude the initiation of intervention services such as the selection and fitting of personal amplification, (i.e., hearing aids, FM systems, and other assistive listening devices) (ASHA, 1991). The ongoing assessment process should be viewed as an intregal part of the management of the hearing-impaired child. Single assessment at a given point in time does not adequately address the problems of progressive or delayed-onset hearing losses. Obviously, newborns and infants at risk for progressive hearing loss must be scheduled and monitored with routine audiologic and otologic evaluations.

DEVELOPMENTAL ASSESSMENT

Because newborns and infants do not generally demonstrate a variety of responses to sound in the clinical environment, the pediatric auditory evaluation should begin with questions for the parent or responsible caregiver. The audiologist should always determine the primary reason for their concern about the infant's hearing. Some parents may have an intuitive belief that their newborn is not responding to sounds appropriately or there may be a significant history of deafness in the family background. Many parents of newborns or infants with lesser degrees of hearing impairment are misled because their child may, in fact, show intermittent appropriate responses to sounds and speech. In some situations, an informal case history will reveal these inconsistent infant responses.

Normal Speech Development

Concurrent with the maturation of auditory functions are the development of speech and language skills (see Table 8–1). Language acquisition occupies a central role in early childhood, and therefore may be used as a simple measure of overall developmental integrity. Although an infant is able to differentiate sounds in the first few months of life, the production of sounds does not develop at the same rate.

Table 8–1. Milestones in speech, language, and hearing development.

Birth–3 Months
 Startles to loud noises
 Calms to familiar voices
 Makes vowel sounds—ooh, ahh
 Squeals, coos, laughs, gurgles

3–6 Months
 Makes variety of sounds, "ba-ba," "ga-ba"
 Enjoys babbling
 Likes sound-making toys
 Changes voice pitch
 Turns eyes and head toward sound

6–9 Months
 Responds to own name
 Imitates speech with nonspeech sounds
 Plays with voice repetition, "la-la-la"
 Understands "no" and "bye-bye"
 Says "da-da" or "ma-ma"
 Listens to music or singing

9–12 Months
 Responds differently to happy or angry talking
 Turns head quickly toward loud or soft sounds
 Jabbers in response to human voice
 Uses two or three simple words correctly
 Gives toys when asked
 Stops in response to "no"
 Follows simple directions

12–18 Months
 Identifies people, body parts, and toys on request
 Turns head briskly to source of sound in all directions
 Can tell you what he or she wants
 Talks in what sounds like sentences
 Gestures with speech appropriately
 Bounces in rhythm with music
 Repeats some words that you say

18–24 Months
 Follows simple commands
 Speaks in understandable two-word phrases
 Recognizes sounds in the environment
 Has a vocabulary of 20 words or more

Source: Reproduced with permission from Presbyterian/St Luke's Community Foundation, Denver, CO.

By the first month, the normal infant "coos" and "gurgles," in addition to crying. By 2 months of age, the infant begins to emit specific sounds more than other noises. Between the ages of 2 and 4 months, the infant seems to focus on the production of vowel-like sounds and true babbling begins. At 5 months, the infant vocal emissions include consonant-vowel combinations. Glottal and labial sounds are heard from the infant by the age of 6 months. At 9 to 10 months, the glottal sounds decrease and alveolar sounds are frequently used.

Babbling ceases at about 6 months of age, and during the next few months, there is undistinguished progress in vocalizing speech sounds. During this period, the mother's feedback of the child's sounds provides the groundwork for the first production of a word. Vocalizations of congenitally deaf infants are identical to those of normal hearing infants until about 5 or 6 months of age. However, the lack of auditory feedback to the deaf infant soon causes vocalization quantity and quality to change (Stoel-Gammon and Otomo, 1986). By 8 months of age, research shows that the spontaneous vocalizations of normal hearing and hearing-impaired infants are clearly different (Kent, Osberger, Netsell, and Hustedde, 1987).

During the second 6 months of life, the infant with normal hearing continues to mimic sounds vocalized by the mother. The sounds of the infant are further imitated by the mother, who in turn adds additional speech improvisations. Soon thereafter the infant now imitates the mother's imitation, and the shaping of the infant's speech pattern is under way. Comprehension of the sound sequence may precede the imitation; sometimes imitation precedes understanding of the meaning of the sound sequence.

The child's first meaningful word is usually uttered around the first birthday and is dependent on a full year of attentive listening activity. Many children are able to repeat "ma-ma" or "da-da" by the age of 9 months. Soon after utterance of the initial word, the child should begin to rapidly build vocabulary. By 18 months the child should have at east a six-word vocabulary and by the age of 2 years should be able to express meaningful two-word sentences. In an intriguing research report, Eilers and Oller (1994) reported that infants with normal hearing produced canonical vocalizations (the production of well-formed syllables) before 11 months of age, whereas infants who were found to be deaf failed to produce canonical syllables until nearly 24 months of age or sometimes well into the third year of life.

Language Screening

It is good clinical practice to include a formal history questionnaire. During the infant's first year of life, completion of a simple questionnaire during the 3-, 6-, and 9-month "well-baby" primary health care office visit can facilitate the early detection of children with impaired hearing (Matkin, 1984). Table 8–2 shows a very simple early detection checklist with four questions related to auditory responsiveness, three questions related to vocal output, and one question that assesses social and motor development to be asked at each "well-baby" visit. Referral to an audiologist or speech-language pathologist should be considered if two or more of the communication questions are answered "No" and the subsequent case history confirms the presence of a delay in the development of preverbal communication behavior.

Developmental language delay is an early sign often associated with hearing loss, so it behooves audiologists to be familiar with administering and interpreting screening tests that include language subtests. There are more than 50 tests of childhood language function, and a full discussion of language screening is beyond the scope of this textbook. However, most of the language tests are not suitable as screening tools for infants and toddlers. Some of the language testing procedures lack age-specific criteria for passing or failing, many have little or no normative data, and few have been validated against other standardized testing instruments.

The Denver Developmental Screening Test (DDST)

The screening test most frequently used by primary care physicians to detect developmental delays during infancy and the preschool years is the *Denver Developmental Screening Test* (Frankenburg and Dodds, 1967). The test yields an overall developmental profile with special emphasis on gross motor, language, fine motor-adaptive, and personal-social skills. It may be administered by trained nonprofessional health aides in 10 to 25 minutes. The test is well-normed on more than 1,000 infants and children that reflect the ethnic, occupational, and economic characteristics of the Denver population. The test includes a gross test for hearing based on the child's response to a loud bell. Although the DDST is frequently used for screening language skills, Walker, Gugenheim, Downs, and Northern (1989) reported poor agreement on the language sector of the DDST with evaluations conducted by qualified speech-language pathologists.

Table 8–2. Simple parent questionnaire for infant development.

QUESTIONS AT 3 MONTHS:

YES	NO		YES	NO	
__	__	1. Jumps (startles) to sudden loud sounds.	__	__	1. Has a special cry when hungry.
__	__	2. Stirs from sleep when there is a loud noise.	__	__	2. Coos when fed and dry.
__	__	3. Stops sucking when there is a sudden new sound.	__	__	3. Laughs.
__	__	4. Smiles at mother.	__	__	4. Holds head up straight while lying on the stomach.

QUESTIONS AT 6 MONTHS:

__	__	1. Turns in the general direction of a new or sudden sound.	__	__	1. Seems to enjoy making sounds with voice, like "baba," "ooh, ooh."
__	__	2. Usually stops crying when mother talks baby.	__	__	2. Chuckles, gurgles, or laughs when. playing.
__	__	3. Enjoys a musical toy.	__	__	3. Makes happy sound when sees is going to be fed.
__	__	4. Reaches out to be is going to be picked up by someone in the family.	__	__	4. Rolls over, either from back to front or from front to back

QUESTIONS AT 9 MONTHS:

__	__	1. Responds to his or her name to "No" and "bye-bye."	__	__	1. Imitates speech but doesn't use real words.
__	__	2. Know if a person's voice sounds friendly or angry.	__	__	2. Seems to be using "own words" to name things.
__	__	3. Looks directly at a new sound or voice.	__	__	3. Makes a lot more and different sounds than a couple of months ago.
__	__	4. Plays peek-a-boo.	__	__	4. Sits well without any help.

Source: "Early recognition and referral of hearing-impaired children" by N. Matkin, 1984, *Pediatrics in Review, 6*(5), p. 153.

The Early Language Milestone Scale (ELM)

Coplan et al. (1982) developed and provided normative data for newborns, infants, and toddlers (0–3 years of age) for a screening test of receptive and expressive language development known as the *Early Language Milestone* (ELM) Scale. The ELM Scale allows for identification of 41 language milestones during the initial 36 months of life in normally developing children. The ELM Scale is a brief assessment tool, requiring 3–6 minutes to administer, with both receptive and expressive items that are specifically age-related. The ELM Scale is reported to yield 97% sensitivity and 93% specificity as a detector of developmentally delayed children. The ELM is based largely on parental report, especially for infants, and the results are only as valid as the accuracy of the parent's recall of developmental milestones.

The Minnesota Child Developmental Inventory (MCDI)

The *Minnesota Child Developmental Inventory* is a more extensive screening instrument used to identify children with developmental delay (Ireton and Thwing, 1972). The MCDI is a 320-item questionnaire that is filled out by the child's primary caregiver. It is composed of eight subtests that evaluate different areas of development including general development, gross motor skills, fine motor skills, expressive language, comprehension-conceptual (language understanding) and comprehension-situation (nonverbal understanding), personal-social, and self-help areas. Children are considered to be functioning within normal developmental limits if their developmental age is greater than 75% of their chronological age. The MCDI identifies children as "borderline delayed" (delay between 25 and 30% of chronological age) and "delayed" (developmental age lower than 70% of chronological age). Apuzzo and Yoshinaga-Itano (1995) administered the MCDI to 69 deaf infants and reported results as a function of infant's age of identification.

When an infant is identified through any standardized screening tool to be functioning significantly below age level, referral must be made for additional testing and evaluation. The referral service will determine if the aberrant screening test finding may be due to problems other than hearing loss. Matkin (1984) suggested that developmental delay in vocabulary, syntax, and phonologic development of 6 months or more is an important possible indicator of bilateral hearing loss. The guideline of a 6 month lag permits the wide variation that may be observed in the normal development of expressive communication. On the other hand, any parental concern for speech and language problems in their young child should be given immediate attention.

Normal Auditory Maturation

Murphy (1962), in England, originally described the auditory maturation process that all normal-hearing infants go though during their early development period. Although considerable variability exists among newborns and infants as to the actual age when each auditory maturation skill is achieved, the knowledgeable observer should be able to identify the presence or absence of age-appropriate responses to sound. Behavioral observation may also be used to corroborate the parent or caregiver's report of the child's auditory behavior, but should not be used as a threshold technique.

During the first 4 months of life, the newborn's behavioral responses to auditory stimuli are limited to reflexive reactions such as arousal from sleep, eye widening, and eye lid blinks which may, or may not, be associated with limb or body startle movements. However, between 4 and 12 months of age, the infant with normal hearing progresses through an orderly auditory matura tion process (Northern and Downs, 1991).

Between 4 and 7 months of age, the normal infant response to sound is a horizontal head turn toward the sound source. At 4 months the head turn is slow and labored, but by 6 months of age the head turn should be definite and brisk. At approximately 7 months of age, the infant should be able to localize to the sound source when it is presented on a lower plane. By 9 months, the baby should be mature enough to perform higher plane localization successfully. And by 12 months of age, the infant with normal hearing should be able to locate the sound source in any plane on either side of the body easily and briskly.

UNCONDITIONED BEHAVIORAL ASSESSMENT PROCEDURES

Evaluation techniques that do not incorporate reinforcement prin ciples are known as unconditioned assessment procedures. These techniques are based on careful observation of some active response to the presence of a sound stimulus. Behavioral observation audiometry may be carried out at crib side, in a pediatrician's office, or in any relatively quiet environment where a skilled observer can present auditory stimuli with known acoustic properties. The unconditioned response may or may not be predefined by some criterion definition, and is often described in terms of reflexive reactions (i.e., startle jerks of arms and/or legs, changes in sucking rhythm, eye blinks, etc.) or change in attending behaviors (i.e., increases or decreases in ongoing activities). An example of an unconditioned behavioral response is the eye-widening response of an infant to the onset of a noise band stimulus in a soundfield, or a full-body startle response observed in a lightly sleeping newborn upon the sudden presentation of a loud acoustic stimulus. Without reinforcement of some type, these unconditioned behavior responses typically show rapid extinction.

Behavioral observation audiometry, or BOA, was the mainstay of clinical audiologic testing of infants and newborns for many years prior to the development of electrophysiologic measures of hearing. Limitations to unconditioned behavioral observation audiometry include rapid habituation of the response which is related to the state of the infant during testing, the parameters of the acoustic stimulus, and the definition of what behavior is accepted as a qualified response. The most significant limitation of BOA, however, is its dependence on subjective judgment by the audiologist as to whether a "qualified response" has occurred. With the application of learning theory concepts taken from the field of psychology, improved methods of behavioral testing of hearing, utilizing response reinforcement paradigms, have been developed and implemented in pediatric audiology (Northern and Downs, 1991).

In pediatric audiology, observation of unconditioned responses is usually conducted with newborns and infants less than 18 months of age. It is necessary that the audiologist be clinically competent in the use of behavioral observation audiometry as a limited hearing screening procedure. BOA is time- and cost-efficient and does not require extensive technical equipment.

Typically, during behavioral observation audiometry, the examiner will use selected bands of noise generated by a small hand-held device, or toys that produce generally low- or high-frequency sounds. No special instrumentation or facility is needed to perform BOA. A trained examiner may perform these measures in a quiet environment with commercially available noisemakers and toys. Because the acoustic environment, the acoustic stimulus, and the infant's response are not under direct control of the examiner, BOA measures are limited and should be considered only estimates of hearing levels and as representing only the response of the better hearing ear.

CONDITIONED BEHAVIORAL RESPONSE TECHNIQUES

Procedures for testing the hearing of children utilizing reinforcers for the elicited action are known as conditioned behavioral response techniques. The procedures are additionally defined by a description of the reinforcer used or the required response which must be observed prior to delivering the reinforcement. The conditioning approach to assessing hearing levels in children is based on a stimulus presentation followed by a specially defined and repeatable active response from the infant or young child. After each acceptable action response, the child's behavior is strengthened through the use of some type of reinforcement. The reinforcement typically is some pleasurable sensory experience or brief play activity.

Behavioral conditioning of infants from birth to 4 months of age to soundfield auditory stimuli is generally agreed not to be feasible. Normally developing infants and young children between 5 months and 24 months age, however, are good candidates for the conditioned behavioral procedures such as visual reinforcement audiometry (VRA), conditioned orientation response (COR) audiometry, visual or tangible reinforced operant conditioned audiometry (VROCA or TROCA), and conditioned play audiometry (CPA). It is important to establish hearing thresholds through conditioned response audiometry with frequency-specific stimuli such as pure tones, FM tones, or narrow bands of noise. Because of the relationship of frequency information between 1500 and 3500 Hz to the perception of speech, the audiologic assessment, at a minimum, should always include threshold measurement at 2000 Hz for each ear when possible. Of course, effective masking of the opposite ear must be utilized as necessary.

Matkin (1977) introduced the descriptor "minimum response level" (MRL) to describe the lowest intensity of an auditory stimulus that produces the expected response during unconditioned or conditioned audiometry with children. Matkin suggested that the use of the term "auditory threshold" implies an exactness of measurement which, in fact, may not be true; whereas the use of the term "minimum response level" implies that improvement in measurement levels may be forthcoming in subsequent evaluation sessions as the infant matures and his or her response skills progress in development.

Visual Reinforcement Audiometry (VRA)

Visual reinforcement audiometry is a powerful assessment technique when conducted by a trained and experienced audiologist.

During the VRA procedure the infant's response behavior can be shaped by the examiner's control of the stimulus-reinforcement paradigm. The audiologist presents calibrated, frequency-specific signals into a controlled acoustic environment. An appropriate sound-treated room or special testing booth with interior dimensions adequate for soundfield measures is essential (i.e., loudspeakers should be at least 1 meter from the infant). The testing system should include adequate animated reinforcing toys.

Visual reinforcement audiometry is the simplest conditioned response procedure used in pediatric audiometry. In this testing paradigm, the infant is required only to detect the auditory stimulus and then respond with a motor head turn in the direction of the reinforcer (Primus and Thompson, 1987). The VRA technique typically utilizes a lighted (or animated) toy, presented at 90° to one side of the infant, that is flashed on and off to reinforce a head-turn response (see Figure 8–1). The expected head-turn response is always in one direction toward the visual object. During training trials, the toy is lighted simultaneously with presentation of the auditory stimulus while the infant's head is turned in the direction of, and the infant is looking at, the rein-

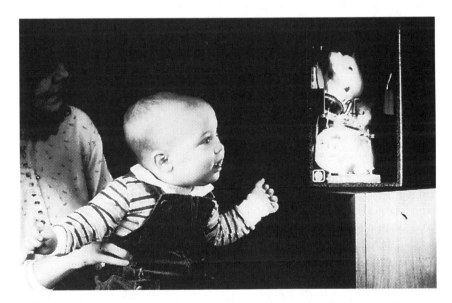

FIGURE 8–1. Visual reinforcement procedure is a simple conditioned response technique. When the infant localizes to the presence of a sound signal, the head turn is reinforced with a lighted toy.

forcer toy. During the training trials, the clinician must be sure that the auditory stimulus is presented loudly enough to be heard easily by the infant. After simultaneously pairing the presentation of the auditory stimulus with the flashing light visual reinforcer through several training trials, the clinician presents the auditory stimulus by itself at a high intensity level and waits for the infant to turn its head toward the toy. When the head turn response occurs, the visual reinforcer quickly is flashed on and off several times to reinforce the infant's head-turn response. Once the visual conditioning is clearly established, and the head-turn response occurs consistently following presentation of the auditory stimulus, subsequent trials are conducted with decreasing intensity levels of the stimulus until the minimal level response of the head turn can be established.

Generally, VRA is conducted in a soundfield environment with calibrated FM pure tones or narrowband noise stimuli. Moore, Thompson, and Thompson (1975) reported success in using the VRA technique in infants as young as 5 months of age. Matkin (1977) achieved 90% success with VRA under earphones in children with normal hearing and hearing impairment between the ages of 12 and 30 months. Moore, Wilson, and Thompson (1977) determined the rank order of visual reinforcers according to their effectiveness in eliciting the VRA head turn response in 12–18 month old infants to be (a) an animated toy, (b) a flashing light, and (c) social approval reinforcement such as exaggerated hand-clapping and facial display of pleasure. In our clinical experience, the VRA evaluation can be extended by using a variety of visual reinforcers or using them together rather than one at a time.

Eilers, Wilson, and Moore (1977) utilized VRA techniques to demonstrate that 1 to 3 month old infants could already discriminate between certain phonemic contrasts in speech sounds. She named the procedure Visually Reinforced Infant Speech Discrimination (VRISD). In a study of 6-month-old infants with normal hearing from the United States and Sweden who were exposed to only their own national language, Kuhl et al. (1992) used the VRISD technique to show that exposure to a specific language in the first 6 months of life alters infants' phonetic perception. These studies underscore the value of the VRA technique in evaluating the hearing of infants.

Conditioned Orientation Response (COR) Audiometry

Conditioned orientation response audiometry places a somewhat higher demand on the response required from the infant. The technique differs from the VRA procedure in the fact that two lighted, or animated, reinforcers are utilized. Each visual, or animated, reinforcer is placed 90° to either side of the infant's midline gaze. The task for the infant is initially to hear the auditory stimulus presentation, localize the source of the stimulus, and respond with a motor head turn toward the side of the stimulus presentation. The clinician reinforces only correct localization head-turn responses by flashing the lighted toy, briefly turning on the animated toy, providing excitatory social approval, or any combination of the visual reinforcers.

The COR training trials are much like the VRA training trials, except that directing the infant's attention to the two stimulus positions initially may require prompting or physical assistance. As the conditioned response requires a two-level task (i.e., detection of the stimulus and appropriate head turn), COR is easier to perform with children in the 9 months to 36 month age range. It is advantageous to keep the stimulus sound source and the reinforcer toy in close proximity so that the pairing of the stimulus and visual reinforcement is in the same plane as the required localization head-turn response.

As children grow older than 12 months of age, more complex tasks can be used to determine their hearing levels. Speech audiometry techniques, visual or tangible reinforcement operant conditioning procedures, or conditioned behavioral activities may be utilized to establish individual threshold audiograms for each ear with frequency-specific information. These pediatric audiometric techniques, however, are beyond the scope of this textbook, because the focus here is within the first year of life.

NONBEHAVIORAL AUDIOMETRIC TECHNIQUES

Early and comprehensive assessment of hearing is essential to the provision of appropriate, individualized intervention strategies for infants and young children with hearing impairment. In fact, an essential component of all infant hearing screening programs is the availability of comprehensive audiologic evaluation facilities staffed by audiologists experienced in pediatric hearing testing.

The 1972 Joint Committee on Infant Hearing Screening pointed out that the high incidence of false-positive and false-negative results obtained through behavioral observation of newborn responses to auditory signals was unacceptable. By 1982, with the advent of early nonbehavioral measures of infant hearing, the Joint Committee recommended the use of behavioral or electrophysiological measurements to accomplish infant hearing screening (see Appendices A and C).

In the 1990 and 1994 versions of the Position Statement on Early Identification of Hearing Loss, the Joint Committee has recommended that only physiologic measures, such as auditory brainstem response (ABR) or otoacoustic emissions (OAE) be utilized in infant hearing screening programs.

The 1994 Position Statement concludes that behavioral observation measures cannot validly and reliably detect hearing loss of 30 dB HL in infants younger than 6 months of age.

The search for objective, nonbehavioral, methods for detecting hearing loss in infants is most interesting. Several innovative programs and ingenious devices have been developed over the years to automate and develop objective infant hearing screening protocols. Although many of the systems have fallen into disuse for a variety of reasons, review of these techniques may suggest future applications based on improved technologies (Swigart, 1986).

Electrodermal Response Audiometry

In the 1940s and 1950s, many clinicians used electrodermal response audiometry (EDR) as an "objective" test for evaluating hearing in children. Electrodermal response audiometry was based on the galvanic skin response and grew out of experimental psychology. The testing technique was based on a conditioning paradigm during which the clinician paired a pure tone and mild electric shock so as to elicit an autonomic change in the sweat glands of the skin. This change in the state of the sweat glands is measured as a reduction in resistance to a small electric current flow between two electrodes taped to the patient's skin. The conditioned autonomic sweat reflex, which involuntarily occurs when the patient "hears" the pure tone stimulus, is easily noted on a single-channel strip chart recorder. Auditory thresholds can be determined at single test frequencies in one ear at a time by judiciously presenting pure tones at decreasing intensities and reinforcing the autonomic galvanic skin response with a mild electric shock.

Although the technique of electrodermal response audiometry was used through the decade of the 1960s to confirm the degree of hearing loss in malingering or noncooperative adults (Goldstein, 1963), the use of EDR as a nonbehavioral technique with infants and children was fortunately set aside as more accurate, less invasive, and more humane objective testing techniques were developed.

Heart Rate Response Audiometry

Another autonomic conditionable response came from experimental psychologists who discovered that change in heart rate could be measured in the presence of auditory stimuli. Zeaman and Wegner (1954, 1956) reported that a brief, moderately loud pure tone would cause a temporary wave-like alteration of the electrocardiogram. In some subjects, the unconditioned heart rate response caused a decelerative type of change, whereas other subjects showed an accelerated heart rate following presentation of an auditory stimulus. The Zeaman and Wegner studies confirmed that changes in heart rate were, in fact, specifically related to the intensity of the auditory signal. Bartoshuk (1962, 1964) examined the cardiac response to sound in neonates. These researchers successfully verified that cardiac acceleration could be reliably observed in 1-, 2-, 3-, and 4-day-old infants. Unfortunately, repeated stimulus presentations, without an easy means of response reinforcement, created cardiac response habituation. Schulman (1970) and Schulman and Wade (1970) conducted research studies on the clinical utilization of heart rate response change as an objective means to identify hearing loss in infants. Schulman was able to obtain reliable cardiac responses with band-limited noise signals of 34 dB SPL in a test time of approximately 20 minutes per infant. Eisenberg (1974) suggested that cardiac responses of audition could be potentially important in infants, but that considerable research was still necessary to define the parameters of the testing technique. With the advent of auditory brainstem response audiometry in the early 1970s, interest in heart rate response as a means to test hearing in infants disappeared.

Respiration Audiometry

Respiration audiometry was developed as a technique for predicting hearing sensitivity by monitoring changes in respiration that occur in response to auditory stimuli. It is a common observation in neonates that sleeping babies often show an increase in respiration rate and amplitude following stimulation by loud sounds. Researchers attempted to quantify this autonomic response with the use of a strain gauge system around the patient's chest (Teel, Winston, Aspinall, Rousey, and Goetzinger, 1967) or a thermistor (a heat-sensing device that changes its electrical resistance in response to a difference in temperature) taped below the patient's nostrils (Hayes and Jerger, 1978). Respiration audiometry was reported to be easy to administer with a simplicity of instrumentation and interpretation of response. Bradford (1975) used pure tone stimulation with respiration audiometry to validate normal hearing in 4- and 12-month-old infants. However, the subjective interpretation of the response proved troublesome for clinicians, and respiration audiometry never caught on as a technique for evaluating hearing in newborns.

The Crib-O-Gram

The Crib-O-Gram was an ingenious automated system for detecting hearing loss in newborns utilizing a motion sensitive transducer placed under the crib mattress to detect any motor activity from the infant stronger than an eye blink or facial grimace including the mild motion created by resting respiration (Simmons and Russ, 1974). The system, developed at Stanford University, was a microprocessor-based, self-cycling, automated program that turned itself on, performed the test, interpreted the results, and then turned off following each complete stimulus presentation and response measurement interval (Jones and Simmons, 1977; Simmons, 1976).

The Crib-O-Gram system monitored the infant's state by measuring crib movement before and after each auditory stimulus presentation (see Figure 8–2). The test stimulus (2000–4000 Hz band-pass noise) was delivered from a transducer placed in the

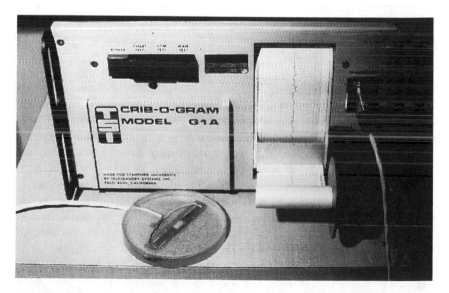

FIGURE 8–2. The Crib-O-Gram was an automated infant hearing screener that operated by monitoring crib movement caused by the baby moving after hearing an auditory stimulus presentation (see text for further explanation).

bassinet and presented 20 or more times over a 7- to 24-hour period. Responses in the form of baby movement (or lack of movement) were analyzed by the microprocessor until a statistically valid decision could be made by the unit regarding whether the baby passed or failed the hearing screening.

The Stanford research group tested more than 12,000 infants with the Crib-O-Gram between 1974 and 1984. Their work established a firm incidence rate for infant deafness of 1:1,000 in the well-baby nursery and 1:52 in the neonatal intensive care nursery. The false-positive rate was 8% for well-babies and 20% for NICU infants (Simmons, McFarland, and Jones, 1979). The Crib-O-Gram had several unique advantages as a system for screening hearing in infants: (a) it was easily operated by minimally trained personnel; (b) it did not interrupt the normal nursery routine; and (c) it was truly an objective hearing screening procedure. Unfortunately, it also had several disadvantages: (a) as an automatic system, it was subject to mechanical failure; (b) the initial cost for the equipment was expensive; (c) an adequate infant response required a high-intensity stimulus greater than 75 dB SPL; and (d) the automated test paradigm was often lengthy for each infant. Although the Crib-O-Gram offered great promise as an automated infant screening system, studies by Wright and Rybak (1983) and Durieux-Smith et al. (1985) showed the device to produce an unacceptably high false-positive rate as well as poor test-retest reliability in repetitive studies of the same infant.

The Auditory Response Cradle

The Auditory Response Cradle was developed in England in 1980 as an automatic, microprocessor-based newborn hearing screening system (Bennett, 1980). More elaborate than the Crib-O-Gram, the Auditory Response Cradle was designed to examine several infant motor responses following programmed auditory stimulus presentations: (a) trunk and limb movements; (b) startle head jerk reflex; (c) changes in respiratory pattern. An 85 dB SPL filtered noise band (2600–4500 Hz) is the auditory stimulus presented to the infant through miniature ear canal probe tips. The automated program presents stimulus trials as well as an equal number of no-sound control trials and then calculates the probability that the infant's motor responses are valid and not unrelated spontaneous movements. When the microprocessor determines a 97% probability rate, the baby is passed as normal hearing. The average length of time for each infant test is reported to be 2 to 10 minutes. More than 5,000 babies had been evaluated with the

Auditory Response Cradle by 1984. Infants with severe hearing loss as well as infants with middle ear disease have reportedly been identified with this hearing screening system while maintaining a low false-positive error rate (Bhattacharya, Bennett, and Tucker, 1984). Apparently well received in England, the Auditory Response Cradle has not been widely used in the United States, perhaps due to the high expense of the equipment.

Acoustic Immittance Measures

Acoustic immittance measurements were introduced into the clinical audiology arena in the early 1970s. Currently, acoustic immittance measurements are an intregal part of every audiology evaluation. By definition, acoustic immittance audiometry is an nonbehavioral objective means of assessing the integrity of the peripheral hearing mechanisms and higher auditory pathways. The acoustic immittance battery of tests is used to categorize the nature of the hearing loss into conductive, cochlear, or brainstem pathology. Acoustic immittance tests are used to determine middle ear pressure, tympanic membrane mobility, Eustachian tube function, integrity and mobility of the middle ear ossicles, and stapedial reflex threshold measurements as well as evaluation of the afferent and efferent auditory pathways.

Acoustic immittance tests have proven especially valuable in the pediatric hearing evaluation, often providing illuminating information in addition to that obtained on the routine audiometric and otologic examinations. The instrumentation requires an air-tight seal of a small probe tip in the external ear canal. The probe tip emits a low frequency tone and measures the sound pressure of the reflected ambient sound energy in the external ear canal. An air pressure system is capable of creating positive, negative, or atmospheric air pressure in the cavity between the probe tip and the tympanic membrane. The technique is relatively simple to conduct, efficient, requires only passive cooperation from the child, and provides a multitude of information regarding the hearing disorder. Current acoustic immittance instrumentation is automated and ranges from automatic microprocessor-based units with data storage capabilities to miniaturized hand-held screening immittance devices (Figure 8–3).

Routine clinical acoustic immittance applications include the tests described below. Although each test provides significant information about the function of the auditory system, the diagnostic power of the measurements is greatly enhanced when the procedures are utilized together and interpreted as a test battery.

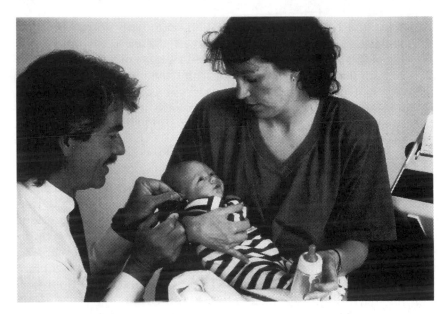

FIGURE 8–3. Acoustic immittance measurements are especially important in pediatric hearing evaluations.

A comprehensive discussion of acoustic immittance measurements is provided by Northern (1995).

- *Tympanometry*—evaluates the integrity and compliance of the tympanic membrane and middle ear system; the technique clearly differentiates the normally mobile system from the nonmobile system; tympanometry also measures middle ear pressure and is especially useful to monitor the pathophysiology of otitis media.
- *Equivalent ear canal volume*—a measure of the volume of air between the immittance probe tip and the tympanic membrane; larger than normal volume is associated with a nonintact tympanic membrane.
- *Acoustic reflex measurements*—measure the contraction of the stapedial muscle when the ear is stimulated with sufficiently loud sound; may be used to establish acoustic reflex thresholds for pure tone and filtered noise band signals; measurements are conducted in the ipsilateral (afferent system) or contralateral (efferent) mode. The acoustic reflex is not measurable in ears with conductive loss and present at reduced sensation levels in ears with cochlear-disorders.

Some controversy exists regarding the use of acoustic immittance measurements in infants as reviewed by Northern (1988). Paradise, Smith, and Bluestone (1976) raised questions about the use of tympanometry when their evaluation of 280 young children showed a high positive correlation (86%) between tympanometry and otoscopy for patients older than 7 months of age but conflicting findings in infants less than 7 months who had confirmed otitis media and yet demonstrated normal tympanograms. Groothuis et al. (1979) found a 92% correlation between otoscopy and tympanometry in infants who were older and younger than 7 months of age. Both studies were flawed, however, by depending on tympanometry only for immittance diagnostic conclusions. Other research studies have confirmed that the acoustic reflex in newborns shows that the prevalence of the infant acoustic reflex increases as probe-tone frequency increases (Northern and Downs, 1991). Nonetheless, the general consensus among clinicians is to use caution when performing immittance measurements with infants younger than 6 months of age.

Auditory Brainstem Response Audiometry

As early as 1939, Davis reported that small changes in electroencephalic activity could be observed in response to auditory stimulation. However, only with the advent of the signal-averaging computer during the 1960s did electroencephalic response audiometry become clinically feasible. The signal-averaging computer algebraically sums the potentials that occur in a fixed time interval following stimulation while "averaging out" random physiologic noise and extraneous electrical activity. This computer enhancement creates an improved signal-to-noise condition which amplifies the specific, time-locked, small magnitude potentials. The physiologic activity is "evoked" with rapid click or filtered noise stimuli presentations. Following multiple stimulus presentations, the computer sums the mean electroencephalographic values obtained during each sampling interval, and waveforms begin to emerge from the baseline physiologic activity. The waveform can be enhanced by increasing the number of stimulus presentations.

In recent years, auditory potentials have been extensively investigated in the auditory and visual modalities using a variety of stimuli and recording techniques. It should be understood that the ABR is, in fact, not a test of hearing per se in the perceptual sense. Therefore, behavioral audiometry and acoustic immittance measures are crucial to complete the pediatric evaluation of hearing sensitivity. In fact, the ABR evoked by click stimuli is greatly influenced by high-frequency hearing loss and therefore limited in providing information regarding auditory sensitivity to frequencies between 1000 and 4000 Hz. Complete information about auditory evoked potentials and their clinical applications may be found in textbooks by Jacobson (1995) and Hall (1992).

Several evoked auditory potentials have been identified by researchers and categorized in terms of their latencies. The shortest latency evoked auditory response occurs prior to 10 msec and reflects the activities of the cochlea, eighth nerve, and brainstem. Hence, these early components are known as the auditory brainstem response (ABR). The ABR presents as a well-defined waveform with five positive direction peaks at latencies between 2 and 10 msec. The ABR is typically a robust response noted for its repeatability and the fact that it is relatively unaffected by the patient's physiological state. Thus, the ABR may be used to provide important clinical information regarding the function and physiology of the auditory system such as site-of-lesion specificity and auditory sensitivity measures.

The evoked ABR waveform is, however, influenced by stimulus parameters such as type, rise-decay time, rate of presentation, and so on. These effects are well-described and therefore predictable to the knowledgeable clinician. For example, the amplitude of the auditory brainstem response is related to the stimulus intensity; the higher the stimulus intensity, the larger the amplitude of the ABR waveform. The growth of wave amplitude is predictably associated with a decrease in response latency of the peak components. As the stimulus intensity is lowered, the waveforms are reduced in amplitude; within 10 to 15 dB of the hearing threshold the composite waveform disappears. In newborns, especially in premature infants, the ABR waveform shows maturational changes. Without adequate normative standards as a function of gestational age, misinterpretation of waveforms can easily occur. Maturation of the infant ABR is completed between 12 and 18 months postterm (Finitzo-Hieber, 1982).

The clinical attributes of the ABR have been well established over the past 25 years. The major disadvantages of ABR measurements are the initial high cost of the equipment, the requirement for a well-trained professional to administer and interpret the tests, and the time consumption of complete data collection. These disadvantages are, however, outweighed by the advantages of ABR testing which include accuracy and reliability of measurement, clinical application in site-of-lesion information, and the determination of hearing sensitivity in difficult-to-test patients. The positive characteristics of the ABR technique make it particularly valuable for evaluating the hearing status of infants.

The evoked auditory brainstem response has become an important component in the evaluation of infants at risk for hearing impairment (Figure 8–4). Reliable ABRs can be recorded from infants as young as 30 weeks gestational age in the newborn intensive care nursery. Conventional ABR testing has been part of the pediatric audiologic test battery for nearly two decades, but the high initial cost of the equipment, the relatively lengthy test time required, and limited access for rural and remote hospitals have limited its utilization. The 1994 Joint Committee on Infant Hearing pointed out that ABR has been recommended for newborn hearing assessment for almost 15 years and has been successfully implemented in both high-risk register and universal hearing screening programs. In many neonatal intensive care units (NICU), ABR is routinely used to screen the hearing of infants (Galambos et al., 1984; Gorga, Reiland, Worthington, and Jesteadt, 1987; Stein et al., 1983).

In newborn hearing programs, the ABR typically is applied as a hearing screening procedure (ASHA, 1989). That is, the infant either "passes" or "fails" the hearing screen based on the presence of an electrophysiologic response to click stimuli at some predefined intensity criteria, usually 30, 40, and/or 60 dB nHL. The

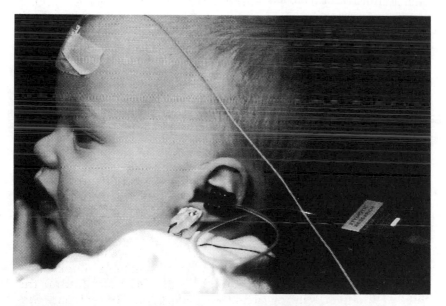

FIGURE 8–4. The auditory brainstem response provides an objective measurement of ear-specific hearing thresholds in infants and young children.

advantages of this approach are that it is a relatively time-efficient procedure and trained volunteers or technicians can conduct the tests without making on-line decisions (Dennis, Sheldon, Toubas, and McCaffee, 1984). For most infants the ABR hearing screening approach is adequate and results in a "pass" on the initial test. In many studies, approximately 80 to 90% of infants "pass" the ABR screen at 30 or 40 dB nHL (Galambos et al., 1984; Hyde et al., 1984; Jacobson and Morehouse, 1984). For infants who fail the single intensity screening test, information is insufficient to predict degree of hearing impairment or the site of dysfunction (Stein et al., 1983). Complete information about the infant's hearing loss is obviously important for appropriate otologic and medical management of the newborn, but is also crucial for the development of effective follow-up habilitation strategies. Accordingly, infants who "fail" the ABR screening test are referred for a complete diagnostic ABR procedure with responses evaluated for threshold and latency measures obtained at a number of different intensity levels. The complete ABR procedure can provide information relevant to both predicted degree of hearing loss and probable site of dysfunction (middle ear, cochlear, or brainstem). Thus, ABR threshold-latency measures as a function of stimulus intensity permit validation of test accuracy and differentiation of auditory disorder from neurologic abnormality (Despland and Galambos, 1980).

The American Speech-Language-Hearing Association (ASHA) developed specific guidelines in 1989 for the audiologic screening of newborns who are at risk for hearing impairment which delineate ABR as the recommended procedure prior to hospital discharge. The guidelines state that "optimally, all newborns should receive audiologic screening to identify the majority of infants who require audiologic evaluation, follow-up, and management" (p. 1).

The ASHA-recommended "pass" criterion for ABR screening is a response from both ears at 40 dB nHL or less. It is important to note that "pass" on ABR screening does not rule out development of hearing impairment in infancy or early childhood. Infants whose responses meet the pass criterion but are at risk for progressive hearing impairment should receive audiologic monitoring on a periodic basis. Infants who do not demonstrate responses at intensity levels of 40 dB nHL should be referred for additional audiologic evaluation and follow-up. Infants who have an ABR response at 40 dB nHL in only one ear should receive audiologic monitoring until either (a) both ears meet pass criterion or (b) stable unilateral hearing impairment is confirmed and follow-up management is initiated.

Automated ABR Infant Screening

During the mid-1980s, an automated ABR system was developed that not only performs the screening test, but also determines the presence of the auditory evoked response. There are several methodological factors that may influence the outcome of ABR infant hearing screening such as earphone placement, collapse of the infant ear canal, muscle artifact, environmental noise, and pass-fail criteria. Peters (1986) described an automated infant screener, known as the Algo-1, based on advanced evoked response technology developed by A. Thornton at the Massachusetts Eye and Ear Infirmary to overcome the problems in ABR infant screening (Figure 8–5).

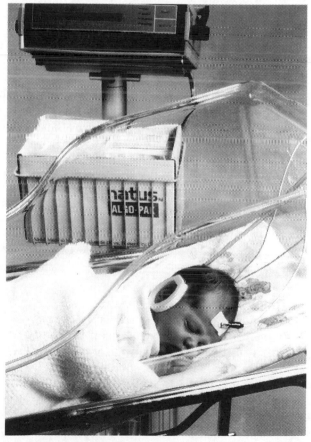

FIGURE 8–5. Automated ABR is commonly used in infant hearing screening programs.

The Algo-I is a battery-operated, microprocessor-controlled instrument, designed solely for infant hearing screening. The computer uses a statistical model for objective detection of the ABR response based on a 35 dB nHL alternating unfiltered click stimulus presented sequentially to each ear. The Algo-I features a number of unique design features such disposable circumaural foam cushion earphones with adhesive backing that seal around the infant's pinnae to reduce environmental noise and automatic artifact rejection systems to control for excessive ambient noise and myogenic interference. The device extracts the desired ABR signal response embedded in the raw EEG activity through a template-matching detection algorithm (Kileny, 1987). If the infant under examination shows an evoked ABR that "matches" the normal ABR template of the Algo-I, a "pass" decision is rendered by the microprocessor; if a suitable match of waveform is not identified by the Algo-I with an extended presentation of stimuli, a "refer for further testing" decision is made by the device.

Peters (1986) presented data from clinical trials with the Algo-I at eight test sites. She reported 94% agreement with the automated ABR system and conventional ABR testing of 304 infant ears; when rigid and strict research protocols were applied in a single clinical site to 136 infant ears, she found 98.5% agreement between results obtained with the two ABR systems. Jacobson et al. (1990) tested 224 stable high-risk infants with automated and conventional ABR and found the automated screener to be a viable alternative to conventional ABR testing. Because trained volunteers can be used to conducted the infant hearing screening, under supervision of an audiologist, the automated ABR screening program is economically efficient (Markowitz, 1990).

Otoacoustic Emissions

Otoacoustic emissions (OAEs) are a relatively recent adjunct to nonbehavioral physiologic-based auditory response measurements. OAEs are low-level "leakage" of acoustic energy associated with the normal hearing process which can be detected with specialized equipment in the external auditory canal. These audiofrequencies are transmitted from the cochlea as a release of sound energy which in some cases is spontaneous, but most likely is evoked in response to external acoustic stimulation. Although the concept of extraneous acoustic energy reflected externally from the cochlea was theorized in 1948 by Thomas Gold, a young English physicist, it was 30 years later when David Kemp (1978) verified the presence of OAEs in the human external ear canal.

Kemp (1978) developed a computerized system which used a sound source and a miniaturized microphone mounted in a probe tip and sealed in the ear canal to measure otoacoustic emissions. Kemp used acoustic transients or clicks as the stimulus and then recorded an acoustic response beginning 5 msec following the onset of click stimulation. Because of his pioneering work, Kemp is credited with the discovery of OAEs which are now sometimes referred to as "Kemp's echoes." Subsequently, numerous research studies have confirmed that OAEs are a preneural by-product of the outer hair cell's active vibration or motility within the cochlea (Kemp, 1979; Kim, 1980). This discovery was especially important because of the long-held belief that the cochlear vibrations transmitted energy only upward through the auditory system. It was Brownell's research (1984, 1990) demonstrating the outer hair cell's active electromotile response that helped explain the mechanics of how OAEs are generated within the cochlea.

From the flurry of research activity which followed the discovery of otoacoustic emissions, two broad classes of OAEs emerged. First, there are *spontaneous emissions* which are present in about 60% of persons with normal hearing (Martin, Probst, and Lonsbury-Martin, 1990). Spontaneous otoacoustic emissions (SOAE) are low-intensity sounds measured in the external ear canal when there is no external sound stimulation. The second category of OAEs involves low-intensity evoked otoacoustic emissions elicited by low-to-moderate levels of acoustic stimulation presented through an ear canal microphone. This category generally includes transient evoked (TEOAEs) and distortion product otoacoustic emissions (DPOAEs). Both of these evoked otoacoustic emissions, TEOAEs and DPOAEs, are used in the hearing screening of infants, although adequate data are not yet available to determine which type is most effective in identifying neonates with hearing loss, or whether both procedures have comparable accuracy (Hall and Chase, 1993).

- *Transient evoked otoacoustic emissions* (TEOAEs) are stable, frequency-dispersive responses to brief acoustic stimulation presented repeatedly, such as clicks or tone pips, that begin 4 to 15 msec after the presentation of the stimuli (Kemp and Ryan, 1993). TEOAEs are easy to record and interpret with only a single stimulation channel that requires inexpensive synchronous averaging instrumentation which has been readily available since the 1970s. The technique samples the noise in the ear canal synchronously with stimulus presentations, and events that are time-locked to the stimuli are preserved in the resulting

averaged response (Glattke and Kujawa, 1991). The TEOAE
recording and measurement technique is the most common procedure used in infant hearing screening. Examples of TOAEs
from infants are shown in Chapter 4 (Figures 4–1, 4–2, and 4–3).

- *Distortion product otoacoustic emissions* are tonal responses
located at precise frequencies determined by two simultaneously presented pure tones with frequencies F1 and F2; the resulting DPOAEs occur at various distortion product frequencies,
including 2f1 – f2, 2f2 – f1, and 3f1 – 2f2 (Lonsbury-Martin and
Martin, 1990). The measurement of DPOAEs requires two separate high-quality stimulus channels and transducers with more
elaborate signal and processing equipment. The use of DPOAEs
to screen the hearing of infants is currently under study in
numerous hospital facilities.

The presence of evoked otoacoustic emissions has proven to
be evidence of a normal functioning cochlea and peripheral hearing system. Otoacoustic emissions are absent in the presence of
conductive hearing impairment and significant sensorineural
hearing loss (Anderson and Kemp, 1979). Cope and Lutman
showed that 80–90% of normally hearing ears produce OAEs, but
that these emissions can seldom be recorded from persons with
hearing loss in excess of 20–30 dB HL. Consequently, Luteman,
Mason, Sheppard, and Gibbin (1989) concluded that the presence
of a click-evoked OAE is a powerful indicator of normal hearing.
Collet et al. (1989) confirmed that subjects with sensorineural
hearing loss never show OAEs when the hearing loss at 1000 Hz
exceeds 40 dB HL. When outer hair cells are structurally damaged
or nonfunctional, otoacoustic emissions cannot be evoked by
acoustic stimuli (Norton, 1993). These findings led Kennedy et al.
(1991) to suggest that the discovery of otoacoustic emissions and
their subsequent application to newborn infants has opened new
avenues to quick and reliable hearing screening.

Interest in the use of OAEs as a technique for screening hearing in infants was first described by the French team of Bonfils,
Uziel, and Pujol (1988). These researchers compared evoked otoacoustic emissions in a sample of 46 infants (mean age of 4.6
months) in whom hearing levels had been evaluated with ABR.
Their subjects were 30 infants with confirmed normal hearing and
16 additional infants with confirmed sensorineural hearing loss.
Otoacoustic emissions elicited with click stimuli of 20 dB HL were
always present when the ABR wave V thresholds were equal to, or
better than, 40 dB HL. In the group of infants with sensorineural
hearing loss, all of whom showed ABR wave V thresholds greater

than 40 dB HL, no OAEs could be identified. Further, the authors reported that the recording of OAEs required approximately 5 minutes per ear, while ABR threshold measurements took an average of 40 minutes. Thus, these early studies suggested that OAEs might be an objective, nonbehavioral, noninvasive, and quick hearing screening procedure which could be used to divide infants accurately into normal hearing and non-normal hearing groups (Figure 8–6).

Other research studies of OAEs as an infant screening procedure followed the report of Bonfils et al. (1988). Stevens et al. (1989,

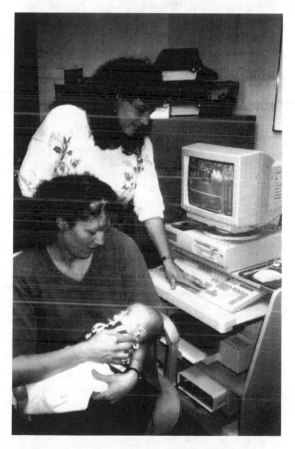

FIGURE 8–6. Evoked otoacoustic emission measurement is an efficient and accurate screening procedure to identify infants with normal hearing from those who might have hearing-impairment.

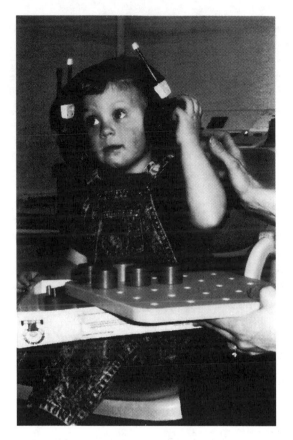

FIGURE 8–7. Hearing testing with young children can also be accomplished through play conditioning techniques.

1990) compared measurements from ABR and OAEs from more than 1,000 infants in NICUs in England. They reported that the evoked otoacoustic emission screen showed test sensitivity of 95% and specificity of 84% when compared with ABR. Stevens et al. concluded that because OAEs are much quicker to measure and yield nearly the same results as ABR, evoked otoacoustic emissions should be used as the primary method for screening infants, with ABR used as a follow-up procedure. Uziel and Piron (1991) collected evoked otoacoustic emissions from normal newborns and infants in NICUs and showed that all ears with no OAEs had ABR thresholds higher than 30 dB HL. Kennedy et al. (1991) reported that OAEs and ABR measurement identified the same babies with sensorineural hearing loss, but that the OAEs more accurately sorted out infants with conductive hearing loss than ABR screening.

In 1993, White and Behrens published a thorough monograph that described in detail the methodology and results of a large infant screening program conducted in Rhode Island. The purpose of their research was to evaluate the feasibility, validity, and cost efficiency of using TEOAEs as a technique for universal newborn hearing screening. Data were reported for 1,850 well-baby and NICU infants born during a 6-month period at the Women and Infants Hospital of Rhode Island. The initial 464 infants were screened using both TEOAE and ABR regardless of results on either test; the following 1,386 infants were screened first with TEOAE, and then only infants who did not pass were screened with ABR (White, Vohr, and Behrens, 1993).

From this sample of 1,850 infants, 11 were identified to have sensorineural hearing loss; 6 infants had bilateral severe-to-profound losses, 4 infants had unilateral severe-to-profound loss, and 1 had a unilateral moderate hearing loss. An additional 37 infants were found to have conductive hearing loss: 31 had bilateral and 6 had unilateral conductive hearing loss. These statistics indicate a prevalence of 5.9 sensorineural hearing losses and 20 conductive hearing losses per 1,000 births. Comparison of TEOAE and ABR results in normal hearing and confirmed sensorineural hearing loss infants between 6 and 12 months of age indicated sensitivity of 100% and specificity of 82% for TEOAEs; ABR screening showed sensitivity of 94% and specificity of 89% (White et al., 1993). The data from the Rhode Island project, according to the principal investigators, demonstrate that EOAE screening of newborns is simple, fast, economical, noninvasive, and accurate in identifying infants with hearing impairments. From a practical viewpoint, the experience of the Rhode Island project revealed the effects of other variables on the success of infant screening. TEOAEs were accomplished in 3.3 minutes if the infants were in deep sleep, but when they were awake or crying the procedure took 5.5 minutes. Infants in deep sleep or dozing state were much more likely to pass the TEOAE screen than infants who were awake or crying. As might be expected, an inverse relationship was found for infants who passed the TEOAE screen and the degree of ear canal obstruction created by debris. Cleaning the infant ear canals of vernix caseosa prior to TEOAE measurement significantly increased the chances for passing the hearing screening (Chang, Vohrn, Norton, and Lekas, 1992). Bergman et al. (1995) evaluated TEOAEs and DPOAEs in a sample of intensive care nursery (ICN) infants with good results. They concluded that

(a) TEOAEs and DPOAEs can be measured in graduates of the ICN with click-evoked ABR thresholds of 30 dB nHL or better and normal middle ear function; (b) both OAE amplitudes and noise amplitudes were larger in newborns compared to older normal-hearing subjects; (c) OAEs in neonates are more easily measured in the higher frequencies, but are difficult to measure at lower frequencies. However, this finding should have little clinical consequence because most educationally significant sensorineural hearing loss involves the higher frequencies; and (d) depending on the stimulus paradigm, both TEOAEs and DPOAEs can be measured very rapidly and are well suited as efficient screening techniques for perinatal hearing loss.

SUGGESTED READINGS

Northern, J., and Downs, M. (1994). *Hearing in Children* (4th ed.). Baltimore, MD: Williams and Wilkins.
   A comprehensive overview, including how-to-test procedures, for evaluating hearing problems in infants and children.
Jacobson, J. T. (Ed.) (1994). *Principles and Applications in Auditory Evoked Potentials.* Needham Heights, MA: Allyn and Bacon.
   This is an extensive textbook on auditory electrical potentials with a section devoted to newborn hearing screening.

CHAPTER 9

Comprehensive Assessment of Infants with Hearing Loss

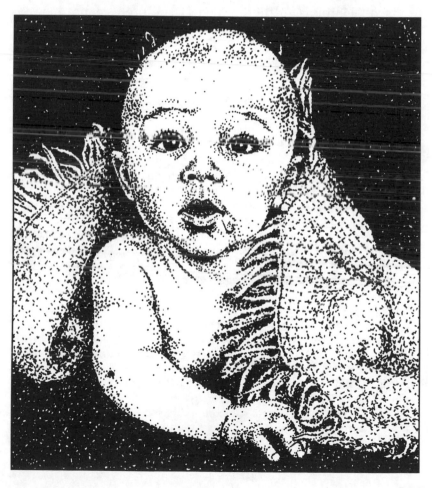

The story of Helen Keller, the young girl born in 1880, who lost her sight and her hearing as a result of a childhood illness, is well known to us all. The life of Helen Keller and her dedicated teacher, Anne Sullivan, who patiently taught Helen to communicate long before the advent of modern electronic technology, is documented in the acclaimed stage play and movie, *The Miracle Worker*, written by William Gibson. Most noteworthy is the famous quote of Helen Keller who said, "Blindness separates people from things, but deafness separates people from people."

Certainly, we have come a long way since the days of Helen Keller, but it has been a long, slow, and laborious journey—and we have not yet come even close to solving the important issues of childhood hearing loss. Much has been studied and written about childhood deafness, but much controversy still exists regarding the "best" solutions to the problems. The professional may be quick to state with confidence what will not work for the newly

---

HELEN KELLER, 1880–1968

Helen Keller is among the most noted American women of achievement. Although totally blind and deaf following a high-fever illness at the age of 19 months, she emerged to become an international role model. Her struggle with life is a stirring story of courage, hard work, and dedication. Born in Alabama, Helen Keller was a frustrated and angry 7-year-old girl who could neither see nor hear. Her famous teacher and lifelong friend, Anne Sullivan, accepted the seemingly hopeless task of educating this handicapped youngster. Under Ms. Sullivan's guidance and teaching, Helen Keller learned to read, write, and ultimately became a strong influence on the lives of others.

She graduated from Radcliffe College in 1904 on her way to becoming an accomplished author, popular lecturer, and political activist. Helen Keller was instrumental in the women's suffrage movement; a friend to several American presidents, industrialists, and entertainers; a popular feature of national news coverage; and a close friend to Alexander Graham Bell, inventor of the telephone in 1876. Overcoming two serious handicaps, Helen Keller traveled tirelessly and used her world-wide fame to bring hope to others with disabilities. "The two most interesting characters of the 19th century," said Mark Twain, "are Napoleon and Helen Keller." Her attitude toward life remains an inspiration to us all as she is often quoted, "Life is either a daring adventure or nothing!"

identified child with hearing loss. However, the same confident professional suddenly equivocates when it comes to recommending what actions that parents should take on behalf of their infant newly identified as deaf. Under these circumstances, is it any wonder that parents who learn that their infant is hearing impaired, don't know where to turn for help?

Prelingual sensorineural hearing impairment represents a diagnostic challenge even to hearing care professionals. It is important to note that hearing loss is a symptom and not a disease. The complex nature of hearing loss in infants makes it increasingly important for a team of professionals to work together, with the family, throughout the assessment and evaluation of the child to reach a diagnosis and formulate a treatment plan. Unfortunately, hearing loss is not an isolated disorder that can be "cured" through applications of modern technology. The treatment and management of hearing loss in infants requires both medical and educational considerations. Solutions are seldom simple and never certain. Assessments and management programs for the families of infants and toddlers with hearing loss involve complex and complicated problems that cannot be managed by a single discipline.

The diagnosis of hearing loss in an infant or young child is not an easy task and requires the cooperative effort of a number of professional specialists. Typically, the parents share their suspicion of hearing loss in their child with the pediatrician or family practice physician. Paradoxically, this can be an exasperating experience which can lead to delay in both the detection and diagnosis process. Primary care physicians commonly have little exposure to the identification and management of pediatric hearing impairment during their training or in their daily clinical practice. Primary care physicians often have crowded waiting rooms, work long hours, and have critical problems to solve. They may interpret parents' concern for their infant's hearing as a result of overprotective behavior and inadvertently delay decisive actions which may affect the family and child for many years.

Parents of children with hearing loss often indict physicians, describing doctors as unwilling to acknowledge their concerns for their child's lack of hearing, failing to perform formal hearing testing, and reluctant to refer the child to an ear specialist or audiologist for further evaluation. These stories are not just from decades past. Many physicians still believe erroneously that hearing in young children cannot be accurately evaluated, parents are not good judges of their infant's lack of response to sound, and young children are likely to outgrow their hearing problems. On average,

9 months pass between the time parents first discuss their concerns about hearing with a primary care physician and referral for audiologic testing. This delay usually occurs because the physician chooses to postpone making a definitive decision and just notes in his chart to follow-up on the parents' concern at the next office visit.

In 1978, parents of hearing-impaired children in Toronto, reported that, although the average age at which they initially suspected hearing loss in their children was 16 months of age, confirmation of hearing loss was delayed 11 to 60 months (Shah, Chandler, and Dale, 1978). Simmons (1980a) reported that 42 babies suspected to have hearing loss at the time of hospital discharge were not fitted with hearing aids until an average age of 22 months. Bergstrom (1984) found that her pediatric patients with hearing loss were suspected to be hearing impaired by their parents at 10 months, confirmed as having hearing impairment by audiologists at an average age of 21 months, and first fitted with hearing aids at 24 months. Elssmann et al. (1987) found the average age of identification of deafness in a group of surveyed parents was approximately 19 months. Audiologists were estimated to have contributed at least a 6-month additional delay between confirmation of the hearing loss and the fitting of hearing aids. The pattern of delay in these reports seemed to be related to (1) delayed action from the responsible physician; (2) infants with multiple medical or social problems in which hearing was only a part of the total concern of the parents; and (3) parental disbelief that their child had a significant hearing problem. The parents of hearing-impaired children often remember with bitter anger the physician who delayed referral of their child for evaluation.

Coplan (1987) reported on the delayed recognition of permanent hearing loss in 46 of 1,000 children referred to his developmental pediatric practice. He found that the mean age of diagnosis of pediatric hearing impairment was a function of the degree of hearing loss. Confirmed diagnosis of profound congenital deafness was at 24 months of age, but lesser degrees of congenital hearing impairment were not diagnosed until a mean age of 48 months. High-risk medical history or physical anomalies associated with embryological abnormalities of the auditory system that should have triggered a prompt search for deafness went unheeded in most cases. Coplan concluded that physicians should not place undue confidence in their ability to detect even major degrees of hearing impairment in infants and young children. Adherence to specific risk criteria, as suggested by the Joint Committee on Infant Hearing (see Chapter 1), regardless of the examiner's subjective impression of how well the infant or child seems to hear, would permit a more timely diagnosis of pediatric hearing impairment (see Table 9–1).

With improved technology to test the hearing of infants, the average age of identification of congenital hearing loss should be decreasing. At the same time, if we have the ability to detect infants with hearing loss accurately, it follows that full assessment and early intervention also should begin sooner. Stein et al. (1990) reported results from two studies of hearing-impaired infants who graduated from the well-baby nursery and an intensive care unit during the years 1980–1982 and 1983–1988. They found that the age of diagnosis of hearing loss for graduates of the intensive care unit was significantly earlier than for graduates of well-baby nursery, but the average age of enrollment in a habilitation program was approximately 20 months for both groups of infants.

Hearing loss in young children is a more common disorder than diabetes mellitus (1.5/1,000), spina bifida (1/1,000), congenital hypothyroidism (0.25/1,000), and phenylketonuria (0.08/1,000). However, the average pediatrician will likely see no more than 10 to 12 children with significant hearing loss in the course of his or her practice lifetime. Primary care physicians who are alert to the early signs of hearing loss in young children, and make the appropriate referrals for evaluation and treatment while providing good ongoing advice and support, can make all the difference to these children and their families.

Fortunately, a cadre of physicians trained and experienced in pediatric otolaryngology may be found in major medical centers. Although hearing loss, per se, is not a disease, the symptom needs

Table 9–1. Causes of hearing impairment in infants.

Prenatal (5%–10%)	Congenital infections (toxoplasmosis, rubella, CMV, herpes, syphilis, chickenpox)
Perinatal (5%–15%)	Prematurity and/or low birthweight, anoxia hyperbilirubinemia, sepsis
Postnatal (10%–20%)	Infection (meningitis, mumps) otitis media, ototoxic medications
Genetic (30%–50%)	Familial or sporadic, syndromic or nonsyndromic
Other (5%)	
Unknown (20%–30%)	

thorough medical evaluation to determine the cause of the hearing loss (see Table 9–1), identify any associated medical or developmental problems, and attempt to predict the chances of recurrence of deafness in future siblings. The medical work-up should include the following considerations: (a) history, including a full pregnancy review; (b) family pedigree, preferably by a qualified genetics counselor; (c) physical examination of the child and possibly other family members; (d) audiometric evaluation of other family members; (e) review of pertinent medical records; (f) laboratory studies as needed; (g) radiographic diagnostic imaging, and (h) scheduled routine medical follow-up as well as developmental speech and language evaluations at appropriate age intervals (Stewart, 1996).

THE COMPREHENSIVE ASSESSMENT

History

A probing history should be carefully obtained from the infant's parents. It is helpful to have both parents present during this part of the evaluation as it is necessary to obtain information from both the mother's and father's side of the family. It is estimated that some 60% of differential diagnoses are concluded from the history-taking portion of the medical examination. A complete history evaluation requires an examiner who is knowledgeable about etiologies of childhood deafness in order to know which history avenues to focus on. Of special importance, the examiner must have a thorough knowledge of the causes and common disorders associated with hearing loss, their clinical manifestations, and modes of treatment available (see Table 9–2).

Family Pedigree

Approximately one half of all congenital deafness is caused by genetic factors. Familial inherited deafness may be present at birth or develop later in childhood and, in many instances, is a progressive-type symptom. Evaluation of the family pedigree, or history, may provide important information about the etiology of the hearing loss and its mode of inheritance. When one or more siblings in the same family are found to have hearing loss and additional relatives such as uncles, aunts, grandparents, or cousins are also noted to have hearing loss, the stage is set for determination of inherited hearing loss. As described more completely later

Table 9–2. Hearing loss indicators.

During First Month of Life

Family history of hereditary childhood sensorineural hearing loss

In utero infection such as cytomegalovirus, rubella, syphilis, herpes, or toxoplasmosis

Craniofacial anomalies including morphological abnormalities of the pinna and ear canal

Birth weight less than 1500 g

Hyperbilirubinemia at a serum level requiring exchange transfusion

Ototoxic medications, including but not limited to the aminoglycosides, as used in multiple courses or in combination with loop diuretics

Bacterial meningitis

Apgar scores of 0 to 4 at 1 minute or 0 to 6 at 5 minutes

Mechanical ventilation lasting 5 days or longer

Stigmata or other findings associated with a syndrome known to include a sensorineural and/or conductive hearing loss

Up to 2 Years of Age

Parent or caregiver concern regarding hearing, speech, language, and developmental delay

Bacterial meningitis or other infections associated with sensorineural hearing loss

Head trauma associated with loss of consciousness or skull fracture

Stigmata or other findings associated with a syndrome known to include a sensorineural and/or conductive hearing loss

Ototoxic medications, including but not limited to aminoglycosides used in multiple courses or in combination with loop diuretics

Recurrent or persistent otitis media with effusion for at least 3 months

Until 3 Years of Age

Family history of hereditary childhood hearing loss

In utero infection, such as cytomegalovirus, rubella, syphilis, herpes, or toxoplasmosis

Neurofibromatosis Type II and neurodegenerative disorders

Recurrent or persistent otitis media with effusion

Anatomic deformities and other disorders that affect eustachian tube function

---

Source: From "The Sounds of Silence" by M. Lotke, 1995, p. 105., *Contemporary Pedia-*

in this chapter, identification of the specific mode of inheritance is often difficult, yet is important information for future generations of the family. Genetic deafness is difficult to identify when the family history is negative, and thus often becomes the diagnosis when no other factors can be identified.

Physical Examination

Although sensorineural deafness is a hidden handicap when it occurs in isolation, the physical examination may uncover significant findings to help identify the cause of the hearing loss. The examiner must be trained to identify features and abnormalities that are associated with childhood deafness. A congenital deformity is an alteration in the shape or structure of a body part that occurs most frequently during the fetal stage. As a general rule, the simpler the malformation, the later the defect occurred during the pregnancy. It is estimated that some 15% of all newborns may have a single simple malformation. When multiple or complex malformations are noted in an infant, the more likely the possibility that a severe problem will be identified.

The physical examination of the infant with hearing loss typically focuses on the head and neck, particularly the ears and facial features. The appearance of an infant's head or face may provide clues to the identification of a condition associated with hearing impairment. Many of the craniofacial syndromes, such as mandibulofacial dysostosis (Treacher-Collins) and trisomy 21 (Down syndrome), include various forms of hearing loss. For example, infants diagnosed with Fetal Alcohol Syndrome (FAS) have a characteristic facial dysmorphology which includes a specific list of features including shortened palpebral fissures, microthalmia (small eyes) and strabismus (crossed eyes), epicanthic folds, maxillary hypoplasia, micrognathia, thin upper lip, hypoplastic philtrum, short upturned nose, flattened nasal bridge, small head, and poorly formed external ears (Gerkin and Church, 1987). Commonly seen pinna anomalies, which may exist in isolation or accompany other deformities, include pre-auricular (supernumerary) tags, sinus tracts or pits, atresia or stenosis of the external ear canal, and abnormally rotated or low-set auricles.

Careful examination of an infant's ears may reveal abnormalities known to be associated in some patients with hearing loss. The external ear develops from six hillocks or tissue thickenings located on both sides of the branchial groove. The ultimate shape and pattern of the convolutions of the auricle, then, are the result of the growth and development of these six centers. This growth process, which occurs between gestational weeks 6 and 20, accounts for the widely divergent forms of the pinna. In fact, the two pinnae on the same infant are likely to not be identical. The presence of significant abnormal variations of the external ear is not necessarily related to the presence of hearing loss in an infant, but when combined with abnormality of the external ear canal makes imperative a thorough evaluation of the structures of the middle and inner ears through radiographic techniques and careful evaluation of the patient's hearing.

Among the most common abnormalities of the external ear is the "small ear" or microtia. The microtic ear can present with wide variation ranging from slight to total absence of the pinna (anotia). Microtia may be described as Type I: the pinna has normal overall dimension and position, but incomplete differentiation; Type II: the auricle is smaller than normal, often located in an abnormal position, and represented by a simple vertical curving ridge of tissue; and Type III: the rudiment(s) of the auricle has no resemblance to any portion of the normal pinna. Although some surgeons may recommend cosmetic surgery to improve the appearance of the congenitally deformed pinna, reconstruction of the auricle requires numerous surgical procedures which, unfortunately, seldom yield an acceptable result.

Abnormal development of the external ear canal often results in a narrowing (stenosis) or complete closure (atresia) of the opening. Stenosis of the ear canal predisposes the patient to cholesteatoma which is difficult to identify early. Atresia of the external ear canal is also classified into three types: Type I atresia is mild and characterized by a small ear canal and nearly normal middle ear; Type II atresia is of medium severity with a bone plug remaining in the medial portion of the external canal; and Type III atresia is a severe deformity in which both the external ear canal and middle ear space are small or totally absent. Surgical correction of minor anomalies is possible, but surgical attempts to correct the more serious anomalies are less likely to be successful and present severe risk to the facial nerve and hearing functions.

Fortunately, most external ear malformations are unilateral with a normally formed opposite ear. The audiologist is responsible for determining the hearing sensitivity for both air- and bone-conducted sound in each ear. It is common medical practice to withhold or postpone surgical correction efforts when the hearing in the opposite ear is within normal limits. When the infant reaches the age of consent, the patient may then make a personal decision as to the merits of corrective surgery. In the case of bilateral atresia, there may be question as to which ear should be operated on. Before any operation is undertaken, however, it is imperative that extensive audiometric evaluation is completed to ensure that bilateral hearing is present in the event of an unexpected tragic result from the attempt at opening one of the external ear canals. Surgical intervention is an important consideration, but should be conducted primarily to construct a sound-conducting mechanism to a normal hearing inner ear, with cosmetic considerations aside. In our experience, the results of surgery for congenital atresia generally have been unsuccessful, resulting in continued stenosis of the external ear canal with little or no improvement in hearing.

Some 427 syndromes that may be associated with hereditary hearing loss have been identified (Gorlin et al., 1995). These syndromes involving hearing loss have been related to conditions of the external ear, the eye, the musculoskeletal system (Cohen and Gorlin, 1955), the skin, the kidney, and the nervous system, as well as abnormalities of metabolism and chromosomes (see Table 9–3). The most obvious syndromes involving some type of hearing loss are associated with craniofacial configurations including position and shape of the eyes, nose, cheeks, and mandible. There are at least 25 hereditary syndromes in which both the auditory and visual systems are involved; therefore ophthalmologic examination is appropriate for all children identified with congenital deafness. The mouth, lips, and teeth should be examined for the presence of abnormalities such as a bifed uvula and submucous or partial cleft palate or lip. An infant with a shortened neck may have a branchial fistula or abnormalities of the vertebrae. Hands and feet are examined for abnormalities of the fingers and toes. The presence of some of these physical signs may be extremely subtle and thus initially observable only to experienced clinicians.

A syndrome is a recognizable pattern of birth defects, which will be obvious in some patients and in others difficult to diagnose. An example of a genetic syndrome that is difficult to diagnose is known by acronym as "CHARGE" syndrome. This syndrome sometimes takes years to identify accurately. The multiple congenital anomalies seen at birth may seem unrelated or not be discovered until later in childhood. CHARGE syndrome's main features include coloboma of the eye, heart defects, atresia of the choanae (nasal passages), retardation of growth, genital hypoplasia causing delayed puberty, and ear malformations which may cause sensorineural and/or conductive deafness.

The examination of the tympanic membrane in the neonate and infant is worthy of mention. The tympanic membrane of the infant is in a different position from that of the toddler and older child. The infant tympanic membrane is more difficult to visualize fully because it is in a more horizontal, rather than vertical, position. The examiner may perceive the eardrum to be smaller and,

Table 9–3. Syndromes that include deafness.

Symptoms	Syndromes
Sensorineural Hearing Loss	
Cardiac	CHARGE syndrome, Jervell Lange-Nielsen
Ophthalmologic	Cockayne's syndrome, Marshall's syndrome, Usher syndrome
Facial	EEC syndrome, fronto-metaphyseal dysplasia, Goldenhar's syndrome, Saethre-Chotzen syndrome, Waardenburg's syndrome I and II
Endocrine/Metabolic	Johanson-Blizzard syndrome, Hunter's syndrome, Hurler syndrome, Maroteaux-Lamy syndrome, Morquio syndrome, Sheie's syndrome, MELAS syndrome, MERRF syndrome
Orthopedic	Klippel-Feil sequence, Levy-Hollister syndrome, Stickler syndrome
Dermatologic	LEOPARD syndrome, Senter syndrome, neurofibromatosis I and II
Chromosomal	Killian/Teschler-Nicola syndrome, Noonan's syndrome, trisomy 13 syndrome, 18q syndrome
Renal	Alport's syndrome, Bartter's syndrome, Epstein's syndrome, autosomal dominant polycystic kidney disease, Bardet-Biedel syndrome, myotonic dystrophy, thalidomide embryopathy, branchio-oto-renal syndrome, Kearns-Sayre syndrome
Conductive Hearing Loss	Achrondopasia, McCune-Albright syndrome, multiple synostosis syndrome, Nager syndrome, orofaciodigital syndrome type II, osteogenesis imperfecta I, otopalatodigital syndrome I and II, scerosteosis, Shprintzen syndrome, Treacher Collins syndrome, other craniosynostosis syndromes or dysostoses.

Source: From "The Sounds of Silence" by M. Lotke, 1995, p. 106. *Contemporary Pediatrics*, *12*(10).

perhaps, retracted because of this angulation when seen in routine otoscopic evaluation. A complete discussion of the proper techniques to be utilized in examining the infant tympanic membrane is presented by Bluestone (1990).

Audiometry

In the search to identify hereditary hearing loss, it is sometimes valuable to obtain threshold audiograms from immediate family members. Family members who deny having hearing problems may be unaware of mild or unilateral sensorineural hearing loss, and their audiometric threshold configuration may also suggest familial origin. Audiograms obtained from family members acknowledged to have hearing impairment may provide clues as to the degree and prognosis of hearing loss in the infant under examination.

Routine audiometric evaluation of young children may reveal an uncommon phenomenon of fluctuating sensorineural hearing loss. A controversial diagnosis of fluctuating hearing loss is a perilymphatic fistula. A fistula is an abnormal opening, usually at the oval or round window, between the inner and middle ear, resulting in the leakage of perilymph. The perilymph leakage may be the cause of vertigo which is also a rare symptom in children. The fistula of the inner ear may occur spontaneously or be associated with exertion or a change in barometric pressure. Because there are no absolute diagnostic tests for the presence of an inner ear fistula, surgical exploration is often recommended. A successful surgical result will stabilize the progressive hearing loss or, in some cases, actually improve hearing (Myer, 1992).

Review of Medical Records

Review of medical records is required because the parents of the hearing-impaired infant may not be aware of all of the medical aspects of the pregnancy, delivery, or birth which may have contributed to the cause of the deafness. The most common prenatal causes of hearing loss are intrauterine infections (i.e., cytomegalovirus [CMV], congenital syndromes, and physical defects associated with prematurity). Perinatal causes of deafness that can be identified from medical records review include hypoxia, hyperbilirubinemia, postnatal infection, ototoxic drug treatments, low birthweight, meconium aspiration, and persistent pulmonary hypertension. Postnatal considerations for the etiology of hearing loss must include bacterial meningitis, cerebral palsy, or other central nervous system disorder. Review of the medical records may reveal some otherwise overlooked high-risk indicator associated with deafness that may provide the etiology of the hearing loss.

Laboratory Studies

The physical examination may lead to a request for laboratory studies to confirm or negate a tentative diagnosis. Laboratory studies tend to add a dimension of accuracy to the art and science of medial diagnosis. Medical laboratory studies provide quantitative numerical results or qualitative descriptive results. Although there is no specific standardized laboratory work-up for congenital deafness, the choice of tests will depend on the physician's lack of concrete evidence to support the diagnosis fully. It is beyond the scope of this textbook to detail the laboratory studies that may be used to discover an underlying etiology for deafness, but a summary of laboratory tests used in otologic diagnosis has been published by White (1996).

An example of the importance of laboratory tests in the diagnosis of deafness can be demonstrated with bacterial meningitis. The initial clinical manifestations of neonatal meningitis are often subtle and deceptive and may be misleading to the primary care physician until the later symptoms of lethargy, fever, and convulsions become more obvious. However, the diagnosis of meningitis requires a lumbar puncture to obtain a small sample of cerebral spinal fluid (CSF). The CSF is sent to the laboratory for culture growths to look for causative agents known to be associated with meningitis, such as *Haemophilus influenzae, Neisseria meningitidis,* or *Streptococcus pneumoniae.* Once the infective agent responsible for the meningitis is identified, the appropriate antibiotic can be administered.

Another example of the need for laboratory work-up can be found in the group of perinatal infections known by the acronym "TORCH" which stands for *Toxoplasmosis, Other* (i.e., syphilis, *rubella, cytomegalovirus, and herpes simplex*). All of these infections may be associated congenital deafness (see Chapter 6). These disorders present with minimal and nonspecific symptoms which require special laboratory tests for conclusive diagnosis. In fact, the evaluation of a congenitally deaf infant for intrauterine infection requires serial antibody studies derived from blood samples. Results are reported in titer values and compared to normal antibody assays for each disease. Cultures for rubella and cytomegalovirus may also be obtained from urine, the nasopharynx, and throat of the infant. At 10 to 12 months of age, these tests are repeated. Persistent elevation of abnormal results is highly suggestive of a previous intrauterine infection. The laboratory studies can help determine whether an intrauterine infection was present during the pregnancy and which specific TORCH disorder is carried by the pediatric patient (Grundfast, 1990).

Radiology

Several types of radiographic studies may also be requested to identify the presence of ossicular anomalies of the external ear canal, middle ear, or cochlea. The newer techniques of computerized tomography (CT) and magnetic resonance imaging (MRI) can clearly identify minute anatomic structures as well as anomalies or genetic defects of the skull and central nervous system. The high-resolution CT scan serves to detect mixed fibrous and bony occlusions and is preferred for examination of the structures of the temporal bone, middle ear ossicles, semicircular canals, facial nerve canal, oval and round windows of the inner ear, and to identify developmental malformations of the cochlea. MRI provides better resolution of soft tissue structures and central nervous system disorders. Results from these radiographic studies can add crucial knowledge to the differential diagnosis of congenital deafness (Rose, 1996).

When the inner ear fails to reach full development during the gestation period, the congenital malformation of the cochlea is known as aplasia. The diagnosis of aplasia is based on computerized tomography (CT) studies of the inner ear. CT is able to show very minor differences in bone density which helps to identify various types of inner ear aplasia. Although wide variation exists in the anatomic abnormalities of the inner ear, four basic classifications of aplasia have been identified:

- *Mondini aplasia* occurs with incomplete development of the membranous and bony labyrinth of the inner ear. Although wide variations exist in this type of aplasia, typically only one and one-half turns of the cochlea are present. Often the middle and apical turns of the cochlea are affected. Many of these patients have minimal residual hearing with additional progressive loss likely during the early years of life. Children with Mondini aplasia are often considered candidates for cochlear implantation.
- *Michel aplasia* is the most severe aplasia, resulting in complete failure of development of the inner ear. There is complete absence of the vestibule, cochlea, and internal auditory meatus.
- Scheibe aplasia is the most common aplasia of the inner ear involving only the membranous labyrinth. Patients may show a normal radiologic result with profound and total deafness.

- *Alexander aplasia* is the least severe anomaly of the inner ear. Only the basal turn of the cochlea is affected, and these patients may show only a high-frequency hearing loss.

Routine Follow-up

When it has been confirmed that an infant has sensorineural hearing loss, routine follow-up is appropriate and necessary. The role of the primary care physician is exactly the same for an infant having hearing impairment as for any other infant with a disability or chronic condition: ongoing medical care and supervision, counseling and providing support to the parents, and appropriate referral for further evaluation. As described in Chapter 10, intervention and management strategies must be agreed upon. Hearing aid fitting is usually accomplished as soon as possible, although it is likely to take 2 to 3 months before amplification is selected and adjusted to the needs of the infant. Repeated medical evaluations may be necessaryito complete the diagnostic work-up and interpret the requested laboratory and radiographic studies. Case history review and additional physical examination may reveal previously overlooked or recently developed symptoms or signs. Routine evaluations may ensure that the latest in management procedures and technology are applied to the pediatric patient with hearing loss.

Continued evaluation of the infant's hearing is necessary to ascertain accurate hearing thresholds or to identify progressive hearing loss. Progressive sensorineural hearing loss is often associated with congenital and familial hearing loss and acquired hearing loss associated with perinatal high-risk indicators. Progressive and continued degeneration of hearing complicates the medical management, hearing aid selection and fitting, changes candidacy for cochlear implant consideration, and ultimately requires redetermination of the individualized educational plan for a child with hearing impairment (Brookhouser, Worthington, and Kelly, 1994). Deposits of bone in the fluid spaces of the cochlea are not uncommon following meningitis or autoimmune diseases. This osteoneogenisis of the inner ear can be the cause of progressive hearing loss and change the intervention plan for a young child from the use of hearing aids to consideration of a cochlear implant.

Routine evaluations are particularly valuable when all the members of the professional team are involved in the work-up of the young child with hearing impairment. The primary care physician and the otolaryngologist can share cooperative decisions regarding the medical management of the young patient. The audiologist and speech-language pathologist can evaluate the communication skills of the child. The classroom teacher or educational specialist can evaluate the performance of the youngster with hearing impairment to monitor academic performance, suggesting areas of weakness in which additional efforts may be required to keep the child on track with the academic progress of equal-aged normal-hearing children. Psychosocial evaluation is useful to determine whether the family or child needs help in adjustment to the social and communication problems associated with deafness. A social worker or psychologist experienced in working with children with hearing loss is an important asset to the medical health team.   Predictions regarding the habilitation potential of infants with hearing impairment should not be made on the basis of audiologic information alone. Multiple variables affect the performance potential of infants and young children with auditory disability, and it is important to note that prelingually deafened infants are not a homogeneous population (Brookhouser and Moeller, 1986).

Routine evaluations should always include at least an otoscopic examination, acoustic immittance tests, otoacoustic emissions, and a current audiogram to check the stability of hearing thresholds. The routine evaluation also provides an opportunity to check for the presence of otitis media and middle ear effusion which can severely compromise the rehabilitation of the infant or child with sensorineural hearing loss. The additional hearing loss created by the presence of middle ear fluid will likely have a deleterious effect on hearing aid performance. Most young children will not be sufficiently aware of the decrease in their hearing due to the overlaid presence of conductive hearing loss. The additional hearing loss will require increased gain from the hearing aid throughout the duration of the otitis media episode. Although the incidence of middle ear effusion in infants with hearing impairment is at least equal to that found in infants with normal hearing, the likelihood of detection of the middle ear problem is considerably less without routine evaluations.

OTITIS MEDIA

Otitis media is a general term used to describe a wide variety of disease conditions of the middle ear. Inflammation of the middle ear can occur as an acute or chronic condition and may, or may not, be accompanied by a watery or mucus-like fluid (middle ear effusion) behind the tympanic membrane. Otitis media is primarily a disorder of childhood characterized by sharp ear pain, high fever, and a bulging red eardrum. However, otitis media may also be present without symptoms and without infection as a long-standing chronic condition with middle-ear fluid that causes conductive hearing loss. Otitis media with effusion is also referred to as noninfected middle ear effusion, secretory otitis media, and serous otitis media. Standardization of the terminology used to describe this disorder of the middle ear is lacking and has continually created confusion in comparing research studies.

Most middle ear disease is a result of Eustachian tube dysfunction. The primary purpose of the Eustachian tube is to equalize pressure in the middle ear space. When the Eustachian tube is abnormally closed, no middle ear ventilation occurs which causes the mucosal lining to begin to secrete fluid. Although the fluid initially is sterile, infants have a number of bacterial agents residing in their nasopharynx which ascend through the Eustachian tube and enter the middle ear causing infection of the middle ear effusion. Otitis media typically is preceded by an upper respiratory infection for several days, followed by sudden onset of fever, irritability, and ear pain.

Otitis media is the most common diagnosis made by primary care physicians for pediatric patients. Middle ear problems occur most frequently during the first 2 years of life and decrease thereafter until the child reaches 5 to 6 years of age. Despite the common occurrence of this disorder, and the volumes of research studies conducted and published, significant uncertainty exists among physicians about the causes, diagnosis, and appropriate treatment of the various forms of otitis media. In fact, because of the lack of scientifically sound data regarding the etiology, pathophysiology, and treatment of otitis media, the U.S. Department of Health and Human Services sponsored development of a Clinical Practice Guideline for Otitis Media with Effusion in Young Children (Stool et al., 1994). The Guideline Study Committee considered results from medical interventions including antibiotic therapy, steroid therapy, and antihistamine/decongestant therapy. They also considered results of surgical interventions, including myringotomy with insertion of tympanostomy tubes, adenoidectomy, and tonsillectomy. The panel evaluated various environmental risk factors and concluded that (a) parents should be encouraged to control infant feeding practices because bottle-fed babies tend to have more otitis media than breast-fed babies; (b) parents should limit passive smoking exposure because of the possibility that freedom from secondary cigarette smoke will decrease a child's risk for otitis media; and (c) research has consistently shown a positive relationship between otitis media with effusion and child care in group facilities.

Widespread variations in practice patterns exist among general physicians and specialists, and questions remain about the appropriateness, effectiveness, and timing of treatment. Otitis media can also resolve spontaneously without treatment, but the length of time required for resolution is variable and unpredictable. Accordingly, after extensive computerized search of all available literature regarding treatment of otitis media, the panel reviewed the data, synthesized the findings, and developed the following treatment guidelines:

- The initial management recommended for middle ear effusion includes observation over time or antibiotic therapy, and control of environmental risk factors. In about 60% of children, middle ear fluid goes away without treatment within 3 months; in 85% of children, middle ear fluid goes away within 6 months without treatment.
- Management when middle ear effusion has persisted for a total of 3 months includes the necessity of hearing evaluation. Middle ear effusion does not go away spontaneously in about 40% of children in 3 months and in about 15% of children in 6 months. If a bilateral hearing deficit is present, the management protocol includes antibiotic therapy *or* bilateral myringotomy with insertion of typmanostomy tubes and control of environmental risk factors.
- Management when middle ear effusion has persisted for 4 to 6 months with a bilateral hearing loss is surgical intervention with bilateral myringotomy and insertion of tympanostomy tubes and control of environmental risk factors. When surgical intervention is conducted to place minute hollow tubes through the tympanic membranes, middle ear fluid is removed and hearing returns to normal immediately.

The panel concluded that certain treatments are not efficacious in helping to improve the middle ear condition of children with otitis media. The medical and surgical treatments that are not recommended include the use of decongestants and/or antihistamines, steroids, or the surgical removal of the tonsils and/or adenoids.

Middle Ear Effusion in Infants and Neonates

Otitis media with effusion occurs commonly in infants and neonates. Routine otoscopy is often difficult to achieve successfully with infants because of the small and narrow external ear canal, the presence of vernix caseosa, and the horizontal position of the tympanic membrane. Balkany et al. (1978) reported results from examination of 125 consecutive infants from the neonatal intensive care unit (NICU) and found middle ear effusion in approximately 30% of this population. The study concluded that otitis media in babies in the NICU is an especially important problem because unrecognized middle ear effusion may act as a focus for dissemination of bacteria into the infant's circulatory and/or central nervous system. Infants with nasotracheal intubation that lasted longer than 7 days had a high presence of middle ear effusion.

Howie, Ploussard, and Sloyer, (1975) drew attention to the "otitis prone" infant, which they described as a baby with an initial episode of otitis media due to Pneumococcus infection before the age of 12 months. These children are often destined to have recurrent bouts of otitis media throughout their childhood, perhaps several episodes each year until the age of 5 or 6 years. There has been substantial concern that early and recurrent otitis media may be linked to developmental problems in children, especially in the domain of abnormal or delayed development of speech and language patterns, cognitive, and educational impairment. The Guidelines Panel questioned the scientific merit of the many studies that correlated speech and language problems in children with otitis media. Otitis media does cause mild to moderate conductive hearing impairment which can fluctuate, remain stable, or alternate with periods of normal or near-normal hearing. It is hypothesized that this hearing loss can adversely affect communication and learning especially during the critical language-learning period of infants.

Although a major emphasis of this textbook is on infants with permanent sensorineural hearing loss, it is likely that many of these babies will also have typical childhood episodes of middle ear effusion and bouts of otitis media. Neonatal patients are unable to describe their symptoms; thus recognition of the disorder depends on accurate examination of well babies, at-risk groups, and recognition of symptoms in infants. When conductive hearing loss from middle ear effusion is overlaid on sensorineural hearing loss, the total degree of hearing impairment is increased. This increased level of hearing loss adversely affects the infant's use of personal amplification (hearing aids) and will likely create additional communication problems in the home and during intervention therapy. Furthermore, the transient nature of conductive hearing loss contributes to the lack of a stable auditory base which normally serves as the foundation of communication.

Early identification and management of hearing loss associated with otitis media is important for optimum developmental outcome. The American Academy of Audiology (1992) recommends a three-stage protocol to identify and manage infants and young children with otitis media:

1. The identification process includes routine audiometric screening of hearing for "at-risk" populations such as the "otitis prone" infants, young children in multi-child day care settings, and infants and children with cleft lip or palate, native Americans, or those with Down syndrome. Those children for whom communication skills are found to be delayed or abnormal should be referred for more assertive medical attention and appropriate communication therapy.
2. The assessment process should include complete audiologic evaluation for infants and children who fail the initial hearing screening procedures, as well as consideration for referral for comprehensive speech and language development evaluation.
3. The management process should include routine audiometric monitoring of hearing sensitivity in children with documented histories of otitis media and accompanying hearing loss.

GENETIC EVALUATION

The explosion of knowledge in medical genetics will expand our understanding of disease and its prevention and treatment. Human genetics is challenging the frontiers of medical science and bioethics with its capacity to alter the basic genetic characteristics of individuals. It is important for hearing health care professionals to continually update their knowledge of human genetics, hereditary disease, and treatment for congenital disorders (Stewart, 1996).

It is estimated that well over half of all cases of childhood deafness have a genetic cause. As recently as 1994, researchers have begun to identify the location of genes involved in hearing impairment. Three recessive genes have been located, one on chromosome 11q, one on chromosome 13q, and one on chromosome 17p. The total number of recessive genes to be discovered is not yet known, but these initial results represent significant advances. In addition, two genes that cause dominant progressive hearing impairment have been located, one on chromosome 1p and another on chromosome 5q. As additional research continues, it is expected that the location of more genes related to hearing impairment will be identified. The practical application of genetics and patterns of inheritance of individual infants is discussed in Chapter 3.

Genetic evaluation is the process through which families at risk for a hereditary disorder or birth defect are evaluated for four reasons: (a) to delineate the diagnosis and/or etiology for the disorder; (b) to estimate the probability of transmitting hereditary disorders to future generations; (c) to outline treatment and management options and to discuss the prognosis for the patient; and (d) to provide options to consider in the event of subsequent pregnancy. Genetic evaluation is typically performed by a team of professionals that includes the child's and/or family's primary care physician; medical or surgical specialists who are managing the presenting condition, such as cardiologists or otolaryngologists; medical geneticists (physicians who specialize in evaluation and diagnosis of hereditary disorders); and genetic associates (non-physician specialists with a postgraduate degree in genetics).

The basis of genetic evaluations is the accurate diagnosis of the suspected condition. For children with newly identified hearing loss, genetic evaluation should be considered even if no specific etiology can be identified. For example, the family of a child with confirmed postmeningitic hearing loss does not require genetic evaluation although they may need reassurance that the hearing loss will not be transmitted to future generations. The family of a child with hearing loss of unknown etiology, however, is an ideal candidate for genetic investigation. If other congenital abnormalities are apparent, genetic evaluation is imperative. In addition, couples with a family history of hereditary disorders may consider genetic investigation prior to conception to identify the risks of transmitting the hereditary disease to their future offspring. We suggest genetic evaluation to anyone asking the following questions about their child with a hereditary disorder: (a) What is it? (diagnosis); (b) What caused it? (etiology); (c) What does it mean? (treatment and management issues); (d) Will it happen again? (recurrence risk); or (e) What can we do in the future to reduce the risk? (options).

Genetic evaluation is a multiple stage process that includes (a) complete review of prenatal, perinatal, medical and developmental histories; (b) construction of a family tree or pedigree; (c) thorough physical examination of the affected individual and observation of other family members; (d) completion of specific diagnostic, laboratory, and cytogenetic evaluations; and (e) family counseling.

It is important for the medical team to examine the infant thoroughly to assess whether the suspected anomaly is an isolated congenital malformation or a component of a broader spectrum of abnormalities. Examination will include assessment of specific physical characteristics such as auricle development, shape, and position;

facial features and symmetry; hand and foot shape and dermal ridge ("fingerprint" pattern); and other common manifestations of congenital abnormalities. The team will also complete a thorough prenatal, birth, medical, and developmental history of the infant. If the infant has obvious dysmorphic features, such as low-set, rotated ears, the geneticist can estimate the gestational interval during which the fetus was affected and search for other signs accordingly (see Table 9–4).

The geneticist may order specific diagnostic, laboratory, and cytogenetic investigations of both the infant and family members depend-

Table 9–4. Diagnostic medical workup of the child with hereditary deafness

History
    Detailed family pedigree
    Maternal prenatal history
    Perinatal and neonatal history
    Subsequent medical history

General Physical Examination
    Generalized congenital bone disorders
    Congenital absence or sparseness of hair and/or nails
    Congenital neurologic deficits
    Ataxia of gait
    Pigmentary disorders
    Congenital heart disease
    Hand anomalies

Concomitant Head and Neck Physical Findings
    Atresia of the external auditory canals
    Malformed external ears
    Facial anomalies, especially of the mandible
    Congenital facial nerve paralysis
    Branchial anomalies
    Heterochromia of the irises
    Increased intercanthal distance
    White forelock in scalp hair
    Retinitis pigmentosa
    Rubella retinopathy
    Congenital cataracts
    Dental anomalies
    Short neck; neck anomalies
    Goiter
    Quality of voice and speech

Routine Laboratory Tests
    Compete blood count
    Urinalysis
    Family audiograms

(continued)

Special Laboratory Tests When Appropriate
Age 1 year and under
Rubella titer
CMV
Immunoglobulin M
Viral cultures of urine, throat, nasopharynx

Special Laboratory Tests When Appropriate
Older than 1 year of age
Electrocardiogram
Protein-bound iodine
Syphilis serology
Serum pyrophosphae and uric acid
Urine mucopolysaccharide screening
Dermatoglyphics
Karyotype, buccal smear
Radiographic diagnostic imaging
Electroretinography
Vestibular testing

Source: Courtesy of LaVonne Bergstrom, M.D.

ing on the suspected condition. For example, in evaluating an infant with cleft palate, bilateral aural atresia, sensorineural hearing loss, and growth retardation whose first or second cousin demonstrates a similar constellation of findings, the medical team may require blood tests to rule out infectious or teratogenetic etiology, computed tomography to assess inner ear development and structure, and cytogenetic study of the infant, cousin, and both sets of parents to investigate chromosomal abnormality. Molecular cytogenetic study of the children and parents may reveal previously unsuspected chromosomal aberrations, such as microdeletions or translocations.

Accurate hearing evaluation is an important component in cases of suspected hereditary hearing loss. In most cases, only the affected infant will demonstrate hearing loss. Nevertheless, his or her siblings and parents should be evaluated by age-appropriate techniques to detect the presence of unsuspected hearing loss. Both the infant and any affected family members should be closely monitored for progression or fluctuation in hearing loss.

As described previously, a family pedigree is a detailed family history of the inheritance of the trait in question. Constructing a family pedigree remains one of the most useful tools of the medical geneticist. Careful investigation of the family history, coupled with thorough examination of the affected child and available family members, may uncover a previously unsuspected hereditary basis for disease.

Genetic evaluation is incomplete without thoughtful and thorough family counseling before, during, and at the completion of the investigation. Before the evaluation, the family's expectations and concerns should be defined to develop realistic expectations of the genetic work-up. Families should be informed that the investigation may not result in a definitive diagnosis of hereditary disease or permit estimation of risk to present or future offspring. During the evaluation, the family should be fully apprised of the role and importance of the various tests and procedures used to arrive at an accurate diagnosis. Because families may wish to know the outcome of every procedure, the relative value of individual tests to the genetic evaluation should be described. Finally, at the conclusion of the evaluation, the family will require detailed discussion of the diagnosis and management of the condition, the probability of transmitting the condition to future offspring or future generations, and mechanisms for future prevention of the disorder.

Kelly (1986) described six elements that the genetic counselor must bring to the counseling session. These are: (a) understanding of the natural history and treatment of the disorder under consideration; (b) understanding of the applicable genetics; (c) understanding of the risk of inheritance in probabilistic terms; (d) understanding the available options; (e) assisting in decision-making; and (f) assisting in implementing the selected option. Although the audiologist and speech-language pathologist can provide diagnostic and treatment information to the evaluation and counseling process, a professional with advanced training in genetics is the appropriate individual to perform family genetic counseling.

Medical geneticists are often asked to counsel parents when the hereditary nature of the hearing loss is known and no other etiology is present. In these cases, the geneticist may employ "odds tables" of predicted recurrence risk for specific hereditary conditions based on family history (e.g., hearing parents with one deaf child and negative family history; hearing parents with one deaf child and positive family history) and predicted frequency of the hereditary condition in the population. Although a definite hereditary diagnosis cannot be made in these cases, the process of genetic evaluation is often of inestimable value to families for informational content and future planning.

Special Considerations in Genetic Evaluation and Counseling

During genetic evaluation and counseling, the geneticist must consider the influence of cultural, religious, and ethical traditions on the family's response to, and benefit from, genetic counseling. Special considerations in the genetic counseling process include (a) preferential marriage, (b) consanguinity, and (c) prenatal diagnosis and ethical dilemmas.

Preferential Marriage

In some communities, individuals with similar traits frequently marry. Marriage of deaf individuals is not uncommon; it is estimated that 90% of deaf adults marry deaf persons. The probability of bearing hearing or deaf offspring may be of interest to these individuals, their families, or their children.

The probability of deaf vs. hearing offspring is dependent on the mode of inheritance in the parents. If both partners in a deaf × deaf marriage have the same recessive hearing loss, the probability of deaf offspring is 100%. If one parent has a dominant hearing loss and the other a recessive loss, the probability of deaf offspring with dominant inheritance is 50%, and the probability of being a carrier for recessive inheritance is 100%. Of course, the genetic basis and gene locus are rarely known, and precise predictions of probability are limited. Genetic counselors who work with deaf couples should acquire a communication system and style, including sign language proficiency, appropriate to their client base and a sensitivity to deaf culture.

Consanguinity

Similar to preferential marriage, consanguinity (marriage between close relatives) represents nonrandom mating and thus nonrandom assortment of genes available to future generations. It is important in clinical genetics because offspring from a consanguineous marriage are at increased risk for autosomal recessive disorders. Because each individual in the population is estimated to carry at least one mutant recessive gene for a serious or lethal abnormality, the likelihood that a couple will transmit two copies of this mutant, recessive gene is increased if they share a common ancestor from whom the gene originated. In general, consanguinity in a family without known genetic disease appears to increase the probability of serious or lethal conditions. In first-degree relationships (incestuous matings, e.g., father-daughter, brother-sister), the risk is marked; in relationships more distant than third degree (e.g., greater than first cousins), the risk is insignificant. In the United States, there are legal restrictions on marriage between relatives; all states ban first-degree marriages.

Prenatal Diagnosis and Ethical Dilemmas

The ability to diagnose certain hereditary conditions in-utero is an important benefit to families at risk for serious genetic disorders. Through prenatal diagnosis, couples can determine the health of their infant for certain conditions before birth. If prenatal diagnosis reveals a healthy fetus, the couple is spared many months of anxiety; if prenatal diagnosis reveals an affected fetus, the couple may elect therapeutic abortion. Therapeutic abortion remains an issue of intense moral and ethical debate. For couples who consider abortion to be unjustifiable under any circumstances, prenatal diagnosis is probably inappropriate. For couples who believe that abortion is justifiable to prevent serious disease and disability, prenatal diagnosis is appropriate if risk of disease is present. Conditions usually considered necessary to justify prenatal diagnosis include increased risk of hereditary or congenital disorder such as increased maternal age, family history of genetic disease, or in-utero exposure to viral infection. Because the procedures are often extremely accurate as a diagnostic test, the option of therapeutic abortion is available to the couple.

Preimplantation diagnosis obviates the need for therapeutic abortion of affected fetuses. It may be an acceptable alternative for couples at risk of transmission of a grave genetic condition for whom elective abortion is not an option. Although not routinely available, preimplantation diagnosis represents the current frontier in prevention of genetic disease.

Most geneticists approach their responsibilities as counselors in a supportive and nondirective manner. Ultimately, it is the family who must decide how to respond to and act on the information provided through genetic evaluation. Prenatal diagnosis is an important tool in diagnosing and preventing genetic disease for selected couples.

SUGGESTED READINGS

Behrman, R., Kliegman, R., and Arvin A. (1996). *Nelson Textbook of Pediatrics* (15th ed.). Philadelphia: W.B . Saunders.
The classic pediatric textbook used in schools of medicine.
Bluestone, C., Stool, S., and Kenna, M. (Eds.) (1996). *Pediatric Otolaryngology* (3rd ed.). Philadelphia: W. B. Saunders.
The authoritative text on the medical diagnosis and treatment of pediatric hearing problems. Section II in Volume I is devoted to otologic considerations in infants and young children.
Bluestone, C., and Klein, J. (1995). *Otitis Media in Infants and Children* (2nd ed.). Philadelphia: W. B. Saunders.
This textbook includes absolutely everything you might want to know about otitis media in infants and children.
Harper, P. (1988). *Practical Genetic Counselling* (3rd ed.). London: Wright Publishers.
A very readable textbook for all health care providers.

CHAPTER 10

Habilitation and Amplication for Infants

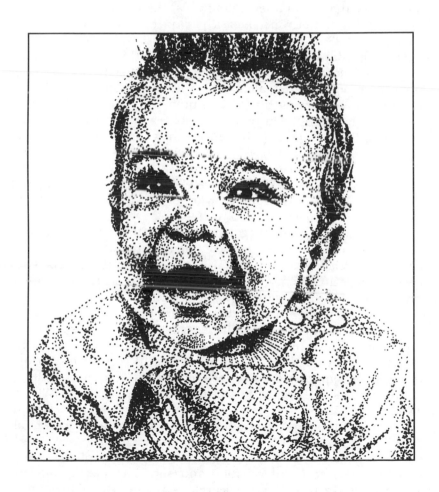

*T*here can be little doubt about the importance of the first 3 years of life to the ultimate successful development of the child. Parents and professionals have long been aware that babies raised by caring adults in stimulating environments are better learners and that these effects can be long lasting. According to a recent Carnegie Report (Carnegie Corporation, 1994), scientists using the latest medical research tools have determined that the brain development that takes place before the age of 1 year is more rapid and extensive than previously realized. Although individual brain cell formation is completed prior to birth, the developing brain maturation is dependent on the environmental influences and experiences that occur early in life.

Radiographic studies using positron emission tomography (PET) show that, from a few initial cells, the prenatal brain develops billions of neurons over a period of just a few months (Chugani, 1993; Chugani, Phelps, and Mazziotta, 1987). The connections (synapses) between the bodies of the brain cells may number as many as 15,000 per neuron. These synapses form the brain's physical "routes" along which learning takes place. In the early months following birth, the number of synapses increases twentyfold to reach the incomprehensible estimate of 1,000 trillion synapses (Kolb, 1989). Although the newborn brain has many more neurons and synapses than it will ever need, as the brain develops, the extraneous connections are eliminated from the dense immature brain. This process of refinement continues until the adolescent years through various episodes of learning and experience (Carnegie Corporation, 1994).

The child of 3 years of age should have attained a high degree of competencies including self-confidence, intellectual curiosity, good social relations, and, perhaps most importantly, the ability to use language to communicate and further the learning process. The deaf infant, without early intervention, will certainly be delayed in all of these normal development processes. The focus of early intervention for infants with hearing impairment is based on preventing delays in oral communication, cognition, and social skills that may result from reduced auditory stimulation. Intervention typically consists of a combined program of educational strategies, therapeutic activities, and sensory aids (Winton and Bailey, 1994)

In one of the most comprehensive studies to date, Levitt et al. (1987) tested each of 120 deaf children annually for a 4-year period. Their data provided strong quantitative evidence of the association between early intervention and superior speech and language skills. In fact, these researchers reported that their most

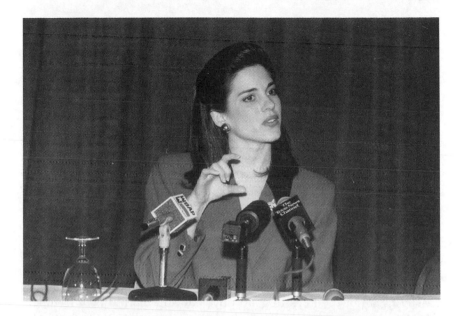

Heather Whitestone, Miss America of 1995, is an exciting example of a successful adult who has met the challenges of a childhood hearing loss. Miss Whitestone lost her hearing as the result of an early episode of meningitis which resulted in a profound bilateral hearing impairment. She graduated from the Central Institute for the Deaf and is a talented ballerina. As Miss America, Heather spread her personal message of *anything is possible* to audiences all over the United States. She attributes her success in life to her positive attitude and strong support team of family and professionals. This outstanding young woman represents the possible success that can be achieved with early diagnosis of hearing impairment and successful habilitation.

important finding was a positive correlation between early intervention and speech and language development, the effects of which persisted well beyond the early years of life.

Although, the importance of early intervention in deaf children cannot be denied, early intervention itself is insufficient to guarantee good speech and language skills. However, the deaf children in the study sample who did not receive special education at an early age consistently scored well below the total group average. The authors of this study concluded that, to intervene effectively, it is necessary to reach the child with hearing impairment as early as possible and to match the program of intervention specifically to the child's individual needs.

EARLY INTERVENTION FOR INFANTS WITH HEARING IMPAIRMENT

As soon as an infant with hearing impairment is identified, the intervention process should begin. Stein and Jabaley (1981) pointed out that the ideal early intervention program must include early diagnosis, comprehensive medical services, productive strategies for language development, and enhancement of the parent-infant bond. Intervention services include everything that professionals, the parent or family members, or the social services staff do to initiate habilitative actions on behalf of the infant with hearing loss. Basically these services are designed to facilitate the child's communicative and social interaction development, but must also include fostering all of the keys to good physical and mental health dependent on an appropriate relationship with the parents or caregivers.

Yoshinaga-Itano (1995) reviewed numerous historical changes that have affected the management of childhood hearing loss in recent years. The age of identification, fortunately, has been steadily decreasing due to improvements in testing technologies and increasing awareness of childhood hearing impairment. In the decade of the 1960s, newborns with profound hearing loss were the most likely to be identified early; however, these are the infants least likely to achieve high success in communication and education. Until the decade of the 1990s, infants with lesser degrees of hearing loss often were not identified until their preschool years, when successful intervention is less likely to be achieved.

There have been vast changes in the choices of educational modes for children with hearing loss. The assessment tools used to measure development have increased in number and improved in quality. School placement decisions and educational service delivery systems have improved and changed dramatically. Advances in technology, such as developments in assistive communication devices, caption decoders, and the use of computers have had a significant impact on the education of children with hearing impairment. Hearing aid technology, as well as hearing aid selection and fitting procedures, have improved significantly, allowing audiologists to achieve greater benefit from personal amplification with younger infants.

Research has shown that babies learn the basics of their native language by the age of 6 months—long before they utter

Learning to speak is so hard for people deaf from infancy because they are trying, without any direct feedback, to mimic sounds they have never heard. Children who learn to speak and then go deaf fare better because they retain some memory of sound. One mother of a deaf child describes the challenge as comparable to learning to speak Japanese from within a soundproof glass booth. And even if a deaf person does learn to speak, understanding someone else's speech remains maddeningly difficult. Countless words look alike on the lips, although they sound quite different. "Mama" is indistinguishable from "papa," "cat" from "hat," "no new taxes" from "go to Texas." Context and guesswork are crucial, and conversation becomes a kind of fast and ongoing crossword puzzle.

From "Deafness as a Culture" by Edward Dolnick, p. 36. *Atlantic Monthly*, September 1993.

"The auditory-linked acquisition of language is unique to human beings because it is a time-locked function, related to early maturational periods in the infant's life. The longer auditory language stimulation is delayed, the less efficient will be the language facility. A baby who is deprived of appropriate language stimulation during the first 3 years of life can never fully attain optimal language function."

"Recent experiments have demonstrated that signed symbols and other visual language forms can be taught to chimpanzees, but in essence it has been on a conditioned basis. This kind of signalization is far removed from the higher conceptualization and syntax of human language. Between the laboriously learned signal response of the chimpanzee and the first voluntary sentence of the 18-month-old baby lies a whole day of creation."

From *Hearing in Children* (First Ed.), 1974, p. v. Baltimore: William and Wilkins Company.

their first words. Newborns are "language universalists": they can learn any sound in any language and distinguish among all the sounds that adults utter. Continued exposure to their native language, however, reduces babies' ability to perceive sounds that are not in that language set. Kuhl and her associates (1992) used computerized speech to generate identical English and Swedish sounds which were presented to 64 six-month-old babies in a double-blind experiment conducted in both the United States and Sweden. The infants showed a significantly stronger preference for and accuracy in identifying the sounds from their own language. This important study demonstrates that linguistic experience during the first 6 months of life already affects infant's perception of speech sounds.

Although the etiologies of hearing loss have changed through the years with medical advances and genetic counseling, the result has been fewer infants with deafness as their only disability, and more infants with multiple disabilities including hearing loss. This situation makes early intervention more complex and difficult to achieve. The optimal approach to early intervention is based on a multidisciplinary professional team evaluation and assessment of the infant with hearing impairment. The multidisciplinary team members share their expertise and perspectives on various issues concerning individual patients. A suggested multidisciplinary team might be composed of individuals with the following training and skills:

1. A physician (i.e., a family practitioner, pediatrician, or otolaryngologist) with experience and expertise in the diagnosis and management of early childhood otologic disorders;
2. A qualified audiologist with experience and expertise in the hearing assessment of infants and young children with hearing loss. The audiologist must also have the knowledge and technical skill to recommend, fit, and manage the wide options of amplification devices currently available which will be appropriate to the child's needs;
3. A speech-language pathologist, a teacher of the deaf and hard-of-hearing, a sign language specialist, or teacher with specialized training in early intervention. These professionals must also have experience and expertise in the assessment of communication skills for infants and young children with hearing loss;
4. Other professionals and specialists may be included on the multidisciplinary team as appropriate to meet the individual habilitation needs of the newborn or young child with hearing impairment and the patient's family. The responsibility for providing the intervention services to the newborn may come from numerous professionals of various specialty areas including special education teachers, counselors, social workers, and early childhood special educators.
5. The multidisciplinary team should always include the parents or caregivers who must be exposed to educational materials and given sufficient information regarding all intervention options available for their newborn. This information should be sufficient to enable the parents or caregivers to make educated

and informed consent decisions when considering and selecting among the intervention choices for their child. Ross (1994) stated that the parents involvement is meant to help them cope with the reality of their child's hearing loss. Ross suggested that a happy child who is able to express and communicate feelings and desires will help alleviate some of the parents' anxieties and guilt, which in turn should have a positive impact on their relationship with the child.

The Role of the Family

The role of parents and family involvement in the newborn with hearing impairment is crucial. The basic components related to early intervention include the following: (a) immediate counseling to support the parents' adaptation to the diagnosis and provide a forum in which they can express and work through their feelings; (b) the infant's impaired auditory reception should be supplemented through the fitting of hearing aids; and (c) encouragement should be given to the early development of a rich symbolic communication system between infants and family members (Greenberg, Calderon, and Kusche, 1984). Early identification and intervention allow the family members to feel that they are doing all they can to assist the child and to bolster the child's sense of being. Such a program provides direct intervention with the child and a psychotherapeutic counseling experience for the parents to help them achieve satisfactory emotional adjustment to the birth of an infant with hearing impairment (First and Palfrey, 1994).

Federal law requires that, when hearing loss is suspected in a newborn or young child, evaluation and early intervention services must be provided in accordance with the Individuals with Disabilities Education Act (IDEA), Part H (birth to 3 years of age) of Public Law 102-119. Formerly known as the Education of the Handicapped Act of 1986 (PL 99-457), the 1990 IDEA version of the law provides for statewide, comprehensive, coordinated multidisciplinary, interagency programs of early intervention services for all children with disabilities and their families. This is typically accomplished by establishing a multidisciplinary evaluation team of professionals to assist in developing an individualized family service plan (IFSP) to define the early intervention program.

The changing roles of the parents and the professional reflect the important fact that the child is always an extension of the family. Traditionally, the professional has acted as an outside expert, who imparted selected information to the parents, and then made critical decisions on behalf of the child. However, in the

1980s, a new awareness developed for the importance of the family in the successful habilitation of the child. The cornerstone of these developments is the recognition that the child cannot be viewed apart from the family, and that the professional's role is to be involved in a collaborative process with the parents to determine what is best for both the child and the family. This change parallels a trend from residential schools for the deaf to more mainstream settings where the family and the home are integral parts of the child's educational and social development. The professional must realize that a family-centered approach to intervention and habilitation is individualized on the basis of each family's resources, priorities, and concerns (Bailey, 1994).

A family-centered treatment philosophy assumes that: (a) social supports affect family functioning; (b) the child's needs are best met by meeting family needs; and (c) families have the right to retain as much control as they desire over the intervention process (Roush and McWilliam, 1994). Thus, intervention is viewed as providing support not only to the child, but also to the child's family and extended family, the family's social network, and the community. For a thorough presentation of the family-based orientation toward children with disabilities and specifically children with hearing loss, the reader is referred to a recent textbook edited by Roush and Matkin (1994).

Changes and revisions in federal legislation reflect the movement toward family-based involvement. For example, when the revision to Part H of Public Law 99-457 was made into Public Law 102-119, authors of the bill changed the term "case manager" to "family service coordinator." States that participate must develop and implement a statewide plan for infant-toddler services. Key elements of the Part H mandate include programs to identify eligible children, comprehensive multidisciplinary assessment, individualized family service plans, public awareness, and designation of a lead state agency. In addition, each state must develop a central directory of services; clearly establish policies for contractual services, funding, and reimbursement; develop procedural safeguards for protection of the family and the child; and establish a comprehensive system of personnel development to ensure the availability of personnel adequately prepared and trained to serve young children with disabilities (Roush and McWilliams, 1994).

The Individualized Family Service Plan (IFSP)

One focus of the Part H portion of the Individuals with Disabilities Education Act (IDEA) is to ensure that the traditional concept of child-centered and professionally directed intervention program is put aside in favor of the family-centered philosophy. Infants and toddlers are uniquely dependent on their families for their survival and nurturing which necessitates a family-centered approach to early intervention. The family-centered framework for habilitation and education of infants and young children with disabilities encourages professionals to work closely with each other and to include the family first and foremost in all decisions.

Numerous regulations surround all aspects of the IFSP, beginning with the evaluation and assessment procedures, assignment of lead agency responsibilities, clear definitions of the early intervention services, general roles of the service providers, time frames for the IFSP to be developed and implemented, and provisions for procedural safeguards and services coordination. Some aspects required in the IFSP are presented below to provide an overview of some of the elements that the plan must include. The IFSP, as required in the statute (Part H Section 1477(d)) must be written and developed by a multidisciplinary team, including the parent(s) or guardian(s). The IFSP must include the following:

- a statement of the infant's or toddler's present levels of development in these developmental areas: cognitive, physical, communication, social or emotional, and adaptive;
- a statement of the vision, hearing, and health status of the infant or toddler;
- a statement of the family's concerns, priorities, and resources related to enhancing the development of the infant or toddler with a disability;
- a statement of the major outcomes expected to be achieved for the child and family; the criteria, procedures, and timeliness to be used to measure progress toward achieving the outcomes;
- a statement of specific early intervention services necessary to meet the unique needs of the infant or toddler and family, including the frequency, intensity, and method of delivering services;
- the projected dates for initiation of the services and the anticipated duration of the services;
- the name of the service coordinator who will be responsible for implementing the plan and coordinating with other agencies and persons.

The IFSP must operate in a way that reflects the diversity of family patterns and structures. Thus, the early intervention systems and strategies must honor the racial, ethnic, cultural, and socioeconomic diversity of families. These principles are known as "cultural competence," which may be defined as a set of congruent behaviors, attitudes, and policies that come together in a system, agency, or professional (practitioner) that can work effectively in cross-cultural situations (Cross, 1988). This concept is held paramount in the establishment of each IFSP and must be respected because American society is composed of people of many colors, cultures, ethnic origins, religions, and beliefs (McGonigel, 1994).

Joint Committee Recommendations for Early Intervention

The 1994 Joint Committee on Infant Hearing recognized the importance of an early intervention program to supplement their recommendation for universal detection of infants with hearing impairment (see Appendix E). Because hearing screening programs are ineffective without appropriate intervention, the Joint Committee recommended that, although the full child evaluation process should be completed within 45 days of referral, intervention services may begin, with parental permission, prior to completion of the diagnostic evaluation.

The 1994 Joint Committee on Infant Hearing outlined the components of an early intervention program for infants with hearing-impairment and their families to include:

1. Family support and information regarding hearing loss and the range of available communication and educational intervention options. Such information should be provided in an objective, nonbiased way to support family choice.
2. Implementation of learning environments and family-centered services consistent with the needs of the child, the family, and their culture.
3. Early intervention services that provide ongoing monitoring of the child's development in all areas, with particular attention to language acquisition and communication skills.
4. Early intervention services that provide ongoing monitoring of the child's medical and hearing status, amplification needs, and development of communication skills.
5. Curriculum planning that integrates and coordinates multidisciplinary personnel and resources so that intended outcomes of the IFSP are achieved.

The Home Intervention Program

Many states have instituted programs to begin intervention as early as possible by working with the parents or guardians in the home. As an example, the Colorado Home Intervention Program

(CHIP) is the responsibility of the State Department of Public Health (Yoshinaga-Itano, 1987). When an infant or young child is identified as hearing-impaired, a staff person visits the family to explain the program and offer support if it is the desire of the parents to become involved in the intervention process. The family is assigned a trained regional facilitator who begins to show the family how to develop the child's skills and facilitates optimum parent-child interaction. The program has four main components: (1) the family is given educational information about hearing, speech and language, and normal child development; (2) the family is shown activities to make their home environment "auditorily rich" so that the infant or young child will benefit from everyday listening; (3) family members are taught skills to help them communicate fully with their child; and (4) the family is taught to encourage and reinforce the young child's spontaneous language.

When the family is comfortable and involved in the home intervention process, assessments of the ongoing activities in the home are videotaped and analyzed for the benefit of the family members. The videotape helps identify the child's skill levels and maps the interactions between the child and members of the family. The videotape is used to monitor the child's development and to help plan a progression of intervention activities to stimulate the child's development further.

Early identification of hearing loss should lead to early intervention. In fact, in Colorado more than one-half of the children who receive services from the Department of Public Health were identified before the age of 1 year, and 80% of the children were identified before the age of 2 years (Yoshinaga-Itano, 1987). The positive effects of early identification and intervention have recently been reported by Yoshinaga-Itano (1995). Children with hearing loss identified between birth and 6 months of age have significantly higher developmental functioning at 40 months of age than children not identified until after 6 months of age. Children with mild and severe sensorineural hearing losses perform similarly at 40 months of age on language functioning and general development when the hearing loss is identified before 6 months of age. Children with profound hearing loss typically perform with significantly lower language function, but with early intervention these children were noted to perform at only 12 to 15 months below their chronological age at 40 months.

The Deaf Culture Movement

Approximately 90% of all deaf children are born to hearing parents, most of whom have never come into contact with a deaf person. The immediate, and most serious problem between hearing parents and the deaf child is communication. The parents usually desire that the child be educated through a communication system that will be as natural as possible—a system which is known as the auditory-oral approach. The system is based on the child's utilization of amplification and assistive listening devices and constant training in speech production and auditory perception.

However, this "auditory-oriented" approach for hearing parents to communicate and educate their deaf child is held in disdain by many deaf adults. During the last few years, deaf adults who depend on communicating primarily through American Sign Language have organized a movement to have deafness recognized as a independent "culture" rather than a medical disability. The deaf culture movement is characterized by its own institutions, organizations, attitudes, and efforts to raise the status of American Sign Language and manual fingerspelling. Deaf culturists criticize all efforts to help deaf children become functional in the "normal" hearing society, including intervention with hearing aids, speech production therapy, and auditory training, as well as precluding cochlear implantation.

Edward Dolnick wrote explicitly about the deaf culture movement in the *Atlantic Monthly* (1993). He pointed out that the view of deafness as a culture is held vehemently by many deaf adults. Because deaf children cannot easily grasp their parents' spoken language, learning to speak presents a monumental challenge. Dolnick described this challenge as "comparable to learning to speak Japanese from within a soundproof glass booth" (p. 39). Therefore, deaf children acquire their sense of cultural identity from their hearing-impaired peers with whom they communicate easily, and fully, through sign language. So strong is the feeling of deaf cultural solidarity that many deaf parents cheer on discovering that their newborn is also deaf. Thus, our well-meaning efforts to integrate deaf children into conventional schools and to help them learn and speak, provokes fierce resistance from activists who favor sign language and argue that the world of deafness is distinctive, rewarding, and worth preserving.

Of course, acceptance of deafness as a heritage similar to some ethnic inheritance is unacceptable to the many professionals who devote their lives to providing services to individuals with hearing-impairment and their families. Public Law 99-547 mandates the identification and treatment of all children with hearing loss. By the age of 5 years, the normal hearing child will have a vocabulary of as many as 26,000 words. At the same age, a deaf child may only have about 200 spoken or signed words. The fact that

American Sign Language has no written form is one reason that the average 16-year-old deaf teenager who relies on sign language reads only at the third- or fourth-grade level (Dolnick, 1993).

However, the deaf cultural movement must be considered fully within the realm of Part H of the Individualized Family Service Plan. The culture of the deaf community, with little awareness from our mainstream society, is no doubt rich and fulfilling to its members. This faction must be taken into account to honor the cultural diversities of families. Although the future of the deaf culture movement is uncertain, it is a force that must be recognized and dealt with by hearing care providers, as well as the parents and families of infants and toddlers with hearing loss. While recognizing the potential benefits of manual communication or "total communication" for some deaf children, as audiologists, we cannot imagine that it can possibly be in the best interests of deaf children to be isolated from the hearing world—for the sake of deaf culture. We also cannot permit any group or individual to make decisions regarding a child's future except the child's parents or guardian. These two tenets are difficult for audiologists to accept and advocate when faced with managing the future of a deaf child born into a family of "deaf culturists."

AMPLIFICATION FOR INFANTS WITH HEARING IMPAIRMENT

Early provision of amplification to assist in speech and language stimulation and development is an important aspect of early intervention. Although many of the guidelines call for the application of intervention procedures to begin no later than 6 months of age, the challenge of meeting such an obligation is daunting. Considering the time involved in initial screening, follow-up screening, referral, and scheduling and completing the diagnostic evaluation, intervention by 6 months of age is a reasonable goal, but it is difficult to achieve. According to Gravel (1995), the nemesis facing audiologists is that early detection is often protracted by repeated evaluation appointments and extended trials with multiple models of hearing aids.

Parental feelings must be considered and dealt with before there can be a successful hearing aid fitting. An important factor which may add to the problem of delayed habilitation is the noted inability of parents to act on professional recommendations. Parental motivation is hampered by the fact that hearing loss is not an obvious handicap, and if the baby's limited auditory behavior does not appear abnormal, parents may find the diagnosis difficult to believe and accept. When infants have serious and chronic health problems following discharge from the hospital, the presence of hearing loss often takes a role of secondary importance (Hayes, 1987).

The fitting of hearing aids on infants has always presented problems for audiologists because of the limited capability to utilize standard behavioral testing techniques. The task is not to be taken casually nor accepted by the inexperienced audiologist. Parents must be made to understand that the hearing aid selection, fitting, and verification process is an ongoing activity to be analyzed and reconsidered by the audiologist at each hearing clinic visit. As more accurate and precise audiometric information is obtained, along with careful observation of the infant's aided behavioral responses noted over time, the audiologist may find it appropriate to modify or adjust the hearing aids (Northern and Downs, 1991).

Traditionally, hearing aids were selected and fit to infants and young children using soundfield measures known as **functional gain measurements**. During the functional gain procedure, sound awareness, minimal response levels, or behavioral localization responses are used with and without hearing aids in the soundfield situation to verify the benefit obtained with amplification. Results with amplification should demonstrate lowered sound awareness and minimal response levels and improved localization of sound at lower intensities. Cooperation from the infant or young child is required for these measurements, and thus testing time can be extensive and test-retest reliability can be questionable. The response variability shown by an infant is often excessive, and the subjective nature of the examiner's task to score objectively the child's behavior under aided and unaided conditions leaves much to be desired in terms of the adequacy of this technique.

Computerized real-ear **probe microphone measurements** are an important objective technique which can be used to fit and adjust hearing aids with infants (Hawkins and Northern, 1992). Probe microphone measurements are obtained by using a soft silicone tube inserted into the ear canal with the hearing aid and earmold in place. The amplified sound is picked up by a probe microphone through the silicone tube and subjected to signal processing by a special purpose computer. The results are presented on a visual display monitor and may be printed out in hard copy. A major advantage of the probe microphone technique is the complete objectivity by which the amplified frequency response and gain of the hearing aid at various volume settings can be determined from the ear canal of the infant. Physiologic differences among infants and young children (i.e., the length, diameter, and shape of the ear canal) are taken into account with the probe microphone measurement system.

Because the infant ear canal presents such a small cavity, it is easy to overamplify with hearing aids. Hearing aid response specifications are required to be determined in a standard, hard-walled cavity of 2 cc in volume. The infant ear canal is often smaller than 0.5 cc, thereby creating an unexpected increase in the hearing aid output as the amplified sound is directed into this small space. The use of real-ear probe microphone systems provides an efficient means to monitor amplified ear canal sound pressure levels so that the volume of the hearing aid can be precisely adjusted to obtain an appropriate amount of gain.

Real-ear probe microphone measures provide quick and efficient objective data regarding ear canal resonance, the aided insertion gain, and overall amplified sound pressure. These measures are critical during the pre-selection, fitting, verification, and post-hearing aid fitting and management of the infant with hearing impairment. In addition, most real-ear probe microphone equipment includes a "listening" system through high fidelity, lightweight earphones so that the amplified sounds of the hearing aid can be heard by the infant's family. Thus, the parents can more fully appreciate exactly how the infant's hearing aids amplify environmental and speech sounds.

Many audiologists use prescriptive hearing aid fitting formulae to adjust and customize the amplification response to the audiometric configuration of the infant's hearing loss whenever possible. This requires data from the unoccluded (open) ear canal of the infant as measured with the probe microphone system. It is well recognized that, as an infant grows older, the ear canal changes in shape, length, and diameter, thereby altering the resonance characteristics of the unoccluded canal. Researchers have measured the typical changes in the real-ear unoccluded response (REUR) of infants and young children (Bentler, 1989; Kruger, 1987). As shown in Figure 10–1, the ear canal frequency response resonance peaks for a newborn at approximately 7200 Hz due to the smaller concha and shorter ear canal length. As the infant's age increases and the canal grows larger and changes shape, the REUR resonant frequency peak decreases in an orderly fashion until it stabilizes at approximately 2700 Hz between 12 and 24 months of age.

The real-ear probe microphone measurement technique is a powerful tool for selecting and fitting hearing aids with infants.

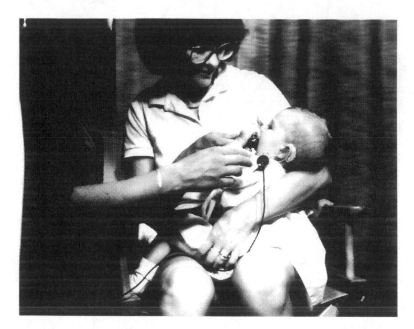

FIGURE 10–1. Probe microphone measurements are essential for the accurate fitting of hearing aids with infants.

Less time is required and improved test results can be obtained efficiently. The measurements may require the aid of an assistant to monitor and hold the silicone tube in place or to distract the infant's attention away from the procedure, so that the data can be collected quickly. Probe microphone measurements provide the audiologist with objective, reliable, and useful data to verify the appropriateness of the hearing aid fitting in infants.

Hearing Aids for Infants and Young Children

An often asked question is how early can an infant be fitted with a hearing aid? The answer is that the infant should be habilitated with a hearing aid as soon as the audiologist is firmly convinced that a significant hearing loss is present in both ears. This may be early in the identification process with the infant, or it may take some time to determine the nature of the hearing loss. Nonetheless, the infant with a hearing loss should be fitted as early as possible with hearing aids, although the process should proceed with special care and deliberation. It is to be understood by all involved with the infant that the evaluation process and the fitting of the hearing aids is a continuing and ongoing process that may take considerable time and require significant changes along the way before the "final" fitting is accomplished. Every hearing aid decision is tentative and subject to change as new information becomes available. For example, if the infant turns out to have a progressive sensorineural hearing loss, then the infant's hearing levels will need routine, periodic monitoring and the hearing aids will likely need continual adjustments to provide the infant with optimal access to acoustical information.

In general, infants are fitted with binaural ear level hearing aids which are available in small sizes to fit behind the ear (BTE). The older style body-type hearing aids, with cord and external receiver, are seldom currently recommended. The BTE hearing aid is custom-fitted and electronically tuned for the specific pattern of hearing loss identified in each ear.

Ear impressions are taken from which soft earmolds are made and fitted to each ear. The earmold may be ordered from a broad assortment of colors and or in cosmetic skin-matching tones. The earmold must fit properly to avoid leakage of the amplified sound which causes acoustic feedback and squeal. Because the pinnae and ear canal of the infant will continue to grow, changing in size and shape, until approximately 9 years of age, it is necessary for earmold impressions be taken several times a year for the first 3 years of life, and at least annually during the child's elementary school years. As the infant's external ear grows each few months, the earmold will begin to have feedback problems. The parents need to be advised that this situation requires an immediate new ear impression and new fabrication of a better fitting earmold. Most infants are fitted with full-shell or full-perimeter (skeleton) type earmolds.

Behind-the-ear hearing aids are usually selected for infants because they offer a wide flexibility of amplified frequency response and gain characteristics. The BTE hearing aid often includes adjustable output controls and has the capability of being coupled to an FM system (see discussion below). The BTE hearing aid may be ordered from the manufacturer with an omni-directional microphone and a specialized compression circuit when appropriate. Although the larger BTE hearing aids may be conspicuous behind the infant's small pinna, some parents actually select the BTE hearing aid cases and earmolds in bright, cheerful colors designed especially for small children.

Some BTE hearing aids are capable of producing dangerously loud output, so the audiologist must give consideration to output limiting adjustments and determining the amplified overall sound pressure level that the hearing aids create in the infant's external ear canal. This is not a trivial issue because high-powered hearing aids potentially may cause further hearing loss. For this reason, some type of automatic gain control and output limiting is necessary for infants and small children who are unable to complain that the hearing aid is violating their comfort levels. Recent developments with programmable, wide dynamic range, compression, and K-amp circuits that provide maximum gain for soft sounds and automatically attenuate loud sounds should be considered with all infant fittings.

Although hearing aids are indeed high-quality amplification devices, it is difficult to achieve sufficient gain in the frequency spectrum above 3000 Hz, thus limiting the ability of the typical infant with hearing loss to hear high-frequency consonants, particularly the fricative sounds. Again, recent advances in hearing aid circuitry and earmold design are improving potential gain realized at the higher frequencies.

Parent counseling is extremely important when attempting to fit hearing aids to infants and young children. Because the parents are responsible for the daily use and care of their infant's hearing aids, it is critical that they be informed completely of the advantages and disadvantages of amplification for their child. Hearing aids do not always meet the expectations of parents, and parents must realize that amplified sound is not a comparable substitute for natural sound. It is important for parents to be counseled regarding realistic expectations from the hearing aids.

Parents should be informed that the hearing aids will amplify all sound in the environment not just the speech signal. This creates a situation with all hearing aids whereby the background noise may be amplified sufficiently to mask out the desired speech the infant needs to hear. This is known as a poor signal-to-noise ratio. For maximum listening of amplified sound, the desired signal should be 15 to 20 dB louder than the background noise. Unfortunately, in our daily circumstances, this optimal signal-to-noise ratio is difficult to achieve without frequency-modulated (FM) assistive listening devices or systems. Most BTE hearing aids may be ordered with direct audio input (DAI) capability for FM use at an additional cost. However, adding the DAI option after the hearing aids have been fit is more costly and will require loaner hearing aids for the child while the hearing aids are returned to the manufacturer for a retrofit procedure.

Most children's hearing aids are ordered with specially designed tamper-proof battery doors and output controls. The small batteries used to provide power for the hearing aids are easily ingested by infants and small children, and parents must be cautioned about the toxicity of the batteries and warned to keep batteries out of reach of their child.

Infants with significant craniofacial disorders and associated bilateral, conductive-type hearing loss are candidates for bone-conduction hearing aids. These hearing aids feature a flat, vibrating surface which is pressed against the mastoid to stimulate the cochlea with amplified sound. Because the problems of these children are immediately obvious at birth, the fitting of the bone conduction hearing aid is often accomplished within the first few weeks of life. Bone conduction hearing aids are recommended and fitted only to children who present with significant conductive hearing loss due to congenital malformations. Certain congenital anomalies, such as external ear canal atresia or microtia of the pinnae, will not be suitable for traditional hearing aid fittings with standard earmolds. Because air-conduction hearing aids produce better amplified sound with less distortion than the bone-conduction hearing aids, bone-conduction hearing aids are used only when necessary. The bone-conduction hearing aid fitting may be temporary until surgical or medical treatment of the infant's conductive hearing loss problem is resolved. Bone-conducted hearing aids also may be selected by the audiologist for infants with chronically draining ears where the traditional earmold may exacerbate the middle ear problem.

Programmable hearing aids offer an interesting option for the amplification flexibility required for infants with hearing loss. Programmable hearing aids typically contain the circuitry for an enormously wide range of frequency response, gain, and output adjustments within the same hearing aid. As more specific information is determined regarding the infant's hearing loss, the audiologist simply reprograms the hearing aid with a computer system to set new electroacoustic characteristics to match the new hearing threshold determinations. The programmable hearing aids, at this time, are generally larger in size than the conventional BTEs and considerably more expensive. It is likely that future developments in technology will make programmable hearing aids more usable with the difficult-to-fit infant population.

Some infants, with small or unusually shaped external ears, present problems in retention of the hearing aids. The audiologist may recommend the use of taupe tape, rubber bands, or some other sticky substance, to be wrapped around the BTE hearing aid case, to make the aid adhere better to the mastoid and skin behind the infant's pinnae. A plastic hook, wire retainer, or helix lock feature may ensure that the hearing aids stay in place. Some parents pin a string or cord to the back of the infant's clothing and connect it to the BTE hearing aid cases or hooks so that the entire amplification system cannot fall off and be lost or broken. Manufacturers offer extended warranties against loss or breakage which are especially valuable for pediatric hearing aid fittings.

Additional in-depth information regarding the selection and fitting of hearing aids on infants and young children has been presented by Northern and Downs (1991) and Northern, Gabbard, and Kinder (1995).

FM Personal Hearing Systems

Hearing aids for amplification of environmental sounds and speech are usually the first intervention the audiologist turns to when hearing loss is identified in an infant. However, we know from years of experience with adults who wear hearing aids that two major problems can limit and interfere with successful amplified listening: (1) background noise and (2) distance from the speaker. Typically, as the speaker moves away from the microphone of the hearing aid, the signal (speech) becomes weaker causing the hearing aid user to turn up the volume which then increases background noise. This creates a situation in which the amplified background noise makes it very difficult to hear and understand the speech of the speaker. One solution to these problems is the radio frequency transmission hearing aid (FM) with the speaker wearing a wireless microphones.

Although initially designed for classroom use for school-age children with significant hearing losses, FM personal hearing aid units are being fitted with increasing frequency to younger children. The FM technology is currently the best means by which to reduce background noise and control speaker distance problems inherent for users of personal amplification. With FM technology, the speaker (parent or teacher) wears a wireless transmitter/microphone, which strengthens reception of the speaker's voice while simultaneously minimizing the interfering effects of background noise. The signal is picked up by the wearer's FM receiver which is coupled to the hearing aids. This effectively puts the speaker's mouth and voice at the listener's ear.

The FM advantage in personal amplification is especially useful in the presence of adverse listening situations. The FM system keeps the microphone near the speaker's mouth, so that the distance between the primary signal (the speaker) and the listener's ears effectively remains at 6 inches—regardless of how far the parent or teacher wearing the microphone moves away from the child with the hearing aids. With the wireless microphone at the speaker's mouth, the background noise is always reduced. This technology effectively increases the signal-to-noise ratio by keeping the primary signal (speech) significantly louder than the interfering environmental noise. Because the listener is not directly connected to the speaker through a hard-wired system, the FM device offers considerable mobility and flexibility.

Traditionally, children's hearing aids were equipped to be dovetailed with a special receiver that plugged in or snapped on to permit FM reception. The child used a body worn receiver that was hard-wired to a behind-the-ear hearing aid. The coupling of the FM system to the personal hearing aid can be electrical or acoustical. Recently, however, technology has improved so that the FM receiver can now be built into the case of the behind-the-ear hearing aid. These special amplification devices can now serve as traditional hearing aids as well as cordless FM systems. Many audiologists considered the FM system to be a secondary personal amplification device to be used by school-age children or adults with special listening needs. However, the FM fitting is somewhat cumbersome for small children and is sometimes unacceptable because of the large body-worn receiver and cord. With the advent of the behind-the-ear hearing aid/FM system, the advantages for use with young children in the early language learning years may prove to be particularly beneficial.

Tactile Aids

Tactile aids are sensory devices that change auditory signals into vibratory or electrical patterns on the skin. Vibrotactile aids are designed to supplement or replace the auditory perception of speech and environmental sounds. Although these devices can provide substantial supplemental cues for understanding speech, research has shown that they cannot replace the information provided by the auditory system. Vibrotactive aids can be useful for providing prosodic cues for speech understanding for some profoundly deaf individuals. These devices are usually reserved for use by children who are so profoundly deaf that they gain little or no benefit from traditional hearing aid amplification.

The development and use of tactile aids to help the deaf with speech perception has been under study since the 1920s. Since that time, numerous designs of tactile devices have been evaluated. Most of the early tactile aids were based on one or two-channel systems. They generated harmonic frequencies that produced an audible distraction to normal hearing persons. Additional limitations of the early tacticle aids included their requirement for a large power supply and their inability to provide fine frequency discrimination.

However, since 1990, truly wearable, commercially produced multichannel tactile aids have available for research and use by deaf children (Weisenberger and Percy, 1994). The most currently utilized vibrotactile device is the Tactaid VII which features a seven-transducer vibratory display attached to a body-worn processor. The encoding strategy of the Tactaid VII delivers energy from the acoustic signal to the seven transducers which are tuned to seven individual filtered frequency bands between 200 Hz and 7000 Hz. The display system of the Tactaid VII is flexible and may be worn at any of several body sites, including the sternum, abdomen, neck or arm. Children are usually fitted to wear the display on their sternum, which has a flat surface area and permits the device to be monitored and adjusted easily if necessary.

Research results obtained with tactile aids and reported during the 1980s were encouraging. Studies were published that showed improvement in their pronunciation of fricative and nasal consonants by children wearing tactile aids (Oller, Payne, and Gavin, 1986); other subjects increased vocalization and sign language skills while using tactile aids (Friel-Patti and Roeser, 1985). Some advocates of vibrotactile aids claim that these devices perform comparably to results obtained with single-channel cochlear implants. Recently, however, in a 2-year study of school-age children who wore a vibrotactile aid and received intensive auditory training showed that the children were unable to recognize recorded words. The study suggested that the vibrotactile aid provided sufficient pattern sequence information to be beneficial to children who are unable to discriminate prosodic (stress or duration) cues in speech. However, the vibrotactile aid did not facilitate the acquisition of speech or spoken language for the children in the study (Geers and Moog, 1994).

Cochlear Implants

Perhaps the most significant technological advance in the treatment of deafness is the highly sophisticated cochlear implant. The early research on cochlear implants was begun in France more than 30 years ago. Cochlear implants have progressed from the single-channel device developed at the House Ear Institute in Los Angeles to the more sophisticated multichannel device developed at the University of Melbourne in Australia in the early 1970s. Since then, cochlear implant technology has evolved to systems that extract pertinent cues from the speech signal and transmit more sound information through multiple electrodes or channels. Designed for profoundly deaf individuals who are unable to obtain benefit from traditional hearing aids, the cochlear implant is surgically inserted through the mastoid bone into the inner ear. The surgery to insert a cochlear implant usually requires 2 to 3 hours and an overnight stay in the hospital. Under general anesthesia, a postauricular skin flap is elevated, a mastoidectomy is performed, and the middle ear is entered. The cochlea is then opened and the electrode is inserted. Following a postoperative healing period of a month to 6 weeks, the device is "tuned" by an audiologist to each child's particular needs.

The cochlear implant device includes several components— some are implanted internally and some are worn externally. The child wears a behind-the-ear device which consists of a micro- phone and transmitting coil on the implanted side. The transmit- ting coil contains a magnet that attracts to another magnet located in the receiver/stimulator under the skin. An external microphone picks up sound and sends it through a cord to a speech processor. The speech processor unit is worn outside the body and functions to change acoustical information into electrical signals. The speech processor selects particular characteristics of the sound, electrical- ly encodes them, and transmits them to the transmitter coil which emits a radio signal. The radio signal is picked up through the skin by the implanted receiver. The receiver/stimulator sends the appropriate electrical signals through the electrode array to stimu- late the nerve endings in the cochlea. The electrode array is made of a microscopic flexible material which allows it to conform to the cochlea's coiled shape. Signals received through the electrode

A cochlear implant relies on the fact that many of the auditory nerve fibers often remain intact in patients with sensorineural deaf- ness. The surviving neurons can be stimulated to fire actively prop- agating nerve impulses by applying external electrical currents of the proper strength, duration, and orientation. Such "evoked poten- tials" arrive at the brain looking just like the impulses generated by acoustic signals that intact hair cells transduce; accordingly the brain interprets them as sound.

In principle, with enough independent channels of stimula- tion, each controlling the activity of a small, local subset of the auditory nerve fibers, one could re-create the normal neural response to acoustic stimuli of any spectral composition. The brain would then process that information in its usual manner and the subject would "hear the "sounds."

From "The Functional Replacement of the Ear" by Gerald E. Loeb, *Scientific American*, February, 1985, p. 106.

montage stimulate the auditory nerve and are perceived as sound by the brain.

The patient receives the electrical stimulations as auditory sensations that vary in pitch and loudness. The specific characteristics of the sounds selected by the speech processor are those thought to be important for understanding speech. The voice pitch defines the rate at which the electrodes are stimulated, while the voice loudness determines the amount of electrical current delivered to each electrode. The sounds from the implant are not like normal hearing, and therefore, each implant patient must undergo a long period of postimplant training. Success with the implant improves with experience over time. Results with congenitally deaf children show continued improvement with the implant over a period of 4 to 5 years.

The initial children's protocol approved by the Food and Drug Administration (FDA) required that candidates for cochlear implants be at least 2 years of age, with profound bilateral sensorineural deafness, normal intelligence, no additional handicaps, and strong evidence of family support. At this time, cochlear implants are intended to be used with profoundly deaf patients who do not benefit from the use of powerful hearing aids. Failure to show progress in auditory development following a substantive trial period with appropriately fitted hearing aids and effective therapy and training is required for all pediatric patients who might be candidates for cochlear implants. To allow appropriate time to meet all of these preselection criteria and medical workup, it is felt that young children should not be implanted prior to 24 months of age (Northern, 1986).

It has been approximately 10 years since the first clinical trials began with cochlear implants in deaf children. The FDA is beginning to relax the initial rigid criteria for implant candidacy. Current results in young deaf children with cochlear implants have exceeded the expectations of most professionals. Surprisingly, postlingually deafened children, especially those deafened from meningitis, are usually able to understand some open-set speech without visual cues with multichannel cochlear implants. These results have been so encouraging that the application of the technology has now been extended to include prelingually deafened children who lost their hearing before developing speech and language.

Increasingly, over the past few years, parents and cochlear implant teams have pressed to implant children earlier than 2 years of age when appropriate diagnostic considerations are met and the children demonstrate lack of auditory development progress with traditional hearing aid amplification. Cohen and Waltzman (1996) describe results obtained in carefully selected children who were implanted prior to the age of 2 years. Initial follow-up demonstrates that all of the children implanted at less than 2 years of age now have some open-set speech understanding. These children were all deafened through meningitis which is often followed by new bone formation in the cochlea (labyrinthitis ossificans). This new ossification growth, if permitted to continue, may obstruct the full insertion of the implant electrode array, and therefore, perhaps preclude optimum benefit.

At the time of this writing, more than 50 infants (below the age of 2 years) from around the world have received multichannel cochlear implants (Cohen and Waltzman, 1966). Surgical techniques require minimal modification because the cochlea is full adult size at birth. Initial progress reviews of these children have shown encouraging results, and there is little doubt that more children will be candidates for cochlear implants at earlier ages.

Consideration of a cochlear implant for an infant or young child is a serious decision. Success with the implant is affected by a number of variables (NIH Consensus Development Conference, 1995). Factors that affect auditory performance with cochlear implants by children include highly variable individual differences due to history of auditory stimulation and general cognitive and linguistic skills, the etiology of the deafness, the age of onset of the hearing loss, the duration of the deafness, the degree of residual hearing, as well as the type of educational placement and home support system. In addition, psychological and social issues may influence successful use of the implant, as well as rehabilitative and educational issues.

Generally, children with onset of deafness at 4 or 5 years of age, and with a short duration of deafness prior to surgical implantation, tend to achieve better success with cochlear implants than do children with early onset of deafness and a relatively long duration of isolation from the world of sound. Nonetheless, recent clinical studies of children with congenital deafness before the age of 3 years, demonstrate comparable levels of benefit from cochlear implants when compared to implanted children with early acquired deafness.

A recent study compared the use of traditional hearing aids, vibrotactile aids, and cochlear implants in matched triad sets of children at the Central Institute for the Deaf over a period of 3 years (Geers and Moog, 1994). Analysis of data showed that the children with cochlear implants outperformed their matched peers. The children with cochlear implants showed significantly faster growth in speech and language acquisition than the matched children wearing the other sensory aids. The researchers reported that the children with cochlear implants were able to identify words based on spectral rather than temporal cues after 1 year of implant use, and progressed within 2 years to show a dramatic increase in perception and production of suprasegmental features as well as vowels. However, it was noted, that this accelerated progress requires at least average intelligence, strong family support, and the child's participation in an intensive auditory-oral education program with daily training.

Presently, cochlear implants are not recommended for infants during the first year of life. It is critical that deafness be proven without doubt, and such documentation is often difficult and takes time to verify at this early age. As early identification of hearing loss become more prevalent, the possibilities for early intervention through hearing aids, FM systems, vibrotactile devices, and cochlear implants will provide wide choices for parents of infants with hearing impairment. These options should be discussed with the parents as soon as the infant's deafness is confirmed. Careful counseling is crucial because parents will have to make critical decisions about their child's future.

The John Tracy Clinic is an internationally noted educational center for preschool deaf children and their parents. The clinic was founded in 1942 by Mrs. Spencer Tracy and named after her congenitally deaf son, John. The clinic is most well-known for their two correspondence courses available to the parents of deaf babies from birth to 2 years of age and to the parents of preschool hearing-impaired children between the ages of 2 to 6 years. The courses are available in English and Spanish. The course is free of charge to parents enrolled in the course, and a bound volume of the complete course is available to professionals working with the deaf.

The courses are aimed at parents to use with their own hearing-impaired infants and young children, and emphasize the importance of early intervention. The home study lessons provide simple exercises based on the stages of language development focused on the whole child. In addition, the programs are aimed at parental attitudes including attention to feelings and emotions. The goal of the John Tracy Clinic Correspondence Course is to encourage, guide, and train the parents of young deaf children with on-site services. Additional information may be obtained by writing to John Tracy Clinic, 806 West Adams Boulevard, Los Angeles, CA 90007.

SUGGESTED READINGS

Maxon, A., and Brackett, D. (1992). *The Hearing Impaired Child: Infancy through High-School Years.* Boston: Andover Medical Publishers.
An interesting overview regarding the management of hearing-impaired children

Martin, F., and Clark, J. (Eds.). (1996). *Hearing Care for Children.* Boston: Allyn and Bacon.
This textbook covers audiologic aspects of pediatric hearing loss including identification, evaluation, counseling, amplification, and intervention.

Schuyler, V., and Rushmer, N. (1987). *Parent-Infant Habilitation.* Portland: Infant Hearing Resource Publishers.
This is an outstanding "how to" textbook aimed at professionals involved with working with hearing-impaired infants and their parents.

References

American Academy of Audiology. (1988). Early identification of hearing loss in infants and children. *Audiology Today, 1*(2), 8–9.

American Academy of Audiology. (1992). Audiologic guidelines for the diagnosis and treatment of otitis media in children. *Audiology Today, 4*, 4.

American Academy of Pediatrics. (1995). Joint Committee on Infant Hearing 1994 position statement. *Pediatrics, 95*(1), 152–156.

American Academy of Pediatrics and the American College of Obstetricians and Gynecologists. (1992). *Guidelines for perinatal care.* Elk Grove Village, IL: American Academy of Pediatrics and American College of Obstetricians and Gynecologists.

American Speech and Hearing Association. (1989). Audiologic screening of newborn infants who are at risk for hearing impairment. *Asha, 31*, 89–92.

American-Speech-Language-Hearing Association. (1991). Guidelines for the audiologic assessment of children from birth through 36 months of age. *Asha, 33*(Suppl. 5), 37–43.

American Speech-Language-Hearing Association. (1994). Joint Committee on Infant Hearing 1994 position statement. *Asha, 36*, 38–41.

Anderson, S., and Kemp, D. (1979). The evoked cochlear mechanical response in laboratory primates. *Archives of Otolaryngology, 224*, 47–54.

Apgar, V. (1953, July/August). A proposal for a new method of evaluating the newborn infant. *Current Research in Anesthesiology and Analgesia, 260.*

Apuzzo, M., and Yoshinaga-Itano, C. (1995). Early identification of infants with significant hearing loss and the Minnesota Child Development Inventory. *Seminars in Hearing, 16*(2), 124–139.

Baily, D. (1994). Foreword. In J. Roush and N. Matkin (Eds.), *Infants and toddlers with hearing loss* (p. xi). Baltimore: York Press.

Balkany, T., Berman, S., Simmons, M., and Jafek, B. (1978) Middle ear effusion in neonates. *Laryngoscope, 88*, 398–405.

Bartoshuk, A. (1962). Human neonatal cardiac acceleration to sound: habituation and dishabituation. *Perceptual Motor Skills, 15*, 15–27.

Bartoshuk, A. (1964). Human neonatal cardiac responses to sound: a power function. *Psychon. Sci., 1*, 151–152.

Bauman, N.M., Kirby-Keyser, L.J., Dolan, K.D., Wexler, D., Gantz, B.J., McCabe, B.R., and Bale, J.F., Jr. (1994). Mondini dysplasia and congenital cytomegalovirus infections. *Journal of Pediatrics, 124*, 71–78.

Bennett, M. (1980). Trials with the auditory response cradle: Headturns and startles as auditory responses in the neonate. *British Journal of Audiology, 14*, 122.

Bent, J.P., III, and Beck, R.A. (1994). Bacterial meningitis in the pediatric population: Paradigm shifts and ramifications for otolaryngology—head and neck surgery. *International Journal of Pediatric Otolaryngology, 30*, 41–49.

Bentler, R. (1989). External ear resonance characteristics in children. *Journal of Speech and Hearing Disorders, 54*(2), 264–268.

Bergman, B., Gorga, M., Neely, S., Kaminski, J., Beauchaine, K., and Peters, J. (1995). Preliminary descriptions of transient-evoked and distortion-product otoacoustic emissions from graduates of an intensive care nursery. *Journal of the American Academy of Audiology, 6*(2), 150–162.

Bergstrom, L. (1984). Congenital hearing loss. In J. Northern (Ed.), *Hearing disorders* (2nd ed., pp. 153–160). Boston: Little, Brown and Co.

Bergstrom, L., Hemenway, W., and Downs, M. (1971). A high risk registry to find congenital deafness. *The Otolaryngology Clinics of North America, 4*, 369.

Bess, F., and Paradise, J. (1994). Universal screening for infant hearing impairment: Not simple, not risk-free, not necessarily beneficial, and not presently justified. *Pediatrics, 93*, 330–334.

Bhattacharya, J., Bennett, M., and Tucker, S. (1984). Long term follow-up of newborns tested with the auditory response cradle. *Archives of Diseases in Children, 59*, 504.

Blake, P.E., and Hall, J.W. (1990). The status of state-wide policies for neonatal hearing screening. *Journal American Academy of Audiology, 1*, 67–74.

Bluestone, C. (1990). Methods of Examination: Clinical Examination. In C. Bluestone, S. Stool, and M. Scheetz (Eds.), *Pediatric otolaryngology* (2nd ed., pp. 111–124). Philadelphia: W.B. Saunders Company.

Bonfils, P., Uziel, A., and Pujol, R. (1988). Screening for auditory dysfunction in infants by evoked oto-acoustic emissions. *Journal of Otolaryngology—Head and Neck Surgery, 114*, 887–890.

Bradford, L. (1975). Respiration audiometry. In L. Bradford (Ed.), *Physiological measures of the audiovestibular system.* New York: Academic Press.

Brookhouser, P., and Moeller, M. (1986). Choosing the appropriate habilitative track for the newly identified hearing-impaired child. *Annals of Otology, Rhinology, and Laryngology, 95*(1), 51–59.

Brookhouser, P., Worthington, D., and Kelly, W. (1994). Fluctuating and/or progressive sensorineural hearing loss in children. *Laryngoscope, 104*, 958–964.

Brownell, W.E. (1984). Microscopic observations of cochlear hair cell motility. *Scanning Electron Microscopy, 3*, 1401–1406.

Brownell, W.E. (1990). Outer hair cell electromotility and otoacoustic emissions. *Ear and Hearing, 11*(2), 82–92.

Carnegie Corporation. (1994). *Starting point.* The report of the Cargegie Task Force on Meeting the Needs of Young Children (pp. 6–10). New York: Author.

Chang, K., Vohr, B., Norton, S., and Lekas, M. (1992). External canal and middle ear status in full term neonates related to evoked otoacoustic emission. [Abstract]. *Pediatric Research, 31,* 89.

Chugani, H. (1993). Positron emission tomography scanning in newborns. *Clinics in Perinatology, 20*(2), 398.

Chugani, H., Phelps, M., and Mazziotta, J. (1987). Positron emission tomography study of human brain functional development. *Annals of Neurology, 22*(4), 495.

Cohen, M.M., and Gorlin, R.J. (1995). Genetic hearing loss associated with musculoskeletal disorders. In R.J. Gorlin, H.V. Toriello, and M.M. Cohen (Eds.), *Hereditary hearing loss and its syndromes* (pp. 141–233). New York: Oxford University Press.

Cohen, N., and Waltzman, S. (1996). Cochlear implants in infants and young children. *Seminars in Hearing, 17*(2), 215–222.

Collet, L., Gartner, M., Moulin, A., Kauffman, I., Disant, F., and Morgon, A. Evoked otoacoustic emissions and sensorineural hearing loss. *Otolaryngology Head and Neck Surgery, 115,* 1060–1062.

Cope, Y., and Lutman, M. (1988). Oto-acoustic emissions. In B. McCormick (Ed.), *Paediatric audiology 0–5 years* (pp. 221–246). London: Taylor and Francis.

Coplan, J. (1987). Deafness: Ever heard of it? Delayed recognition of per manent hearing loss. *Pediatrics, 79*(2), 206–212.

Coplan, J., Gleason, J.R., Ryan, R., Burke, M., and Williams, M. (1982). Validation of an early language milestone scale in a high-risk population. *Pediatrics, 70,* 677–683.

Cross, T. (1988). Cultural competence continuum. *Focal Point, 3*(1), 1–4.

Cunningham, G. (1971). *Conference on newborn hearing screening: Proceedings, summary and recommendations.* Washington, DC: A.G. Bell Association for the Deaf.

Dahle, A.J., and McCollister, F.P. (1988). Audiological findings in children with neonatal herpes. *Ear and Hearing, 9,* 256–258.

Dahle, A.J., McCollister, F.P., Stagno, S., Reynolds, D.W., and Hoffman, H.E. (1979). Progressive hearing impairment in children with congenital cytomegalovirus infection. *Journal of Speech and Hearing Disorders, 44,* 220–229.

Davis, P.A. (1939). Effects of acoustic stimuli on the waking human brain. *Journal of Neurophysiology, 2,* 444–499.

Deliac, P., Demarquez, J.L., Barberot, J.B., Sandler, B., and Paty, J. (1990). Brainstem auditory evoked potentials in icteric fullterm newborns: alterations after exchange transfusion. *Neuropediatrics, 21,* 115–118.

Dennis, J.M., Sheldon, R., Toubas, P., and McCaffee, M. (1984). Identification of hearing loss in the neonatal intensive care unit population. *American Journal of Otology, 5*(3), 201–205.

Despland, P., and Galambos, R. (1980). The auditory brainstem response (ABR) is a useful diagnostic tool in the intensive care nursery. *Pediatric Research, 14,* 154–158.

Dodge, P.R., David, H., Feigin, R.D., Holmes, S.J., Kaplan, S.L., Jubelirer, D.P., Stechenberg, B.W. and Hirsh, S.K. (1984). Prospective evaluation of hearing impairment as a sequela of acute bacterial meningitis. *New England Journal of Medicine, 311,* 869–875.

Dolnick, E. (1993). Deafness as a culture. *The Atlantic Monthly, 272*(3), 37–53.

Downs, M.P., (1986). The rationale for neonatal hearing screening. In E.T. Swigart (Ed.), *Neonatal hearing screening* (pp. 3–16). San Diego: College-Hill Press.

Downs, M.P., and Silver, H.K. (1972). The A.B.C.D.'s to H.E.A.R.: Early identification in nursery, office and clinic of the infant who is deaf. *Clinical Pediatrics, 11,* 563–566.

Downs, M.P., and Sterritt, G.M. (1964). Identification audiometry for neonates. A preliminary report. *Journal of Auditory Research 4*(1), 69–80.

Durieux-Smith, A., Picton, T., Edwards, C., Goodman, J., and MacMurray, B. (1985). The Crib-O-Gram in the NICU: an evaluation based on brain stem electric response audiometry. *Ear and Hearing, 6,* 20.

Eilers, R., and Oller, K. (1994). Infant vocalizations and the early diagnosis of severe hearing impairment. *The Journal of Pediatrics, 124*(2), 199–203.

Eilers, R., Wilson, W., and Moore, J. (1977). Developmental changes in speech discrimination in infants. *Journal of Speech and Hearing Research, 20*(4), 766–779.

Eisenberg, R. (1975). Cardiotachometry. In L. Bradford (Ed.), *Physiological measures of the audio-vestibular system.* New York: Academic Press.

Elmer-Dewitt, P. (1994, January 17). The genetic revolution. *Time, 143,* 46–53.

Elssman, S., Matkin, N., and Sabo, M. (1987). Early identifidcation of congenital sensorineural hearing impairment. *The Hearing Journal, 40*(9), 13–17.

Elverland, H.H., and Torbergsen, T. (1991). Audiologic findings in a family with mitochondiral disorder. *American Journal of Otology, 12,* 459–465.

Ewing, I.R., and Ewing, A.W.F. (1944). The ascertainment of deafness in infancy and early childhood. *Journal of Laryngology and Otology,* 309–333.

Ewing, I.R., and Ewing, A.W.G. (1947). *Opportunity and the deaf child.* London: University of London Press.

Feightner, J. (1992). Screening in the 1990s: Some principles and guidelines. In F. Bess and J. Hall (Eds.), *Screening children for auditory function.* Nashville, TN: Bill Wilkerson Center Press.

Finitzo, T. (1995). Stewardship in universal hearing detection programs. *Audiology Today, 7*(5), 25.

Finitzo-Heiber, T. (1982). Auditory brainstem response: its place in infant audiological evaluations. *Seminars in Hearing, 3,* 76—87.

Finitzo-Hieber, T., McCracken, G.H., Jr., and Brown, K.C. (1985). Prospective controlled evaluation of auditory function in neonates given netilmicin or amikacin. *Journal of Pediatrics, 106,* 129–136.

Finitzo-Hieber, T., McCracken, G.H., Jr., Roeser, R.J., Allen, D.A., Chrane, D.F., and Morrow, J. (1979). Ototoxicity in neonates treated with gentamicin and kanamycin: results of a four-year controlled follow-up study. *Pediatrics, 63,* 443–450.

First, L.R., and Palfrey, J.S. (1994). The infant or young child with developmental delay. *New England Journal of Medicine, 330*(7), 478–483.

Fowler, K.B., Stagno, S., Pass, R.F., Britt, W.J., Boll, T.J., and Alford, C.A. (1992). The outcome of congenital cytomegalovirus infection in relation to maternal antibody status. *New England Journal of Medicine, 326,* 663–667.

Frankenburg, W., and Dodds, J. (1967). The Denver developmental screening test. *Journal of Pediatrics, 71*(2), 181.

Frankenburg, W., and North, A. (1974). *A guide to screening: EPSDT-Medicaid.* American Academy of Pediatrics in cooperation with Social and Rehabilitative Service, U.S. Department of Health, Education and Welfare.

Friel-Patti, S., and Roeser, R. (1985). Evaluating changes in the communication skills of deaf children using vibrotactile stimulation. *Ear and Hearing, 4,* 31–40.

Froding, C.A. (1960). Acoustic investigation of newborn infants. *Acta Otolaryngologica, 52,* 31–41.

Galambos, R., Hicks, G., and Wilson, M. (1982). Hearing loss in graduates of a tertiary intensive care nursery. *Ear and Hearing, 3*(1), 87–90.

Galambos, R., Hick, G., and Wilson, M. (1984). The auditory brainstem response reliably predicts hearing loss in graduates of a tertiary intensive care nursery. *Ear and Hearing, 5*(4), 254–260.

Geers, A., and Moog, J. (1994). Effectiveness of cochlear implant and tactile aids for deaf children: The sensory aids study at the Central Institute for the Deaf. *The Volta Review, 96,* 5.

Gerkin, K., and Church, M. (1907). Fetal alcohol syndrome and hearing loss. *Seminars in Hearing, 8*(2), 89–92.

Glattke, T., and Kujawa, S. (1991) Otoacoustic emissions. *American Journal of Audiology, 1,* 29–49.

Gleich, L.L., Urbina, M., and Pincus, R.L. (1994). Asymptomatic congenital syphilis and auditory brainstem response. *International Journal of Pediatric Otolaryngology, 30,* 11–13.

Gold, T. (1948) Hearing II. The physical basis of the action of the cochlea. *Proceedings of the Royal Society British, 135,* 492–498.

Goldstein, R. (1963). Electrophysiologic audiometry. In J. Jerger (Ed.), *Modern developments in audiology* (pp. 168–190). New York: Academic Press.

Goodhill, V. (1967). Auditory pathway lesions resulting from Rh incompatibility. In F. McConnell and P.H. Ward (Eds.), *Deafness in childhood* (pp. 215–228). Nashville, TN: Vanderbilt University Press.

Gorga, M., Reiland, J., Worthington, D., and Jesteadt, W. (1987). Auditory brainstem responses from graduates of an intensive care nursery: Normal patterns of response. *Journal of Speech and Hearing Research, 30*, 311–318.

Gorlin, R.J. (1995). Genetic hearing loss associated with endocrine and metabolic disorders. In R.J. Gorlin, H.V. Toriello and M.M. Cohen (Eds.), *Hereditary hearing loss and its syndromes* (pp. 318–354). New York: Oxford University Press.

Gorlin, R., Toriello, H., and Cohen, M. (1995). *Hereditary hearing loss and its syndromes.* New York: Oxford University Press.

Gorlin, R.J., Wester, D.C., and Carey, J.C. (1995). Genetic hearing loss associated with renal disorders. In R.J. Gorlin, H.V. Toriello and M.M. Cohen (Eds.), *Hereditary hearing loss and its syndromes* (pp. 234–256). New York: Oxford University Press.

Gravel, J. (1995). Meeting the challenges of children with hearing loss. *Hearing Instruments, 46*(6), 5.

Gregg, N.M. (1941). Congenital cataract following German measles in the mother. *Transactions of the Ophthalmologic Society of Australia, 3*, 35–46.

Greenberg, M., Calderon, R., and Kusche, C. (1984). Early intervention using simultaneous communication with deaf infants: The effect on communication development. *Child Development, 55*, 607–616.

Groothuis, J.R., Sell, S.H.W., Wright, P.F., and Altemeier, W. (1979). Otitis media in infancy: tympanometric findings. *Pediatrics, 63*, 435–442.

Grundfast, K. (1990). Hearing loss. In C. Bluestone and S. Stool (Eds.), *Pediatric otolaryngology* (2nd ed., pp. 203–229). Philadelphia: W.B. Saunders.

Hall, J. W., III. (1992) *Handbook of auditory evoked responses.* Needham, MA: Allyn & Bacon.

Hall, J. W., III, and Chase, P. (1993). Answers to 10 common clinical questions about otoacoustic emissions today. *The Hearing Journal, 46*(10), 29–34.

Hall, J.W., III, Kripal, J.P., and Hepp, T. (1988). Newborn hearing screening with auditory brainstem response: measurement problems and solutions. *Seminars in Hearing, 9*(1), 15–32.

Hardy, J.B., Dougherty, A., and Hardy, W.G. (1959). Hearing responses audiologic screening in infants. *Journal of Pediatrics, 55*, 382–390.

Harrison, M. (Ed.) (1994). Total quality management: application to audiology. *Seminars in Hearing, 15*, 4.

Hawkins, D., and Northern, J. (1992). Probe-microphone measurements with children. In H.G. Mueller, D.B. Hawkins, and J.L. Northern (Eds.), *Probe microphone measurements: Hearing aid selection and assessment* (pp. 159–182). San Diego: Singular Publishing Group.

Hayes, D. (1987). Problems in habilitation of hearing-impaired infants. *Seminars in Hearing, 8*(2), 181–185.

Hayes, D. (1994). Hearing loss in infants with craniofacial anomalies. *Otolaryngology—Head and Neck Surgery, 110*, 39–45.

Hayes, D., and Jerger, J. (1978). Response detection in respiration audiometry. *Archives of Otolaryngology, 104*, 183–185.

Healthy People 2000. (1990). U.S. Department of Health and Human Services, Public Health Service (DHHS Publication No. PHS 91-50213). Washington, DC: U.S. Government Printing Office.

Hendricks-Munoz, K., and Walton, J.P. (1988). Hearing loss in infants with persistent pulmonary hypertension. *Journal of Pediatrics, 81,* 650–659.

Hicks, T., Fowler, K., Richardson, M., Dahle, A., Adams, L., and Pass, R. (1993). Congenital cytomegalovirus infection and neonatal auditory screening. *Journal of Pediatrics, 123,* 779—782.

Holtzman, N. (1992). What drives neonatal screening programs? *The New England Journal of Medicine, 323,* 495.

Hosford-Dunn, H., Johnson, S., Simmons, F.B., Malachowski, N., and Low, K. (1987). Infant hearing screening: Program implementation and validation. *Ear and Hearing, 8*(1), 12–20.

Howie, V., Ploussard, J., and Sloyer, J. (1975) The "otitis-prone" condition. *American Journal Diseases of Children, 129,* 676–679.

Hung, K.L. (1989). Auditory brainstem responses in patients with neonatal hyperbilirubinemia and bilirubin encephalopathy. *Brain and Development, 11,* 297–301.

Hutchin, T.P., and Cortopassi, G.A. (1995). Mitochondria and risk for deafness. *American Journal of Audiology, 4,* 12–14.

Hyde, M., Riko, K., Corbin, H., Moroso, M., and Alberti, P. (1984). A neonatal hearing screening program using brainstem electric response audiometry. *Journal of Otolaryngology, 13,* 49–54.

Hyde, M., Riko, K., and Malizia, K. (1990). Audiometric accuracy of the click ABR in infants at risk for hearing loss. *Journal of the American Academy of Audiology, 1,* 59–66.

Ireton, H., and Thwing, E. (1972). *The Minnesota Child Development Inventory.* Minneapolis: University of Minnesota, MN.

Jacobson, J. (Ed.). (1994). *Principles and applications in auditory evoked potentials.* Needham Heights, MA: Allyn and Bacon.

Jacobson, J., and Jacobson, C. (1987). Application of test performance characteristics in newborn auditory screening. *Seminars in Hearing, 8*(2), 133–141.

Jacobson, J.T., Jacobson, C.A., and Spahr, R.C. (1990). Automated and conventional ABR screening techniques in high-risk infants. *Journal of the American Academy of Audiology, 1,* 187–195.

Jacobson, J.T., and Morehouse, C. (1984). A comparison of auditory brainstem response and behavioral screening of high risk and normal newborn infants. *Ear and Hearing, 5,* 247–253.

Jerger, J.F., and Hayes, D. (1976). The cross-check principle in pediatric audiometry. *Archives of Otolaryngology, 102,* 614-620.

Johnson, J., Mauk, G., Takekawa, K., Simon, P., Sia, C., and Blackwell, P. (1993). Implementing a statewide system of services for infants and toddlers with hearing disabilities. *Seminars in Hearing, 14*(1), 105-119.

Joint Committee on Infant Hearing. (1994). Position statement. *Audiology Today, 6*(6), 6–9.

Jones, F., and Simmons, F. (1977). Early identifcation of significant hearing loss: the Crib-O-Gram. *Hearing Instruments, 28,* 8–10.

Keller, H. (1954). *The story of my life.* Garden City, NY: Doubleday.

Kelly, T.E. (1986). *Clinical genetics and genetic counseling* (2nd ed.). Chicago: Yearbook Medical Publishing.

Kemp, D. (1978). Stimulated acoustic emissions from within the human auditory system. *Journal of the Acoustical Society of America, 64*(5), 1386–1391.

Kemp, D. (1979). Evidence of mechanical non-linearity and frequency selective wave amplification in the cochlea. *Archives of Otolaryngology, 224,* 37–45.

Kemp D., and Ryan, S. (1993). The use of transient evoked otoacoustic emissions in neonatal hearing screening programs. *Seminars in Hearing, 14*(1), 30–45.

Kennedy, C. , Kimm, D., Cafarelli, D., Evans, P., Hunter, M., Lenton, S., and Thornton, R. (1991). Otoacoustic emissions and auditory brainstem response in the newborn. *Archives of Disease in Childhood, 64,* 1124–1129.

Kent, R., Osberger, M., Netsell, R., and Hustedde, C. (1987). Phonetic development in identical twins differing in auditory function. *Jounal of Speech and Hearing Disorders, 52,* 64–75.

Kileny, P.R. (1987). Algo-I automated infant hearing screener: preliminary results. *Seminars in Hearing, 8*(2), 125–131.

Kim, D. (1980). Cochlear mechanics: implications of electrophysical and acoustical observations. *Hearing Research, 2,* 297–317.

Kolb, B. (1989). Brain development, plasticity, and behavior. *American Psychologist, 44*(9), 1203–1212.

Koop, C.E. (1993). We can identify children with hearing impairment before their first birthday. *Seminars in Hearing, 14*(1), 1–2.

Kruger, B. (1987). An update on the external ear canal response in infants and young children. *Ear and Hearing, 8,* 333–336.

Kuhl, P., Williams, K., Lacerda, F., Stevens, K., and Lindblom, B. (1992). Linguistic experience alters phonetic perception in infants by 6 months of age. *Science, 255,* 606–608.

Levitt, H., McGarr, N., and Geffner, D. (1987). Development of language and communication skills in hearing-impaired children. *ASHA Monographs,* No. 26. Rockville, MD: American Speech-Language-Hearing Association.

Lindner, R. (1992). What drives neonatal screening programs: A response. *New England Journal of Medicine, 326*(7), 494–495.

Loeb, G. (1985, February). The functional replacement of the ear. *Scientific American,* p. 106.

Lonsbury-Martin, B., and Martin, G. (1990) The clinical utility of distortion product emissions. *Ear and Hearing, 11,* 144–154.

Lotke, M. (1995). The sounds of silence. *Contemporary Pediatrics, 12*(10), 104–130.

Luteman, M., Mason, S., Sheppard, S., and Gibbin, K. (1989). Differential diagnostic potential of otoacoustic emissions: A case study. *Audiology, 28,* 205–210.

Mahoney, T.M. (1984). High-risk hearing screening of large general newborn populations. *Seminars in Hearing, 5*(1), 25–36.

Mahoney, T.M., and Eichwald, J.G. (1987). The ups and "DOWNS" of high-risk screening: The Utah statewide program. *Seminars in Hearing, 8*, 155–163.

Margolis, R., and Thornton, A.R. (1991). Spreadsheet systems for tracking audiology patients. *Audiology Today, 3*(4), 24–26.

Markides, A. (1976). The effect of hearing aid use on the user's residual hearing. *Scandinavian Audiology, 5*, 205–210.

Markowitz, R.K. (1990). Cost effectiveness comparisons of hearing screening in the neonatal intensive care unit. *Seminars in Hearing, 11*(2), 161–166.

Marlowe, J. (1993). Screening all newborns for hearing impairment in a community hospital. *American Journal of Audiology, 2*(1), 22–25.

Marron, M.J., Crisafi, M.A., Driscoll, J.M., Jr., Wung, J.T., Driscoll, Y.T., Fay, T.H., and James, L.S. (1992). Hearing aid neurodevelopmental outcome in survivors of persistent pulmonary hypertension of the newborn. *Pediatrics, 90*, 392–396.

Martin, G., Probst, R., and Lonsbury-Martin, B. (1990). Otoacoustic emissions in human ears: Normative findings. *Ear and Hearing, 11*(2), 106–120.

Matkin, N. (1977). Assessment of hearing sensitivity during the preschool years. In F. Bess (Ed.), *Childhood deafness* (pp. 127–134). New York: Grune and Stratton.

Matkin, N.D. (1984). Early recognition and referral of hearing-impaired children. *Pediatrics in Review, 6*(5), 151–155.

Matkin, N., and Carhart, R. (1966). Audiological patterns characterizing hearing impairment due to Rh incompatibility. *Archives of Otolaryngology, 84*, 502–512.

Mauk, G.W., and Behrens, T.R. (1993). Historical, political, and technological context associated with early identification of hearing loss. *Seminars in Hearing, 14*(1), 1–17.

Mauk, G.W., White, K.R., Mortensen, L.B., and Behrens, T.R. (1991). The effectiveness of screening programs based on high-risk characteristics in early identification of hearing impairment. *Ear and Hearing, 12*, 312–319.

Maxon, A., White, K., Behrens, T., and Vohr, B. (1995). Referral rates and cost efficiency in a universal newborn hearing screening program using transient evoked otoacoustic emissions. *Journal American Academy of Audiology, 6*(4), 271–277.

McCollister, F.P., Simpson, L.C., Dahle, A.J., Pass, R.F., Fowler, K.B., Amos, C.S., and Boll, T.J. (1996). Hearing loss and congenital symptomatic cytomegalovirus infection: A case report of multidisciplinary longitudinal assessment and intervention. *Journal American Academy of Audiology, 7*, 57–62.

McConnell, F., and Liff, S. (1975). The rationale for early identification and intervention. *Otolaryngologic Clinics of North America, 8*(1), 77–87.

McGonigel, M. (1994). The individualized family service plan. In J. Roush and N. Matkin (Eds.), *Infants and toddlers with hearing loss* (pp. 99–112). Baltimore: York Press.

Mencher, G.T. (1976). *Early identification of hearing loss. Proceedings from the 1974 Nova Scotia Conference on Early Identification of Hearing Loss* (pp. 1–207). Basel, Switzerland: S. Karger AG.

Moore, J.M., Thompson, G., and Thompson,M. (1975). Auditory localization of infants as a function of reinforcement conditions. *Journal of Speech and Hearing Disorders, 40,* 29–34.

Moore, J.M., Wilson, W.R., and Thompson, G. (1977). Visual reinforcement of head-turn responses in infants under twelve months of age. *Journal of Speech and Hearing Disorders, 42,* 328–334.

Morton, N.E. (1991). Genetic epidemiology of hearing loss. *Annals of the New York Academy of Sciences, 630,* 16–31.

Murphy, K. (1962). Development of hearing in babies. *Child Family, 1*(1), 1–13.

Myer, C. (1992). Fluctuating hearing loss in children. *American Journal of Audiology, 1*(2), 25–26.

Nakamura, H., Takada, S., Shimabuku, R., Matsuo, M., Matsuo, T., and Negishi, H. (1985). Auditory nerve and brainstem responses in newborn infants with hyperbilirubinemia. *Pediatrics, 75,* 703–708.

National Institutes of Health Consensus Statement (1993). Early identification of hearing loss in infants and young children: Consensus development conference on early identification of hearing loss in infants and young children. Vol. 11(1), 1–3.

National Institutes of Health. (1995). Consensus Development Conference Statement: Cochlear implants in adults and children. Washington, DC

Naulty, C.M., Weiss, I.P., and Herer, G.R. (1986). Progressive sensorineural hearing loss in survivors of persistent fetal circulation. *Ear and Hearing, 7,* 74–77.

Nield, T.A., Schrier, S., Ramos, A.D., Platzker, A.C.G., and Warburton, D. (1986). Unexpected hearing loss in high-risk infants. *Pediatrics, 78,* 417–422.

Northern, J. (1986). Selection of children for cochlear implantation. *Seminars in Hearing, 7*(4), 341–347.

Northern, J. (1988). Recent developments in acoustic immittance measurements in children. In F. Bess (Ed.), *Hearing impairment in children* (pp. 176–189). Parkton, MD: York Press.

Northern, J. (1995). Acoustic immittance measurements. In J. Northern (Ed.), *Hearing Disorders* (3rd ed., pp. 57–72). Needham, MA: Allyn & Bacon.

Northern, J., and Downs, M. (1991). *Hearing in children* (4th ed.). Baltimore, MD: Williams and Wilkins Co.

Northern, J., Gabbard, S.A., and Kinder, D. (1995). Pediatric considerations in selecting and fitting hearing aids. In R.E. Sandlin (Ed.), *Handbook of hearing aid amplification: Part II, Clinical considerations and fitting practices* (pp.113–132). San Diego: Singular Publishing Group.

Northern, J., and Hayes, D. (1994). Universal screening for infant hearing impairment: Necessary, beneficial and justifiable. *Audiology Today, 6*(2), 10–13.

Norton, S. (1993). Application of transient evoked otoacoustic emissions to pediatric populations. *Ear and Hearing, 14,* 64–73.

Nwaesei, C.G., Van Aerde, J., Boyden, M., and Perlman, M. (1984). Changes in auditory brainstem responses in hyperbilirubinemic infants before and after exchange transfusion. *Pediatrics, 7,* 800–803.

Oller, K., Payne, S., and Gavin, W. (1986). Tactile speech perception by minimally trained deaf subjects. *The Volta Review, 88,* 21–36.

Pappas, D. (1983) A study of the high-risk registry for sensorineural hearing impairment. *Archives of Otolaryngology—Head and Neck Surgery, 91,* 41–44.

Paradise, J.L., Smith, C., and Bluestone, C.D. (1976). Tympanometric detection of middle ear effusion in infants and young children. *Pediatrics, 58,* 198–206.

Perlman, M., Fainmesser, P., Sohmer, H., Tamari, H., Wax, Y., and Pevsmer, B. (1983). Auditory nerve-brainstem evoked responses in hyperbilirubinemic neonates. *Pediatrics, 72,* 658–664.

Peters, J.G. (1986). An automated infant screener using advanced evoked response technology. *Hearing Journal, 3,* 25–30.

Primus, M.A., and Thompson, G. (1987). Response and reinforcement in operant audiometry. *Journal of Speech and Hearing Disorders, 52,* 294–299.

Raffin, M., and Matz, G. (1994). Letter to the editor. *Pediatrics, 94*(6), 952.

Raynor, D.B. (1993). Cytomegalovirus infection in pregnancy. *Seminars in Perinatalogy, 17,* 394–402.

Rose, J. R. (1996) Medical imaging in otologic diagnosis. In J. Northern (Ed.), *Hearing disorders* (3rd ed., pp. 111–125). Needham Heights, MA: Allyn & Bacon.

Rosetti, L.M. (1990). *Infant-toddler assessment: An interdisciplinary approach.* Boston: College-Hill Press.

Ross, M. (1994). The child is the focus, not the approach. *Hearing Instruments, 45*(10, Suppl. 2), 4.

Roush, J., and Matkin, N. (1994). *Infants and toddlers with hearing loss.* Baltimore: York Press.

Roush, J., and McWilliams, R.A. (1990). A new challenge for pediatric audiology: Public law 99-457. *Journal of the American Academy of Audiology, 1,* 196–208.

Roush, J., and McWilliam, R. (1994). Family-centered early intervention: Historical, philosophical, and legislative issues. In J. Roush and N. Matkin (Eds.), *Infants and toddlers with hearing loss* (pp. 3–121). Baltimore: York Press.

Salamy, A., Eldredge, L., and Tooley, W.H. (1989). Neonatal status and hearing loss in high-risk infants. *Journal of Pediatrics, 114,* 847–852.

Schulman, C. (1970). Heart rate response habituation in high-risk premature infants. *Psychophysiology, 6,* 690–694.

Schulman, C., and Wade, G. (1970). The use of heart rate in the audiological evaluation of non-verbal children: Clinical trials on an infant population. *Neuropaediatric, 2,* 197–205.

Schulman-Galambos, C., and Galambos, R. (1979). Brainstem evoked response audiometry in newborn hearing screening. *Archives of Otolaryngology, 105,* 86–90.

Schumacher, R.E., Spak, C., and Kileny, P.R. (1990). Asymmetric brain stem auditory evoked responses in infants treated with extracorporeal membrane oxytgenation. *Ear and Hearing, 11,* 359–362.

Sell, E.J., Gaines, J.A., Gluckman, C., and Williams, E. (1985). Persistent fetal circulation neurodevelopmental outcome. *American Journal of Diseases in Children, 139,* 25–28.

Shah, C., Chandler, D., and Dale, R. (1978). Delay in referral of children with impaired hearing. *Volta Review, 80,* 207.

Shimizu, H., Walters, R.J., Proctor, L.R., Kennedy, D.W., Allen, M.C., and Markowitz, R.K. (1990). Identification of hearing impairment in the neonatal intensive care unit population: Outcome of a five-year project at the Johns Hopkins Hospital. *Seminars in Hearing, 11,* 150–160.

Simmons, F., McFarland, W., and Jones, W. (1979). An automated hearing screening technique for newborns. *Acta Otolaryologica, 87,* 1.

Simmons, F., and Russ, F. (1974). Automated newborn hearing screening, the Crib-O-Gram. *Archives of Otolaryology, 100,* 1.

Simmons, F.B. (1976). Automated hearing screening test for newborns: The crib-o-gram. In G. Mencher (Ed.), *Early identification of hearing loss* (pp. 171–180). Basel: Karger.

Simmons, F.B. (1980a). Diagnosis and rehabilitation of deaf newborns, part II. *Asha, 22,* 475.

Simmons, F.B. (1980b). Patterns of deafness in newborns. *Laryngoscope, 90,* 448–453.

Stagno, S., Reynolds, D.W., Amos, C.S., Dahle, A.J., McCollister, F.P., Mohindra, I., Ermocilla, R., and Alford, C.A. (1977). Auditory and visual defects resulting from symptomatic and subclinical congenital cytomegaloviral and toxoplasma infections. *Pediatrics, 59,* 669–678.

Stein, L. (1995). On the real age of identification of congenital hearing loss. *Audiology Today, 7*(1), 10–11.

Stein, L.K., and Boyer, K.M. (1994). Progress in the prevention of hearing loss in infants. *Ear and Hearing, 15,* 116–125.

Stein, L., Clark, S., and Kraus, N. (1983). The hearing-impaired infant: patterns of identification and habilitation. *Ear and Hearing, 4*(5), 232–236.

Stein, L., and Jabaley, T. (1981). Early identification and parent counseling. In L. Stein, E. Mindel, and T.Jabaley (Eds.), *Deafness and mental health* (pp. 23–35). New York: Grune & Stratton.

Stein, L., Jabaley, T., Spitz, R. Stoakley, D., and McGee, T. (1990). The hearing-impaired infant: Patterns of identification and habilitation revisited. *Ear and Hearing, 11*(3), 201–205.

Stevens, J., Webb.H., Hutchinson, J., Connell, J., Smith, M., and Buffin, J. (1989). Click evoked otoacoustic emissions compared with brainstem electric response. *Archives of Disease in Childhood, 64,* 1105–1111.

Stevens, J., Webb, H., Hutchinson, J., Connell, J., Smith, M., and Buffin, J. (1990). Click evoked otoacoustic emissions in neonatal screening. *Ear and Hearing, 11,* 128–133.

Stewart, J. (1996) Congenital deafness. In J. Northern (Ed.), Hearing disorders (3rd ed., pp. 189–198). Needham Heights, MA: Allyn & Bacon.

Stoel-Gammon, C., and Otomo, K. (1986). Babbling development of hearing impaired and normally hearing subjects. *Journal of Speech and Hearing Disorders, 51*(1), 33–41.

Stool, S., Berg, A. Berman, S. et al. (1994) *Otitis media with effusion in young children. Clinical practice guideline*, Number 12. AHCPR Publication No. 94-0622. Rockville, MD: Agency for Health Care Policy and Research, Public Health Service, U.S. Department of Health and Human Services.

Strauss, M. (1985). A clinical pathologic study of hearing loss in congenital cytomegalovirus infection. *Laryngoscope, 95*, 951–962.

Swigart, E.T. (1986). *Neonatal hearing screening.* San Diego: College-Hill Press.

Tan, K.L., Skurr, B.A., and Yip, Y.Y. (1992). Phototherapy and the brainstem auditory evoked response in neonatal hyperbilirubinemia. *Journal of Pediatrics, 120*, 306–308.

Teel, J., Winston, M., Aspinall, K., Rousey, C., and Goetzinger, C. (1967). Thresholds of hearing by respiration using a polygraph. *Archives of Otolaryngology, 86*, 66–68.

Thelin, J.W., Mitchell, J.A., Hefner, M.A., and Davenport, S.L. (1986). CHARGE syndrome. Part II. Hearing loss. *International Journal of Pediatric Otolaryngology, 12*, 145–163.

Toriello, H.V. (1995). Genetic hearing loss associated with renal disorders. In R.J. Gorlin, H.V. Toriello, and M.M. Cohen (Eds.), *Hereditary hearing loss and its syndromes* (pp. 368–412). New York: Oxford University Press.

Turner, R. (1991). Modeling the cost and performance of early identification protocols. *Journal American Academy of Audiology, 2*(4), 195–205.

Turner, R. (1992a). Comparison of four hearing screening protocols. *Journal American Academy of Audiology, 3*(3), 200–207.

Turner, R. (1992b). Factors that determine the cost and performance of early identification protocols. *Journal American Academy of Audiology, 3*(4), 233–241.

U.S. Department of Health and Human Services, Public Health Service (1990). *Healthy People 2000: National health promotion and disease prevention objectives.* Washington, DC: Government Printing Office.

Uziel, A., and Piron, J. (1991). Evoked otoacoustic emissions from normal newborns and babies admitted to an intensive care baby unit. *Acta Otolaryngolica* (Stockholm), (Suppl. 482), 85–91.

Van Almen, P., Allen, L., Adkins, T., Anderson, K., Blake-Rahter, T., English, K., and DeConde Johnson, C. (1994). Letter to the editor. *Pediatrics, 94*(6), 957.

Walker, D., Gugenheim, S., Downs, M., and Northern, J. (1989). Early language milestone scale and language screening of young children. *Pediatrics, 83*(2), 284–288.

Walton, J.P., and Hendricks-Munoz, K. (1991). Profile and stability of sensorineural hearing loss in persistent pulmonary hypertension of the newborn. *Journal of Speech and Hearing Research, 34*, 1362–1370.

Wedenberg, E. (1956). Auditory tests on newborn infants. *Acta Otolaryngologica, 46*, 446–461.

Weisenberger, J., and Percy, M. (1994). Use of the Tactaid II and Tactaid VII with children. *The Volta Review, 96*(5), 41–57.

White, J.D. (1996). Laboratory diagnosis of otologic disease. In J. Northern (Ed.), *Hearing disorders* (3rd ed., pp. 99–110). Needham Heights, MA: Allyn & Bacon.

White, K., and Behrens, T. (Eds.). (1993). The Rhode Island Hearing Assessment Project: Implications for universal newborn screening. *Seminars in Hearing, 14*(1), 1–122.

White, K.R., Vohr, B.R., and Behrens, T.R. (1993). Universal newborn hearing screening using transient evoked otoacoustic emissions: Results of the Rhode Island Hearing Assessment Project. *Seminars in Hearing, 14*(1), 19–29.

White, K., and Maxon, A. (1995). Universal screening for infant hearing impairment: Simple, beneficial and presently justified. *International Journal of Pediatric Otolaryngology, 32*, 205.

Williamson, W.D., Demmler, G.J., Percy, A.K., and Catlin, F.I. (1992). Progressive hearing loss in infants with asymptomatic congenital cytomegalovirus infection. *Pediatrics, 90*, 862-866.

Winton, P., and Bailey, D., Jr. (1994). Becoming family centered: strategies for self-examination. In J. Roush and N. Matkin (Eds.), *Infants and toddlers with hearing loss* (pp. 24–39). Baltimore: York Press.

Wright, L., and Rybak, L. (1983). Crib-O-Gram (COG) and ABR: Effect of variables on test results. *Journal of the Acoustical Society of America, 74*(Suppl. 1), 540.

Yoshinaga-Itano, C. (1987). Aural habilitation: A key to the acquisition of knowledge, language and speech. *Seminars in Hearing, 8*(2), 169–174.

Yoshinaga-Itano, C. (1995). Efficacy of early identification and early interventiion. *Seminars in Hearing, 16*(2), 115–123.

Zeaman, D., and Wegner, N. (1954). The role of drive reduction in the classical conditioning of an autonomically mediated response. *Journal of Experimental Psychology, 48*, 349–354.

Zeaman, D., and Wegner, H. (1956). Cardiac reflex to tones of threshold intensity. *Journal of Speech and Hearing Disorders, 21*, 71–75.

APPENDIX A

Statement on Neonatal Screening for Hearing Impairment (November, 1970)

In recognition of the need to identify hearing impairment as early in life as possible, auditory screening programs have been implemented in newborn nurseries throughout the country. Review of data from the limited number of controlled studies which have been reported to date has convinced us that results of mass screening programs are inconsistent and misleading.

To determine whether mass screening programs for newborn infants should indeed be instituted, intensive study of a number of variables is essential. These should include stimuli, response patterns, environmental factors, status at the time of testing, and behavior or observers. Furthermore, confirmation of results obtained in the nursery must await data derived from extended follow-up studies which involve quantitative assessment of hearing status.

In view of the above considerations and despite our recognition of the urgent need for early detection of hearing impairment, we urge increased research efforts, but cannot recommend routine screening of newborn infants for hearing impairment.

Supplementary Statement Of Joint Committee on Infant Screening
(July, 1972)

In light of the urgent need to detect hearing impairment as early as possible, a 1970 statement of the Joint Committee urged further investigation of screening methods but discouraged routine hearing screening which is not research oriented. In consonance with that statement, and in view of the information that application of high risk data can increase the detectability of congenital hearing impairment perhaps as much as tenfold, the Committee considers it appropriate to make additions to the 1970 statement.

The Committee recommends that, since no satisfactory technique is yet established that will permit hearing screening of all newborns, infant AT RISK for hearing impairment should be identified by means of history and physical examination. These children should be tested and followed-up as hereafter described.

I. The criterion for identifying a newborn as AT RISK for hearing impairment is the presence of one or more of the following:
   A. History of hereditary childhood hearing impairment.
   B. Rubella or other nonbacterial intrauterine fetal infection (e.g., cytomegalovirus infections, Herpes infection).
   C. Defects of ear, nose, or throat. Malformed, low-set or absent pinnae; cleft lip

or

    palate (including submucous cleft); any residual abnormali-
ty of the otorhinolaryngeal system.

D. Birthweight less than 1500 grams.

E. Bilirubin level greater than 20 mg/100 ml serum.

II. Infants falling in this category should be referred for an
indepth audiological evaluation of hearing during their first
two months of life and, even if hearing appears to be normal,
should receive regular hearing evaluations thereafter at office
or well-baby clinics. Regular evaluation is important since
familial hearing impairment is not necessarily present at birth
but may develop at an uncertain period of time later.

APPENDIX B

Conference on Newborn Hearing Screening

Proceedings Summary & Recommendations

San Francisco International Airport
Hilton Inn
California
February 23, 24, 25, 1971

Conference Sponsors

Maternal and Child Health Service
Health Services and Mental Health Administration
Public Health Service
Department of Health, Education and Welfare
Rockville, MD 20852

Bureau of Maternal and Child Health
California State Department of Public Health
2151 Berkeley Way
Berkeley, CA 94704

This report is reprinted with permission of the sponsors
and is available from
The Alexander Graham Bell Association for the Deaf
3417 Volta Place, N.W.
Washington, DC 20007

NEWBORN HEARING SCREENING RECOMMENDATIONS

I would like to preface these recommendations by saying that we were most fortunate to have had the opportunity to assemble such a qualified and experienced group of professionals from a broad spectrum of disciplines. I believe that we have gone far toward accomplishing the conference objectives and the proceedings of this conference will be a most valuable resource for others who will consider this same subject in the future.

The formulation of general statements and recommendations was perhaps the most difficult task facing the Conference. In selecting the participants we made a deliberate effort to include both proponents and opponents of mass newborn screening and realized that as a result the differences of opinion and the broad spectrum of points of view represented would not be conducive to unanimity of conclusions.

But the situation is not at all bleak; while we found the diversity we expected, we also found some broad areas of agreement. The statements listed under "Recommendations" were then submitted to the assembled group and approved after general discussion. Participants were given an opportunity to review the written recommendations subsequent to the meeting. The following statements represent the final recommendations of the conference.

George C. Cunningham

RECOMMENDATIONS

I. A high risk population can and should be identified by prenatal history and postnatal physical assessment of the infant. As a first step a registry should contain the following groups.

Prenatal High Risk Procedure

1. All infants with a family history of childhood deafness in some member of the immediate family, i.e., father, mother, or sibling.
2. All infants whose mothers have had rubella documented or strongly suspected during any period of pregnancy.

3. All infants with a family history of congenital malformations of the external ear, cleft lip or palate.
4. All infants with a family history of deafness in other relatives, with onset in childhood.

POSTNATAL

5. All infants found to have a structural abnormality of the external ear, cleft lip or palate, including bifid uvula.
6. All infants having bilirubin values of 20 mg/100 mg or more, who had exchange transfusions are at high risk of bilirubin encephalopathy.
7. All infants under 1,500 grams.
8. All infants with abnormal otoscopic findings.

(It was suggested that Groups 1, 2 and 5 would be referred to an otologic-audiologic testing center for more elaborate workup by available methods, such as evoked potential, cardiac response audiometry and followed by periodic followup evaluations including consecutive tests.)

II. While from the standpoint of preventive, therapeutic and rehabilitative intervention there is little special advantages to detecting congenital deafness in the first few days of life, and acknowledging that screening test validity and accuracy are improved if screening is deferred to a later age, the possibility of screening all newborns should be seriously considered if: (1) one or more relatively reliable and inexpensive auditory screening techniques are available, and (2) it can be shown this procedure yields significant number of cases that would be missed or not detected until after the optimal period for intervention if an alternate program were selected for screening based on delayed testing alone.

III. An auditory screening technique, if it is to be applicable to all infants, must be simplified so as to meet the following criteria as far as possible. It should
   1. Require a minimal investment in new personnel, training, time and equipment;
   2. Detect a significant number of infants with impaired hearing that would not be detected by high risk screening alone;
   3. Have an acceptably low rate of false negatives (missed cases) and false positives;
   4. Have a screening criteria that is clearly pass or fail

whether by subjective judgment, e.g., awakens versus does not awaken, or by instrument results, e.g., red light, green light, amber light.

IV. Because of limited resources available to the health delivery system, an analysis of the net cost versus net benefit of any proposed newborn screening program and the relative priority for this investment of resources must be considered. Data should be assembled and developed that could be used to illustrate the net advantage to the individual and society of early case finding before early detection can be recommended as a high priority item for health funds. In consideration of these cost factors the screening of only high risk registry infants should be analyzed and might be acceptable as an alternative to universal screening.

V. Regardless of what is done in the nursery, followup including reexamination by a suitably reliable technique must be part of the recommended program for all infants during the first year of life.

VI. Parents and all health and educational personnel should be encouraged to refer all suspected children as they can be tested at any age. There is no age too young for detection or for rehabilitation. In implementing this recommendation an assessment of resources available for services to those detected and referred should first be made.

VII. The Conference recommends that greater effort be made to train those responsible for the care of infants in the evaluation of the ear with the pneumatic otoscopic and encourages such evaluations of infants and toddlers. Such evaluation should include a brief history and an appropriate test of auditory function performed with simple equipment by suitably trained personnel. Screening programs should be designed to utilize the skills and resources of public health agencies in assuring completeness of followup.

VIII. All screening procedures should be viewed as part of comprehensive health care and ultimately coordinated into an efficient multifaceted screening and health surveillance and maintenance program.

IX. Areas identified as promising possibilities for research efforts that could contribute to the decision to screen and to the design of the screening program are:
1. Validation of the cribogram approach on a large sample in several institutions with appropriate followup;
2. Validation of a simple awakening response to a specified standard stimulus (90 dB fluctuating 2,000-3,000 Hz, noise at 14 inches) with appropriate followup;

3. Simplification of the instrumental (objective) approach to screening;
4. Long-term periodic testing of a high risk population prospectively to ascertain the frequency of acquired deafness;
5. Efforts should be made to identify conditions which are associated with a high risk of hearing problems to be added to the high risk registry; criteria of high risk should be refined by a continuing investigation of the correlation between selected phenomena and hearing defects;
6. Evaluation should be made of the usefulness and reliability of vestibular testing in the nursery and during infancy;
7. There should be epidemiological studies of the incidence and clinical significance of conductive losses in the first year of life;
8. The effectiveness of genetic counseling in various settings on family size should be evaluated;
9. Evaluation of the available hearing evaluation tests for early infancy (4 to 8 months) should be carried out and a simple practical procedure recommended and promoted.

APPENDIX C

Joint Committee on Infant Hearing Position Statement 1982

Early detection of hearing impairment in the affected infant is important for medical treatment and subsequent educational intervention to ensure development of communication skills.

In 1973, the Joint Committee on Infant Hearing Screening recommended identifying infants at risk for hearing impairment by means of five criteria and suggested follow-up audiological evaluation of these infants until accurate assessments of hearing could be made. Since the incidence of moderate to profound hearing loss in the at-risk infant group is 2.5% to 5%, audiologic testing of this group is warranted. Acoustic testing of all newborn infants has a high incidence of false-positive and false-negative results and is not universally recommended.

Recent research suggests the need for expansion and clarification of the 1973 criteria. This 1982 statement expands the risk criteria and makes recommendations for the evaluation and treatment of the hearing-impaired infant.

I. IDENTIFICATION
A. Risk Criteria
The factors that identify those infants who are AT RISK for having hearing impairment include the following:
1. A family history of childhood hearing impairment.
2. Congenital perinatal infection (e.g., cytomegalovirus, rubella, herpes, toxo-plasmosis, syphilis).
3. Anatomic malformations involving the head or neck (e.g., dysmorphic appearance, including syndromal and nonsyndromal abnormalities, overt or submucous cleft palate, morphologic abnormalities of the pinna).
4. Birthweight less than 1500 gm.
5. Hyperbilirubinemia at level exceeding indications for exchange transfusion.
6. Bacterial meningitis, especially from *H. influenzae*.
7. Severe asphyxia, which may include infants with Apgar scores of 0-3 who fail to institute spontaneous respiration by 10 minutes and those with hypotonia persisting to 2 hours of age.

B. Screening Procedures
The hearing of infants who manifest any item on the list of risk criteria should be screened, preferably under supervision of an audiologist, optimally by 3 months of age, but not later than 6 months of age. The initial screening should include the observation of behavioral or electro-

physiological response to sound.* If consistent electro-physiological or behavioral responses are detected at appropriate sound levels, the screening process will be considered complete except in those cases in which there is a probability of a progressive hearing loss (e.g., family history of delayed onset, degenerative disease, intra-uterine infections). If results of an initial screening of an infant manifesting any risk criteria are equivocal, the infant should be referred for diagnostic testing.

II. **DIAGNOSIS FOR INFANTS FAILING SCREENING**
   A. Diagnostic evaluation of an infant under 6 months of age includes:
      1. General physical examination and history including:
         a. Examination of the head and neck
         b. Otoscopy and otomicroscopy
         c. Identification of relevant physical abnormalities
         d. Laboratory tests such as urinalysis and diagnostic tests for perinatal infections.
      2. Comprehensive audiological evaluation:
         a. Behavioral history
         b. Behavioral observation audiometry
         c. Testing of auditory evoked potentials, if indicated.
   B. After the age of 6 months, the following are also recommended:
      1. Communication skills evaluation
      2. Acoustic immittance measurements
      3. Selected tests of development

III. **MANAGEMENT OF THE HEARING-IMPAIRED INFANT**
Habilitation of the hearing-impaired infant may begin while the diagnostic evaluation is in process. The Committee recommends, however, that whenever possible, the diagnostic process should be completed and habilitation begun by the age of 6 months. Services to the hearing-impaired infant under 6 months of age include:
   A. Medical Management
      1. Reevaluation
      2. Treatment

---

    3. Genetic evaluation and counseling when indicated

B. Audiologic Management

    1. Ongoing audiological assessment

    2. Selection of hearing aid(s)

    3. Family counseling

C. Psychoeducational Management

    1. Formulation of an individualized educational plan

    2. Information about the implications of hearing impairment

After the age of 6 months, the hearing-impaired infant becomes easier to manage in a habilitation plan but he or she will require the services listed above.

APPENDIX D

Joint Committee on Infant Hearing 1990 Position Statement

The following expanded position statement was developed by the Joint Committee on Infant Hearing and approved by the American Speech-Language-Hearing Association (ASHA) Legislative Council (LC 40-90) in November 1990. Joint Committee member organizations that approved this position statement and their respective representatives who prepared this statement include the following: American Speech-Language-Hearing Association—Fred H. Bess, chair, Noel D. Matkin, and Evelyn Cherow, ex officio; American Academy of Otolaryngology-Head and Neck Surgery—Kenneth M. Grundfast, co-chair; American Academy of Pediatrics—Allen Erenberg and William P. Potsic; Council on Education of the Deaf (A.G. Bell Association for the Deaf, American College of Educators of the Hearing Impaired, Convention of American Instructors of the Deaf, and the Conference of Educational Administrators Serving the Deaf)— Lita Aldridge and Barbara Bodner-Johnson; Directors of Speech and Hearing Programs in State Health and Welfare Agencies—Thomas Mahoney. Consultants: Alan Salamy and Gregory J. Matz. Ann L. Carey, 1988-1990 vice president for professional and governmental affairs, was the ASHA monitoring vice president.

I. Background

The early detection of hearing impairment in children is essential in order to initiate the medical and educational intervention critical for developing optimal communication and social skills. In 1982, the Joint Committee on Infant Hearing recommended identifying infants at risk for hearing impairment by means of seven criteria and suggested follow-up audiological evaluation of these infants until accurate assessments of hearing could be made (ASHA, 1982). In recent years, advances in science and technology have increased the chances for survival of markedly premature and low birth weight neonates and other severely compromised newborns. Because moderate to severe sensorineural hearing loss can be confirmed in 2.5% to 5.0% of neonates manifesting any of the previously published risk criteria, auditory screening of at-risk newborns is warranted (Hosford-Dunn, Johnson, Simmons, Malachowski, & Low, 1987; Jacobson and Morehouse, 1984; Mahoney & Eichwald, 1987; Stein, Ozdamar, Kraus, & Paton, 1983). Those infants who have one or more of the risk factors are considered to be at increased risk for sensorineural hearing loss.

Recent research and new legislation (P.L. 99-457) suggest the need for expansion and clarification of the 1982 criteria. This 1991 statement expands the risk criteria and makes recommendations for the identification and management of hearing-impaired neonates and infants. The Joint Committee recognizes that the performance characteristics of these new risk factors are not presently known; further study and critical evaluation of the risk criteria are therefore encouraged. The protocols recommended by the Committee are considered optimal and are based on both clinical experience and current research findings. The Committee recognizes, however, that the recommended protocols may not be appropriate for all institutions and that modifications in screening approaches will be necessary to accommodate the specific needs of a given facility. Such factors as cost and availability of equipment, personnel and follow-up services are important considerations in the development of a screening program (Turner, 1990).

II. **Identification**

A. Risk Criteria: Neonates (birth - 28 days)

The risk factors that identify those neonates who are at-risk for sensorineural hearing impairment include the following:

1. Family history of congenital or delayed onset childhood sensorineural impairment.
2. Congenital infection known or suspected to be associated with sensorineural hearing impairment such as toxoplasmosis, syphilis, rubella, cytomegalovirus and herpes.
3. Craniofacial anomalies including morphologic abnormalities of the pinna and ear canal, absent philtrum, low hairline, etcetera.
4. Birth weight less than 1500 grams (~3.3 lbs.).
5. Hyperbilirubinemia at a level exceeding indication for exchange transfusion.
6. Ototoxic medications including but not limited to the aminoglycosides used for more than 5 days (e.g., gentamicin, tobramycin, kanamycin, streptomycin) and loop diuretics used in combination with aminoglycosides.
7. Bacterial meningitis.
8. Severe depression at birth, which may include infants with Apgar scores of 0-3 at 5 minutes or those who fail to initiate spontaneous respiration by 10 minutes or those with hypotonia persisting to 2 hours of age.
9. Prolonged mechanical ventilation for a duration equal to or greater than 10 days (e.g., persistent pulmonary hypertension).
10. Stigmata or other findings associated with a syndrome known to include sensorineural hearing loss (e.g., Waardenburg or Usher's Syndrome).

B. Risk Criteria: Infants (29 days - 2 years)
   The factors that identify those infants who are at-risk for
   sensorineural hearing impairment include the following:
   1. Parent/caregiver concern regarding hearing, speech,
      language and/or developmental delay.
   2. Bacterial meningitis.
   3. Neonatal risk factors that may be associated with pro-
      gressive sensorineural hearing loss (e.g., cytomegalo-
      virus, prolonged mechanical ventilation and inherited
      disorders).
   4. Head trauma especially with either longitudinal or
      transverse fracture of the temporal bone.
   5. Stigmata or other findings associated with syndromes
      known to include sensori-neural hearing loss (e.g.,
      Waardenburg or Usher's Syndrome).
   6. Ototoxic medications including but not limited to the
      aminoglycosides used for more than 5 days (e.g., gen-
      tamicin, tobramycin, kanamycin, streptomycin) and
      loop diuretics used in combination with aminoglycosides.
   7. Children with neurodegenerative disorders such as
      neurofibromatosis, myoclonic epilepsy, Werdnig-
      Hoffman disease, Tay-Sach's disease, infantile
      Gaucher's disease, Nieman-Pick disease, any meta-
      chromatic leukodystrophy, or any infantile demyelinat-
      ing neuropathy.
   8. Childhood infectious diseases known to be associated
      with sensorineural hearing loss (e.g., mumps, measles).

III. **Audiologic Screening Recommendations for Neonates &
Infants**
   A. Neonates
      Neonates who manifest one or more items on the risk
      criteria should be screened, preferably under the supervi-
      sion of an audiologist. Optimally, screening should be
      completed prior to discharge from the newborn nursery
      but no later than 3 months of age. The initial screening
      should include measurement of the auditory brainstem
      response (ABR) (ASHA, 1989). Behavioral testing of new-
      born infants' hearing has high false-positive and false-neg-
      ative rates and is not universally recommended. Because
      some false-positive results can occur with ABR screening,
      ongoing assessment and observation of the infant's audito-
      ry behavior is recommended during the early stages of inter-
      vention. If the infant is discharged prior to screening, or if
      ABR screening under audiologic supervision is not available,

the child ideally should be referred for ABR testing by 3 months of age but never later than 6 months of age.

The acoustic stimulus for ABR screening should contain energy in the frequency region important for speech recognition. Clicks are the most commonly used signal for eliciting the ABR and contain energy in the speech frequency region (ASHA, 1989). Pass criterion for ABR screening is a response from each ear at intensity levels 40 dB nHL or less. Transducers designed to reduce the probability of ear-canal collapse are recommended.

If consistent electrophysiological responses are detected at appropriate sound levels, then the screening process will be considered complete except in those cases where there is a probability of progressive hearing loss (e.g., family history of delayed onset, degenerative disease, meningitis, intrauterine infections or infants who had chronic lung disease, pulmonary hypertension or who received medications in doses likely to be ototoxic). If the results of an initial screening of an infant manifesting any risk criteria are equivocal, then the infant should be referred for general medical, otological, and audiological follow-up.

B. Infants

Infants who exhibit one or more items on the risk criteria should be screened as soon as possible but no later than 3 months after the child has been identified as at risk. For infants less than 6 months of age, ABR screening (see II A.) is recommended. For infants older than 6 months, behavioral testing using a conditioned response or ABR testing are appropriate approaches. Infants who fail the screen should be referred for a comprehensive audiological evaluation. This evaluation may include ABR, behavioral testing (> 6 months) and acoustic immittance measures (see ASHA, 1989 Guidelines, for recommended protocols by developmental age).

IV. **Early Intervention for Hearing-Impaired Infants and Their Families**

When hearing loss is identified, early intervention services should be provided, in accordance with Public Law 99-457. Early intervention services under P.L. 99-457 may commence before the completion of the evaluation and assessment if the following conditions are met: (a) parental consent is obtained, (b) an interim individualized family service plan (IFSP) is developed, and (c) the full initial evaluation process is completed within 45 days of referral.

The interim IFSP should include the following:

A. The name of the case manager who will be responsible for both implementation of the interim IFSP and coordination with other agencies and persons;

B. The early intervention services that have been determined to be needed immediately by the child and the child's family.

These immediate early intervention services should include the following:

1. Evaluation by a physician with expertise in the management of early child-hood otologic disorders.

2. Evaluation by an audiologist with expertise in the assessment of young children, to determine the type, degree, and configuration of the hearing loss, and to recommend assistive communication devices appropriate to the child's needs (e.g., hearing aids, personal FM systems, vibrotactile aids).

3. Evaluation by a speech-language pathologist, teacher of the hearing-impaired, audiologist, or other professional with expertise in the assessment of communication skills in hearing-impaired children, to develop a program of early intervention consistent with the needs of the child and preferences of the family. Such intervention would be cognizant of and sensitive to cultural values inherent in familial deafness.

4. Family education, counseling and guidance, including home visits and parent support groups to provide families with information, child management skills and emotional support consistent with the needs of the child and family and their culture.

5. Special instruction that includes:

   a. the design and implementation of learning environments and activities that promote the child's development and communication skills.

   b. curriculum planning that integrates and coordinates multidisciplinary personnel and resources so that intended outcomes of the IFSP are achieved; and,

   c. ongoing monitoring of the child's hearing status and amplification needs and development of auditory skills.

V. **Future Considerations for Risk Criteria**

Because of the dynamic changes occurring in neonatal-prenatal medicine, the committee recognizes the forthcoming research may result in the need for revision of the 1990 risk register. For example, the committee has concerns about the possible ototoxic effects on the fetus from maternal drug abuse; however, present data are insufficient to detrermine whether the fetus or neonate are at risk for hearing loss. In addition, yet-to-be-developed medications may have ototoxic effects on neonates and infants. Therefore, the committee advised clinicians to keep apprised of published reports demonstrating correlations between maternal drug abuse and ototoxicity and between future antimicrobial agents and ototoxicity. Clinicians should also take into account the possible interactive effects of multiple medications administered simultaneously. Finally, the committee recommends that the position statement be examined every 3 years for possible revision.

References

American Speech-Language-Hearing Association. (1989). Guidelines for audiologic screening of newborn infants who are at-risk for hearing impairment. *Asha*, 31, (3), 89-92.

Early intervention program for infants and toddlers with handicaps: Final regulations. *Federal Register*, 54, No. 119, pp. 26306-26348, June 22, 1989.

Hosford-Dunn H, Johnson S, Simmons B, Malachowski N and Low L (1987). Infant hearing screening: Program implementation and validation. *Ear and Hearing* 8:12 20.

Jacobson J and Morehouse R (1984). A comparison of auditory brainstem response and behavioral screening in high risk and normal newborn infants. *Ear and Hearing* 5(4), 245-253.

Joint Committee on Infant Hearing (1982). Position statement. *Asha* 24(12), 1017-1018.

Mahoney TM and Eichwald JG (1987). The ups and "downs" of high risk hearing screening: The Utah statewide program. In K.P. Gerkin and A. Amochaev (Eds.), *Seminars in Hearing* 8(2), 155-163.

Stein L, Ozdamar O, Kraus N and Paton J (1983). Follow-up of infants screened by auditory brainstem response in the neonatal intensive care unit. *Journal of Pediatrics* 63, 447-453.

Turner RG (1990). Analysis of recommended guidelines for infant hearing screening. *Asha* 32(9), 57-61.

Suggested Reading

Early Intervention

Early intervention program for infants and toddlers with handicaps: Final regulations. *Federal Register*, 54, No. 119, pp. 26306-26348, June 22, 1989.

Levitt H, McGarr N and Geffner D (1987). Development of language and communication skills in hearing impaired children. *Asha* (Monograph No. 26). Rockville, MD: American Speech-Language-Hearing Association.

Ling D (1981). Early speech development. In G. Mencher and S.E. Gerber (Eds.), *Early management of hearing loss* (pp. 310-335). New York: Grune and Stratton.

McFarland WH and Simmons FB (1981). The importance of early intervention with severe childhood deafness. *Pediatric Annals* 9:13-19.

A Report to the Congress of the United States. (1988). The Commission on Education of the Deaf: Toward equality: Education of the deaf.

Early Identification of Hearing Impairment in Neonates and Infants

Alberti P, Hyde M, Riko K, Corbin H and Fitzhardinge P (1985). Issues in early identification of hearing loss. *Laryngoscope* 95(4), 373-381.

American Academy of Pediatrics (1986). Committee on Fetus and Newborn. Use and abuse of the Apgar score. *Pediatrics* 78:1148.

American Speech-Language-Hearing Association (1989). Guidelines for audiologic screening of newborn infants who are at-risk for hearing impairment. *Asha* 31(3), 89-92.

American Speech-Language-Hearing Association (1990). Guidelines for infant hearing screening - Response to Robert G. Turner's analysis. *Asha* 32(9), 63-66.

Bergman I, Hirsch RP, Fria TJ, Shapiro SM, Holzman I and Painter MJ (1985). Cause of hearing loss in the high-risk premature infant. *Journal of Pediatrics* 106:95-101.

Bess FH (Ed) (1988). *Hearing impairment in children.* Parkton, MD: York Press.

Brummett RE (1981). Ototoxicity resulting from the combined administration of potent diuretics and other agents. *Scandinavian Audiology* Supplement 14:215-224.

Brummett RE, Fox KE, Russell NJ and Davis RR (1981). Interaction between aminoglycoside antibiotics and loop-inhibiting diuretics in the guinea pig. In S Lerner, G Matz and J Hawkins (Eds), *Aminoglycoside ototoxicity* (pp. 67-77), Boston: Little, Brown.

Brummett RE, Traynor J, Brown R and Himes D (1975). Cochlear damage resulting from kanamycin and furosemide. *Acta Otolaryngologica* 80:86-92.

Church MW and Gerkin KP (1988). Hearing disorders in children with fetal alcohol syndrome: Findings from case reports. *Pediatrics* 82:147-154.

Coplan J (1987). Deafness: Ever heard of it? Delayed recognition of permanent hearing loss. *Pediatrics* 79:206-213.

Elssman S, Matkin N and Sabo M (1987). Early identification of congenital sensorineural hearing impairment. *The Hearing Journal* 40:13-17.

Gerkin KP (1984). The high risk register for deafness. *Asha* 26(3), 17-23.

Gerkin KP and Amochaev A (Eds) (1987). Hearing in infants: Proceedings from a national symposium. *Seminars in Hearing* 8:77-187.

Gorga M, Reiland J, Beauchaine K, Worthington D and Jesteadt W (1987). Auditory brainstem responses from graduates of an intensive care nursery: Normal patterns of response. *Journal of Speech and Hearing Research* 30:311-318.

Gorga M, Kaminski JR and Beauchaine KA (1988). Auditory brainstem responses from graduates of an intensive care nursery using an insert earphone. *Ear and Hearing* 9:144-147.

Halpern J, Hosford-Dunn H and Malachowski N (1987). Four factors that accurately predict hearing loss in 'high risk' neonates. *Ear and Hearing* 8:21-25.

Hendricks-Munoz KD and Walton JP (1988). Hearing loss in infants with persistent fetal circulation. *Pediatrics* 81(5), 650-656.

Hosford-Dunn H, Johnson S, Simmons B, Malachowski N and Low L (1987). Infant hearing screening: Program implementation and validation. *Ear and Hearing* 8:12-20.

Hyde M, Riko K, Corbin H, Moroso M and Alberti P (1984). A neonatal hearing screening research program using brainstem electric response audiometry. *Journal of Otolaryngology* 13:49-54.

Jacobson J and Morehouse R (1984). A comparison of auditory brainstem response and behavioral screening in high risk and normal newborn infants. *Ear and Hearing* 5(4), 245-253.

Joint Committee on Infant Hearing (1982). Position statement. *Asha* 24(12), 10171-1018.

Kahlmeter O and Dahlager JI (1984). Aminoglycoside toxicity-A review of clinical studies published between 1975 and 1982. *Journal of Antimicrobial Chemotherapy* 13 (suppl. A), 9-22.

Kaka J, Lyman C and Kllarskl D (1984). Tobramycin-furosemide interaction. *Drug Intelligence and Clinical Pharmacy* 18:235-238.

Lary S, Briassoulis G, DeVries L, Dubowitz L and Dubowitz V (1985). Hearing threshold in preterm and term infants by auditory brainstem response. *Journal of Pediatrics* 107:593-599.

Mahoney TM and Eichwald JG (1987). The ups and "downs" of high risk hearing screening: The Utah statewide program. In KP Gerkin and A Amochaev (Eds), *Seminars in Hearing* 8(2), 155-163.

Matkin ND (1984). Early recognition and referral of hearing impaired children. *Pediatrics in Review* 6:151-158.

Matz G (1990). Clinical perspectives on ototoxic drugs. *Annals of Otology, Rhinology and Laryngology* 99:39-41.

Naulty CM, Weiss IP and Herer GR (1986). Progressive sensorineural hearing loss in survivors of persistent fetal circulation. *Ear and Hearing* 7:74-77.

Nield TA, Schrier S, Ramos AD, Platzker ACG and Warburton D (1986). Unexpected hearing loss in high-risk infants. *Pediatrics* 78:417-422.

Northern JL and Downs MP (1984). *Hearing in Children* (3rd ed). Baltimore: Williams and Wilkins.

Salamy A, Eldridge L and Tooley WH (1989). Neonatal status and hearing loss in high-risk infants. *Journal of Pediatrics* 114:847-852.

Schwartz DM, Pratt RE and Schwartz JA (1989). Auditory brainstem responses in preterm infants: Evidence of peripheral maturity. *Ear and Hearing* 10:14-22.
Stein L, Ozdamar O, Kraus N and Paton J (1983). Follow-up of infants screened by auditory brainstem response in the neonatal intensive care unit. *Journal of Pediatrics* 63:447-453.

Surgonski N, Shallop J, Bull MJ and Lemons JA (1987). Hearing screening of high risk newborns. *Ear and Hearing* 8:26-30.

Turner RG (1990). Analysis of recommended guidelines for infant hearing screening. *Asha* 32(9), 57-61.

Diagnosis and Management

Bess FH (Ed) (1988). *Hearing impairment in children.* Parkton, MD: York Press.

Clark TC and Watkins S (1985). The SKI* Hi model: Programming for hearing impaired infants through home intervention. Logan, UT: SKI* Hi Institute.

Dodge PR, Davis HD, Feigin RD, Holmes SJ, Kaplan SL, Jubelirer DP, Stechenberg GW and Hirsh SK (1984). Prospective evaluation of hearing impairment as a sequela of acute bacterial meningitis. *The New England Journal of Medicine* 311:869-874.

Fitzgerald MT and Bess FH (1982). Parent/infant training for hearing impaired children. *Monographs in Contemporary Audiology* 3:1-24.

Gravel JS (Ed) (1989). Assessing auditory system integrity in high-risk infants and young children. *Seminars in Hearing* 10:213-290.

Hosford-Dunn H, Simmons BF, Winzelberg J and Petroff M (1986). Delayed onset hearing loss in a two-year-old. *Ear and Hearing* 7:78-82.

Matkin ND (1988). Key considerations in counseling parents of hearing-impaired children. In RF Curlee (Ed), *Seminars in Speech and Language* 9(3), 209-222.

Mencher GT and Gerber SE (1981). *Early management of hearing loss*. New York: Grune and Stratton.

Ross M and Giolas TG (Eds) (1978). *Auditory management of hearing impaired children*. Baltimore: University Park Press.

Thompson G and Wilson WR (1984). Clinical application of visual reinforcement audiometry. In T Mahoney (Ed), *Seminars in Hearing* 5:85-89.

Thompson M, Atcheson J and Pious C (1985). *Birth to three: A curriculum for parents, parent trainers, and teachers*. Seattle, WA: University of Washington Press.

United States House of Representatives 99th Congress, 2nd session. Report 99-860. *Report Accompanying the Education of the Handicapped Act Amendments of 1986*.

APPENDIX E

NIH Concensus Statement

Early Identificaiton of Hearing Impairment in
Infants and Young Children

Volume 11, Number 1
March 1-3, 1993

NATIONAL INSTITUTES OF HEALTH
Office of the Director

Introduction

There is a clear need in the United States for improved methods and models for the early identification of hearing impairment in infants and young children. Approximately 1 of every 1,000 children is born deaf. Many more are born with less severe degrees of hearing impairment, while others develop hearing impairment during childhood. Reduced hearing acuity during infancy and early childhood interferes with the development of speech and verbal language skills. Although less well documented, significantly reduced auditory input also adversely affects the developing auditory nervous system and can have harmful effects on social, emotional, cognitive, and academic development, as well as on a person's vocational and economic potential. Moreover, delayed identification and management of severe to profound hearing impairment may impede the child's ability to adapt to life in a hearing world or in the deaf community.

The most important period for language and speech development is generally regarded as the first 3 years of life and, although there are several methods of identifying hearing impairment during the first year, the average age of identification in the United States remains close to 3 years. Lesser degrees of hearing loss may go undetected even longer. The result is that for many hearing-impaired infants and young children, much of the crucial period for language and speech learning is lost. There is general agreement that hearing impairment should be recognized as early in life as possible, so that the remediation process can take full advantage of the plasticity of the developing sensory systems and so that the child can enjoy normal social development.

During the apst 30 years, infant hearing screening has been attempted with a number of different test methods, including cardiac response audiometry, respiration audiometry, alteration of sucking patterns, movement or startle in response to acoustic stimuli, various behavioral paradigms, and measurement of acoustic reflexes. For the past 15 years, auditory brain stem response (ABR) audiometry has been the method of choice. More recently, attention has turned to the measurement of evoked otoacoustic emissions (EOAE), which shows promise as a fast, inexpensive, noninvasive test of cochlear function. Each method is effective in its own way, but technical or interpretative limitations have impeded widespread application. Moreover, these approaches vary in their sensitivity, specificity, and predictive value in identifying hearing impairment.

Until now, most neonatal screening programs have focused on infants who satisfy one or more of a number of criteria for inclusion in a "high-risk register." However, the use of high-risk criteria (HRC) to limit the population being screened excludes approximately 50 percent of infants with hearing impairment. The preferred screening test method for HRC children has come to be ABR, combined with auidologic followup and/or diagnostic ABR for those infants who fail the screening protocols. Despite the relatively good predictive efficiency of ABR, its cost, time requirements, and technical difficulties have discouraged the general application of this method in screening the far larger newborn population not meeting the HRC.

On March 1-3, 1993, the National Institute on Deafness and Other Communication Disorders, together with the Office of Medical Applications of Research of the National Institutes of Health convened a Consensus Development Conference on the Early Identification of Hearing Impairment in Infants and Young Children. Cosponsors of the conference were the National Institute of Child Health and Human Development and the National Institute of Neurological Disorders and Stroke. The conference brought together specialists in audiology, otolaryngology, pediatrics, neonatology, neurology, speech and hearing sciences, speech-language pathology, health care administration, epidemiology, education, counseling, nursing, and other health care areas, as well as representation from the public. Following 1-1/2 days of presentations by experts in relevant fields and discussion by the audience, an independent consensus panel weighed the scientific evidence and prepared a draft statement in response to the following key questions:

- What are the advantages of early identification of hearing impairment and the consequences of late identification of hearing impairment?
- Which children (birth through 5 years) should be screened for hearing impairment and when?
- What are the advantages and disadvantages of current screening methods?
- What is the preferred model for hearing screening and followup?
- What are the important directions for future research?

What Are the Advantages of Early Identification of Hearing Impairment and the Consequences of Late Identification of Hearing Impairment?

The primary justification for early identification of hearing impairment in infants relates to the impact of hearing impairment on speech and language acquisition, academic achievement, and social/emotional development. The first 3 years of life are the most important for speech and language acquisition. Consequently, if a child is hard of hearing or deaf at birth or experiences hearing loss in infancy or early childhood, it is likely that child will not receive adequate auditory, linguistic, and social stimulation requisite to speech and language learning, social and emotional development, and that family functioning will suffer. The goal of early identification and intervention is to minimize or prevent these adverse effects.

The consequences of hearing impairment are many. Animal studies show that early auditory deprivation interferes with the development of neural structures necessary for hearing. Human infants with hearing loss, particularly those with sensorineural impairments, may experience similar disruptions that will have a direct impact on language acquisition. Significant hearing loss interferes with the development of phonological and speech perception abilities needed for later language learning, e.g., meaningful language at the word, phrase, and sentence levels. These impairments in communication skills can lead to poor academic performance (especially reading), and ultimately, to limitations in career opportunities.

The degree and type of hearing impairment impact on a child's development. Other factors can further exacerbate the consequences of hearing impairment. For example, some children have additional sensory disabilities and/or associated neurological disorders that further interfere with perceiving and processing information. Environmental factors, such as the quality of language input provided by the parents, can either facilitate or impede communication skills. Socioeconomic-related factors, such as the lack of access to health care, other associated health problems, high-risk populations, and social stresses, also may exacerbate the consequences of deficits. Early identification and intervention can address these factors, thus minimizing their effects.

Over the past two decades, advances in technology have provided ever-improving opportunities to identify hearing impairments in infants soon after birth. Consequently, the systematic evaluation of the effects of earlier identification and earlier intervention can now be conducted. Because such data are not presently available, it is difficult to evaluate fully the effectiveness of early identification and intervention on language development. There are, however, a wide range of clinical observations, a number of descriptive studies, and a few statistically controlled, nonrandomized trials that support the benefits of early identification and intervention.

The benefits to be gained from early intervention may vary, depending on the severity and type of hearing impairment. Children with sensorineural hearing loss who receive early amplification, when indicated, and a comprehensive habilitation program may show improved speech and language skills, school achievement, self-esteem, and psychosocial adaptation when compared to hearing-impaired children who do not receive amplification until 2 to 3 years of age. The advantages of early intervention can only be attained when the appropriate services are available and accessible to these children and their families.

Which Children (Birth Through 5 Years) Should Be Screened for Hearing Impairment and When?

Answering the questions of who should be screened and when presents us with a practical dilemma. It is clear that the earliest possible identification of hearing-impaired infants is optimal for effective intervention to improve communication skills, language development, and behavioral adjustment. Identification of all children with hearing impairment at birth is ideal. As a practical matter, the cost of universal screening has been prohibitive. Attempts have been made to limit costs by focusing neonatal testing on those at highest risk. Unfortunately, research shows that this approach misses 50 percent of children who are eventually diagnosed with severe to profound hearing impairment. In spite of current screening programs, the average diagnosis of hearing impairment remains constant at about 2-1/2 years of age. In order to meet the goal of the Joint Committee on Infant Hearing to identify and initiate treatment by 6 months of age and to more completely identify hearing-impaired infants, we must dramatically change our approach to screening.

Some changes can be made in auditory screening procedures that would have a minimal effect on cost but would increase identification rate. Data have shown that infants admitted to the neonatal intensive care unit (NICU) have an increased risk of significant bilateral sensorineural hearing loss (1-3 percent); the addition of other neonatal high-risk factors does not add significantly to the identification of hearing loss. *Consequently, we recommend that all infants admitted to the NICU be screened for hearing loss prior to discharge.* To improve the accuracy and efficiency of the test, screening should take place as close to discharge as possible. Infants in the well-baby nursery with diagnoses of craniofacial anomalies, family history of hearing loss, and diagnosis of intrauterine infection comprise a special high-risk category. Thus, they should be screened using the same protocol and followup vigilance as the NICU population.

In addition to screening all NICU babies, we strongly recommend that universal screening be implemented for all infants within the first 3 months of life. Recent data suggest that this will virtually complete our identification of newborns with hearing impairment. Even though we recommend universal screening within the first 3 months, as a practical matter this is most efficiently achieved by screening prior to discharge from the well-baby nursery. The disadvantages of hospital well-baby screening, such as missed screening because of early discharge and the possibility of higher false-positive rate, are outweighed by the accessibility of all newborns to testing at this time. The addition of screening in the well-baby nursery and as a part of well-baby care will increase cost. The benefit, however, is likely to be high. For well-baby screening to be cost effective, we recommend techniques that are rapid, reliable, highly sensitive, specific, and easily administered by trained and supervised personnel. Infants who are not screened in the hospital should be screened by 3 months of age.

Identification of hearing impairment must be seen as imperative for all infants and as an important adjunct to child health care. Since 20-30 percent of children who subsequently have hearing impairment will develop hearing loss during early childhood, an ever-vigilant pluralistic approach must be taken to hearing screening and identification of young children. The first approach must include the eliciting and acknowledging of parental concern regarding hearing loss and/or speech and language acquisition. At present 70 percent of children with acquired hearing impairments are initially identified by parents. *Parental concern about hearing should be sufficient reason to initiate prompt formal hearing evaluation.* Another necessary approach includes ongoing evaluation of speech and language development at routine child health supervision visits using formal assessment tools. Failure to attain appropriate language milestones, especially during the first 18 months of life, should result in prompt referral for further hearing evaluation.

Several causes of acquired hearing loss during early childhood have been described. For example, bacterial meningitis has been associated with a 5-30 percent incidence of profound hearing loss. *We recommend that all children recovering from bacterial meningitis be referred for diagnostic audiologic assessment, ideally prior to discharge from the hospital.* Other risk factors for acquired or progressive hearing loss, for which diagnostic hearing evaluation should be considered include, but should not be limited to, significant head trauma with persistent symptoms referable to hearing or balance, viral encephalitis or labyrinthitis, excessive noise exposure, exposure to ototoxic drugs, perinatal cytomegalovirus (CMV) infection, familial hearing impairment, infants with chronic lung disease or diuretic therapy, and infants with repeated episodes of otitis media with persistent middle ear effusion.

Since new cases of hearing impairment can arise in early childhood, school entry screening procedures should be extended to all private and public school students. School entry screening represents an additional universal approach for the identification of hearing impairment in America's children. Schools must make appropriate referral for audiologic followup and educational intervention.

What Are the Advantages and Disadvantages of Current Screening Methods?

Ideally, all children who have significant hearing impairment will be detected prior to the development of speech and language so that appropriate intervention might maximize their potential for normal development. An ideal screening method would also be readily available at modest cost with complete specificity and sensitivity. Unfortunately, no such screening method is currently available. Each of the current screening methods, while offering advantages, also has disadvantages.

High-risk criteria (Joint Committee on Infant Hearing, 1990), which identify approximately 9 percent of newborns, encompass half of the children who are subsequently found to have hearing impairment; approximately 1-3 percent of HRC babies have significant bilateral sensorineural hearing loss. Identificaiton of HRC babies can be performed routinely using existing hospital-based health care mechanisms at modest cost. Although lacking in sensitivity, the HRC has been used as a first stage for other screening strategies. The use of HRC to screen for hearing impairment has many disadvantages. The principal disadvantage is taht 50 percent of newborns with congential hearing deficits are not in the HRC group and are missed by this screen. Children who are not born in larger hospitals may not be routinely identified as being at risk. Another disadvantage of this screen is that followup is not optimal in most programs currently in use, thus only a small proportion of cases are identified.

Auditory brainstem responses can be used to screen for hearing impairment in newborns, since ABR's do not require a voluntary response and can be done without sedation. This screening test is highly sensitive; nearly all children born with significant congenital hearing deficits could be detected in the newborn nursery using ABR and can be referred for further evaluation. However, over-referral is a problem, since there are false-positive ABR's in babies with normal hearing. In the NICU setting, for every child with significant hearing impairment who is detected, approximately six babies are referred for followup. In the well-baby nursery, where the prevalence of hearing impairment is far lower, for every child with significant hearing impairment, more than 100 babies are referred. This high referral rate may cause undue parental anxiety. Since ABR screening and followup are expensive and required trained personnel, this method has been applied principally to newborns who are at highest risk for hearing impairment (those in the NICU or the HRC). Newer automated ABR technology and innovative analysis schemes may diminish costs.

Evoked otoacoustic emissions represent a newer type of newborn screening method that offers potential additional benefits. Like the ABR, this technique could be applied to all newborns prior to hospital discharge. The measurement of EOAE can be performed in the newborn nursery with less skilled personnel in a shorter time than conventional ABR and without the need for scalp electrodes. The sensitivity of EOAE in the detection of congenital hearing impairment is very high, but newborn EOAE testing tends to have more false-positives when compared to ABR, especially during the first 48 hours of life. Nevertheless, the use of EOAE in the detection of hearing impairment in well babies could be a more cost-effective way of detecting early hearing impairments. Over-referral may be a major problem.

Behavioral testing (such as visual reinforcement audiometry or conditioned orienting response), usually at 6 months of age or later, may be used to detect hearing impairment reliably in almost all infants prior to the acquisition of speech and language. This method would minimize the problems of over-referral and "labeling" that are inherent in the newborn screening methods. Identified infants could begin timely rehabilitation or intervention, and later onset hearing impairments could be detected. Several disadvantages of this strategy exist: (1) traditional behavioral audiometry in a 6-month-old infant requires skilled personnel and is time-consuming; (2) unlike newborn testing, the evaluation of older infants requires reasonable access to a testing facility; (3) testing is most difficult in developmentally delayed infants who are at highest risk; and (4) some hearing impairments would not be treated until after 1 year of life because of a lack of lead time to implement intervention. There are new versions of behavioral audiometry that may eliminate some or all of these objections, but these new techniques remain to be validated in large samples.

These new behavioral techniques may provide appropriate methods for use in organized hearing screening programs beyond the neonatal period.

Public and professional education. Presently, as many as 70 percent of infants and children with hearing impairment are identified because of parental concern about their child's hearing. Efforts to educate parents about signs of hearing impairment by brochures and posters in prenatal clinics and physician's offices are simple and inexpensive. Public service announcements should be used. Professional societies should be encouraged to issue position papers on the importance and current recommended methods of identification. The effectiveness of these strategies has not been extensively evaluated.

Professional education involves calling attention to (1) neonatal risk factors for hearing impairment (the HRC), (2) risk factors for acquired hearing impairment, (3) early behavioral signs of hearing impairment, and (4) the ineffectiveness of crude measures of hearing sensitivity such as hand clapping, which are useless and misleading. In order to be effective, regular professional education and continuing professional education activities at regular intervals will likely be necessary to make health care providers alert and the health system responsive to identifying children with hearing impairment. Such ongoing continuing education programs have been developed by several professional organizations. Continuing professional education has begun in Colorado and Arizona, and guidelines for child health supervision have been developed by the American Academy of Pediatrics and the American Academy of Family Practice. This strategy for professional education is inexpensive and utilizes the current health care system. Ongoing developmental surveillance by attentive and educated primary health providers would likely identify those children with acquired hearing impairment. The principal disadvantage of such a system is that children do not consistently receive medical surveillance. Finally, this method may not identify children with hearing deficits before 1 year of age.

What Is the Preferred Model for Hearing Screening and Followup?

The principal goal of an early identification program is to identify hearing impairment present at birth, in order to effect appropriate intervention as early as possible. *In order to detect those children born with moderate, severe, and profound hearing impairment, we recommend universal newborn screening.* Because of the accessibility of babies in the newborn nursery, such screening is best accomplished prior to hospital discharge.

The screening of all newborn babies presents special problems in cost feasibility. There are approximately 4 million live births each year in the United States. Given an incidence of hearing impairment of 0.1 percent per year (i.e., 1 in every 1,000 live births) then 3,996,000 babies who are screened will have normal hearing sensitivity. It is vital that these babies be identified rapidly, and at minimal cost.

The panel identified two techniques-EOAE and ABR-as showing maximal promise as universal screening tools for the newborn. As noted earlier, each has its unique advantages and disadvantages. Weighing the evidence presented, the panel felt that EOAE shows best promise as a rapid, cost-effective means of quickly discharging all babies with normal auditory systems. In keeping with its high sensitivity, however, the EOAE lacks adequate specificity. It fails a relatively large number of babies whose hearing sensitivity is, in fact, normal. In order to prevent the majority of these "false alarms" from burdening the system for followup diagnostic evaluation, a second or confirmatory screen seems desirable. The panel felt that this goal would be best achieved by a second-stage ABR screen of all babies who fail the EOAE screen. Thus the preferred model for universal screening begins with an initial screen by EOAE. All babies who pass this screen are discharged. All babies who fail, however, are rescreened by ABR. Babies who pass the ABR screen are discharged but should be flagged for rescreen at 3-6 months. Babies who fail the ABR screen are referred for diagnostic evaluation. The purpose of the followup diagnostic evaluation is twofold: (1) to verify the existence and to determine the type and severity of hearing impairment and (2) to initiate a remediation program for the child and family.

It should be emphasized that only a small percentage of the total number of babies screened experiences both stages of the total screening process. If the specificity of the EOAE screen is taken as 90 percent, then 90 percent of the babies screened are discharged after the first (EOAE) stage. Only the 10 percent who fail the EOAE stage will undergo the second, ABR, stage. The roles of the two stages, EOAE and ABR, are viewed as complementary. The first, EOAE, rapidly and inexpensively rules out significant hearing impairment (99.9 percent of all babies), but has limited specificity. The second, ABR, appears to require more time and effort, but has the potential to identify failure with better specificity.

Although this two-stage screening process is recommended, the panel is aware that many clinics and hospitals have already successfully implemented universal screening programs based on ABR alone. The panel encourages such sites to continue these programs. The procedure detailed above is recommended, however, as an apparently cost-feasible approach to mass screening for those teams contemplating the initiation of a universal screening program.

It must be recognized that not all hearing impairment in infancy and early childhood will be present at birth. A significant number of infants and children will develop hearing impairment during the first years of life. Such losses may be acquired as a result of medical conditions or may result from progressive hereditary etiologies.

The detection of late onset or progressive losses must rely on a pluralistic approach. Screening at birth is best accomplished before the baby leaves the hospital, but during the next 2 to 3 years there is no single comparable site that can serve as the optimal location for identification. It should be noted, however, that, in some locales, hearing screening programs are in place through day-care and head-start programs. Education of parents or other primary caretakers, medical and nursing personnel, and all other professionals who have opportunity to observe the child must be relied upon to recognize factors that place the child at high risk for hearing impairment and behavioral signs of a possible change in hearing status, in order to refer for appropriate audiologic assessment. School entry, to include both public and private resources, will continue to provide an additional opportunity for universal identification of childrne with significant hearing impairment.

Finally, it should be recognized that a critical component of any screening program is a database system. Such a database is important for tracking the progress of infants and children identified by the program and for ongoing monitoring of all aspects of the performance of the screening program.

What Are the Important Directions for Future Research?

- Conduct large-scale studies on efficacy of early identification and intervention.
  Examples include:
  - Controlled trials of screening by audiologists versus trained nonprofessionals or volunteers.
  - Controlled trials of the influence of different settings (NICU, special test environment) on the effectiveness of screening procedures.
  - Comparison of early intervention with later intervention for different levels of hearing loss and types of intervention.

APPENDIX F

Joint Committee on Infant Hearing 1994 Position Statement

This 1994 Position Statement was developed by the Joint Committee on Infant Hearing. Joint committee member organizations that approved this statement and their respective representatives who prepared this statement include the American Speech-Language-Hearing Association (Allan O. Diefendorf, Ph.D., Chair; Deborah Hayes, Ph.D.; and Evelyn Cherow, M.A., ex officio); the American Academy of Otolaryngology-Head and Neck Surgery (Patrick E. Brookhouser, M.D. and Stephen Epstein, M.D.); the American Academy of Audiology (Terese Finitzo, Ph.D. and Jerry Northern, Ph.D.); the American Academy of Pediatrics (Allen Erenberg, M.D. and Nancy Roizen, M.D.); and the Directors of Speech and Hearing Programs in State Health and Welfare Agencies (Thomas Mahoney, Ph.D. and Kathie J. Mense, M.S.).

POSITION STATEMENT

The Joint Committee on Infant Hearing endorses the goal of universal detection of infants with hearing loss as early as possible. All infants with hearing loss should be identified before 3 months of age, and receive intervention by 6 months of age.

I. BACKGROUND

In 1982, the Joint Committee on Infant Heairng recommended identification of infants at risk for hearing loss in terms of specific risk factors and suggested follow-up audiologic evaluation until an accurate assessment of hearing could be made (Joint Committee on Infant Hearing, 1982; American Academy of Pediatrics, 1982). In 1990, the Position Statement was modified to expand the list of risk factors and recommend a specific hearing screening protocol.

In concert with the national initiative *Healthy People 2000* (U.S. Department of Health and Human Services, Public Health Service, 1990), which promotes early identification of children with hearing loss, this 1994 Position Statement addresses the need to identify *all* infants with hearing loss.

The prevalence of newborn and infant hearing loss is estimated to range from 1.5 to 6.0 per 1,000 live births (Watkin, Baldwin and McEnery, 1991; Parving, 1993; White and Behrens, 1993). Risk factor screening identifies only 50% of infants with significant hearing loss (Pappas, 1983; Elssman, Matkin and Sabo, 1987; Mauk, White, Mortensen and Behrens, 1991). Failure to identify the remaining 50% of children with hearing loss results in diagnosis and intervention at an unacceptably late age.

This 1994 Position Statement:

1. endorses the goal of unviersal detection of infants with hearing loss and encourages continuing research and development to

improve techniques for detection of and intervention for hearing loss as early as possible;

2. maintains a role for the high-risk factors (hereafter termed indicators) described in the 1990 Position Statement, and modifies the list of indicators associated with sensorineural and/or conductive hearing loss in newborns and infants;

3. identifies indicators associated with late-onset hearing loss and recommends procedures to monitor infants with these indicators;

4. recognizes the adverse effects of fluctuating conductive hearing loss from persistent or recurrent otitis media with effusion (OME) and recommends monitoring infants with OME for hearing loss;

5. endorses provision of intervention services in accordance with Part H of the Individuals with Disabilities Education Act (IDEA); and

6. identifies additional considerations necessary to enhance early identification of infants with hearin gloss.

II. CONSIDERATIONS FOR DETECTING HEARING LOSS IN INFANTS

A successful infant hearing program must detect hearing loss that will interfere with normal development of speech and oral language. Because normal hearing is critical for speech and oral language development as early as the first 6 months of life (Kuhl, Williams, Lacerda, Stephens and Lindbloom, 1992), it is desirable to identify infants with hearin gloss before 3 months of age.

Facilities or agencies that implement infant hearing programs must develop protocols to achieve identification of all infants with hearing loss. To gain access to most infants, the Joint Committee on Infant Hearing recommends the option of evaluating infants before discharge from the newborn nursery. For infants discharged early or delivered at an alternative birthing site, it is desirable to have their hearing assessed before 3 months of age.

Concern for hearing should not stop at birth. Some childrne may develop delayed-onset hearing loss. For infants identified with indicators associated with delayed-onset hearing loss (see Sections III B and III C, below), ongoing monitoring and evaluation will be necessary (ASHA, 1991).

A. Technical Considerations

Hearing loss of 30 dB HL and greater in the frequency region important for speech recognition (approximately 500 through 4000 Hz) will interfere with the normal development of speech and language. Techniques used to assess hearing of infants must be capable of detecting hearing loss of this degree in infants by age 3 months and younger. Of the various approaches to newborn hearing assessment currently available, two *physiologic measures* (auditory brainstem response [ABR] and otoacoustic emissions [OAE]) show good promise for achieving this goal.

ABR has been recommended for newborn hearing assessment for almost 15 years (Schulman-Galambos and Galambos, 1979) and has been successfully implemented in both risk register and universal newborn hearing screening programs (Galambos, Hicks and Wilson, 1982, 1984; Kileny, 1987; Amochaev, 1987; Hyde, Riko and Malizia, 1990). Follow-up studies of infants screened by this technique demonstrate acceptable identification of infants with hearing loss (Stein, Ozdamar, Kraus and Paton, 1983; Kileny and Magathan, 1987).

More recently, OAEs have been introduced for risk register and assessment of newborn hearing (Bonfils, Uziel and Pujol, 1988; Stevens et al., 1989, 1990; Kennedy et al., 1991; White and Behrens, 1993). Follow-up studies of infants screened by this technique are limited but suggest that OAEs can identify infants with hearing loss of approximately 30 dB HL and greater (Kennedy et al., 1991).

Specific characteristics of test performance for ABR and OAE have not been fully defined in universal infant hearing detection applications. Because direct comparisons of ABR and OAE test performance are not currently available, the Joint Committee on Infant Hearing recommends that each team of health care professionals responsible for the development and implementation of infant hearing programs evaluate and select the technique that is most suitable for their care practices. New technologies or improvements to existing technologies that substantially enhance infant hearing assessment should be incorporated into existing programs as appropriate.

Each of the two physiologic measures has its advantages and disadvantages; both procedures outperform behavioral assessment in newborn hearing detection applications. *Behavioral measures*, including automated behavioral techniques, cannot validly and reliably detect the criterion hearing loss of 30 dB HL in infants less than 6 months of age (Jacobson and Morehouse, 1984; Durieux-Smith, Picton, Edwards, MacMurray and Goodman, 1987; Hosford-Dunn, Johnson, Simmons, Malachowski and Low, 1987). However, for infants 6 months developmental age and older, conditioned behavioral techniques provide reliable and valid measures of hearing sensitivity (ASHA, 1991).

Other professionals as appropriate for the individual needs
child and family.

team will develop a program of early intervention services
SP) based on the child's unique strengths and needs and
tent with the family's resources, priorities, and concerns
to enhancing the child's development. This multidiscipli-
eam must include the parent/caregiver. Team planning
be cognizant of and sensitive to the range of available com-
ation and educational choices, and parents should be given
ent information regarding all options to enable them to exer-
formed consent when selecting their child's program.
onents of an early intervention program for children with
g loss and their families should include:
Family support and information regarding hearing loss and
nge of available communication and educational interven-
ptions. Such information must be provided in an objective,
ased way to support family choice. It is recommended to use
mer organizations and persons who are deaf or hard-of-
g to provide such information. Professional, consumer, state
community-based organizations should be accessed to pro-
ongoing information regarding legal rights, educational mate-
support groups and/or networks, and other relevant
rces for children and families.
Implementation of learning environments and services
ned with attention to the family's preferences. Such services
ld be family-centered and should be consistent with the
s of the child, the family, and their culture.
Early intervention activities that promote the child's develop-
t in all areas, with particular attention to language acquisition
communication skills.
Early intervention services that provide ongoing monitoring
e child's medical and hearing status, amplification needs, and
lopment of communication skills.
Curriculum planning that integrates and coordinates multi-
plinary personnel and resources so that intended outcomes of
FSP are achieved.

ADDITIONAL CONSIDERATIONS

uccessful programs for identifying infants with hearing loss
characterized by commitment and support from health care
inistrators, physicians, audiologists, families and caregivers,
a community educated about the importance of hearing and
nt development. Because of the dynamic changes in technolo-
nd in education and health care policy, the Joint Committee

B. Personnel

Teams of professionals, including audiologists, physicians (otolaryngologists and pediatricians), and nursing personnel, are often
involved in establishing infant hearing programs. Audiologists
should supervise infant hearing assessment programs. Personnel
appropriate to the infant hearing program who are trained and
supervised by an audiologist may conduct some aspects of the
infant hearing program (National Institutes of Health, 1993).

C. Implementation

Conditions that permit implementation and/or conversion to a
universal infant hearing program, as well as timelines to initiate
such programs, vary by program and location. However, program
development and specific timelines should be established by each
program to move toward the Joint Committee's goal. Pending
development of programs to identify **all** infants with hearing loss,
the Joint Committee on Infant Hearing recommends that programs based on indicators and currently in operation continue to
provide assessment services to identified infants. The section that
follows lists indicators associated with sensorineural and/or conductive hearing loss in neonates (Section III A) and infants
(Section III B). On implementation of universal infant hearing programs, these indicators may be used to aid in the etiologic diagnosis of hearing loss as well as to identify those infants who develop
health conditions associated with hearing loss and who therefore
require ongoing hearing monitoring.

D. Cost/Benefit Analysis

Cost/benefit analysis of infant hearing programs should
include consideration of direct cost of identification, assessment
and intervention. In addition, it may be valuable to determine the
cost savings that accompany early detection and subsequent
management of the child with hearing loss. Each infant hearing
program should develop a cost/benefit analysis associated with its
specific protocol. The results of cost/benefit analysis vary widely
because of differences in protocol, location, geographic and economic considerations, and other factors.

III. INDICATORS ASSOCIATED WITH SENSORINEURAL AND/OR CONDUCTIVE HEARING LOSS:

A. **For use with neonates (birth through age 28 days) when universal screening is not available.**
   1. Family history of hereditary childhood sensorineural hear-
      ing loss.

2. In utero infection, such as cytomegalovirus, rubella, syphillis, herpes, and toxoplasmosis.
3. Craniofacial anomalies, including those with morphological abnormalities of the pinna and ear canal.
4. Birth weight less than 1,500 grams (3.3 lbs).
5. Hyperbilirubinemia at a serum level requiring exchange transfusion.
6. Ototoxic medications, including but not limited to the aminoglycosides, used in multiple courses or in combination with loop diuretics.
7. Bacterial meningitis.
8. Apgar scores of 0-4 at 1 minute or 0-6 at 5 minutes.
9. Mechanical ventilation lasting 5 days or longer.
10. Stigmata or other findings associated with a syndrome known to include a sensorineural and/or conductive hearing loss.

B. For use with infants (age 29 days through 2 years) when certain health conditions develop that require rescreening.

1. Parent/caregiver concern regarding hearing, speech, language, and/or developmental delay.
2. Bacterial meningitis and other infections associated with sensorineural hearing loss.
3. Head trauma associated with loss of consciousness or skull fracture.
4. Stigmata or other findings associated with a syndrome known to include a sensorineural and/or conductive hearing loss.
5. Ototoxic medications, including but not limited to chemotherapeutic agents or aminoglycosides, used in multiple courses or in combination with loop diuretics.
6. Recurrent or persistent otitis media with effusion for at least 3 months.

C. For use with infants (age 29 days through 3 years) who require periodic monitoring of hearing.

Some newborns and infants may pass initial hearing screening but require periodic monitoring of hearing to detect delayed-onset sensorineural and/or conductive hearing loss. Infants with these indicators require hearing evaluation at least every 6 months until age 3 years, and at appropriate intervals thereafter.

Indicators associated with delayed-onset sensorineural hearing loss include:

1. Family history of hereditary childhood hearing loss.
2. In utero infection, such as cytomegalovirus, rubella, syphilis, herpes, or toxoplasmosis.

---

3. Neurofibromatosis Type II and neu

Indicators associated with conductive l

1. Recurrent or persistent otitis medi
2. Anatomic deformities and other di eustachian tube function.
3. Neurodegenerative disorders.

IV. EARLY INTERVENTION

When hearing loss is identified, evaluatic tion services should be provided in accorda Individuals with Disabilities Education Act Law 102-119 (formerly PL 99-457). A multic will be completed to determine eligibility an ing an individualized family service plan (IF early intervention program. Because specifi eligibility are not uniform from state to state users and service providers should contact Access Projects (RAP) coordinators for inforn

The full evaluation process should be con of referral. However, intervention services m completion of the evaluation if parental/care obtained and an interim IFSP is developed. S intervention services that might be offered be full evaluation of all developmental areas inc amplification, support, and information to pa ing loss and the range of intervention altern

The interim IFSP should include the name nator who will be responsible for both implen im IFSP and coordination of activities among persons.

The multidisciplinary evaluation and assess identified with hearing loss should be performe fessionals working in conjunction with the par professionals may include, depending on the n

1. A physician with expertise in the manag hood otologic disorders.
2. An audiologist with expertise in the asse and young children to determine type, degree, and configuration of hearing loss, and to recor devices appropriate to the child's needs (e.g., h al FM systems, vibrotactile aids, and/or cochle
3. A speech-language pathologist, audiologi specialist, and/or teacher of children who are hearing with expertise in the assessment and i munication skills.

on Infant Hearing recommends consideration of the following factors to facilitate establishment and maintenance of infant hearing programs:

1. Development of a uniform state and national database incorporating standardized technique, methodology, reporting, and system evaluation. This database will enhance (including efficacy and cost/benefit analysis), continuous quality improvement, and public policy development.

2. Development of a tracking system to insure that newborns and infants identified with or at risk for hearing loss have access to evaluation, follow-up, and intervention services.

3. Systematic evaluation of techniques for identification and assessment, and intervention for hearing loss in infants. Replication and ongoing assessment of current programs will assist in evaluating the efficacy of infant hearing programs and widespread acceptance of the benefits of early identification of infants with hearing loss.

4. Ongoing refinement of current indicators associated with sensorineural and/or conductive hearing loss.

5. Outcome studies to investigate the impact of early identification on the degree of literacy and communication competence achieved and to establish factors that contribute to outcome.

6. Continued research into the prevention of hearing loss in newborns and infants.

REFERENCES

American Academy of Pediatrics (1982). Position statement 1982-Joint Committee on Infant Hearing. *Pediatrics* 70:496-497.

American Speech-Language-Hearing Association (1991). Guidelines for the audiologic assessment of children from birth through 36 months of age. *Asha* 33 (Suppl. 5), 37-43.

Amochaev A (1987). The infant hearing foundation: A unique approach to hearing screening of newborns. In K Gerkin and A. Amochaev (Eds), Hearing in infants: Proceedings of the national symposium (pp. 165-168). *Seminars in Hearing*, 8.

Bonfils P, Uziel A and Pujol R (1988). Screening for auditory dysfunction in infants by evoked otoacoustic emissions. *Archives of Otolaryngology-Head and Neck Surgery* 114:887-890.

Durieux-Smith A, Picton T, Edwards C, MacMurray B and Goodman J (1987). The Crib-o-gram in the NICU: An evaluation based on brainstem electric response audiometry. *Ear and Hearing* 6:20-24.

Elssman S, Matkin N and Sabo M (1987, September). Early identification of congenital sensorineural hearing loss. *Hearing Journal* 40(9), 13-17.

Galambos R, Hicks G and Wilson M (1982). Hearing loss in graduates of a tertiary intensive care nursery. *Ear and Hearing* 3:87-90.

Galambos R, Hicks G and Wilson M (1984). The auditory brainstem response reliably predicts hearing loss in graduates of a tertiary intensive care nursery. *Ear and Hearing* 5:254-260.

Hosford-Dunn H, Johnson S, Simmons B, Malachowski N and Low K (1987). Infant hearing screening: Program implementation and validation. *Ear and Hearing* 8:12-20.

Hyde M, Riko K and Malizia K (1990). Audiometric accuracy of the click ABr in infants at risk for hearing loss. *Journal of the American Academy of Audiology* 1:59-66.

Jacobson J and Morehouse R (1984). A comparison of auditory brainstem response and behavioral screening in high risk and normal newborn infants. *Ear and Hearing* 5:254-253.

Joint Committee on Infant Hearing (1982, December). Position statement. *Asha* 24:1017-1018.

Kennedy C, Kimm L, Dees D, Evans P, Hunter M, Lenton S and Thornton A (1991). Otoacoustic emissions and auditory brainstem responses in the newborn. *Archives of Disease in Childhood* 66:1124-1129.

Kileny P (1987). ALGO-1 automated infant hearing screener: Preliminary results. In K Gerkin and A Amochaev (Eds), Hearing in infants: Proceedings of the national symposium (pp. 125-131). *Seminars in Hearing*, 8.

Kileny P and Magathan M (1987). Predictive value of ABR in infants and children with moderate to profound hearing loss. *Ear and Hearing* 8:217-221.

Kuhl PK, Williams KA, Lacerda F, Stephens KN and Lindbloom B (1992). Linguistic experience alters phonetics perception in infants by six months of age. *Science* 255:606-608.

Mauk GW, White KR, Mortensen LB and Behrens TR (1991). The effectiveness of screening programs based on high-risk characteristics in early identification of hearing loss. *Ear and Hearing* 12:312-319.

National Institutes of Health (1993). *Early identification of hearing loss in infants and young children: Consensus development conference on early identification of hearing loss in infants and young children.*

Pappas DG (1983). A study of the high-risk registry for sensorineural hearing loss. *Archives of Otolaryngology-Head and Neck Surgery* 91:41-4.

Parving A (1993). Congenital hearing disability: epidemiology and identification: A comparison between two health authority districts. *International Journal of Pediatric Otolaryngology* 27:29-46.

Schulman-Galambos C and Galambos R (1979). Brainstem evoked response audiometry in newborn hearing screening. *Archives of Otolaryngology* 105:86-90.

Stein L, Ozdamar O, Kraus N and Paton J (1983). Follow-up of infants screened by auditory brainstem response in the neonatal intensive care unit. *Journal of Pediatrics* 103:447-453.

Stevens J, Webb H, Hutchinson J, Connell J, Smith M and Buffin J (1989). Click evoked otoacoustic emissions compared to brainstem electric response. *Archives of Disease in Childhood* 64:1105-1111.

Stevens J, Webb H, Hutchinson J, Connell J, Smith M and Buffin J (1990). Click evoked otoacoustic emissions in neonatal screening. *Ear and Hearing* 11:128-133.

U.S. Department of Health and Human Services, Public Health Service (1990). *Healthy People 2000: National health promotion and disease prevention objectives.* Washington, DC: U.S. Government Printing Office.

Watkin P, Baldwin M and McEnergy G (1991). Neonatal at risk screening and the identification of deafness. *Archives of Disease in Childhood* 66:1130-1135.

White KR and Behrens TR (Eds) (1993). The Rhode Island hearing assessment project: Implications for universal newborn hearing screening. *Seminars in Hearing* 14:1-119.

SUGGESTED READINGS

Early Identification of Hearing Loss in Neonates and Infants

Alberti P, Hyde M, Riko K, Corbin H and Fitzhardinge P (1985). Issues in early identification of hearing loss. *Laryngoscope* 95:373-381.

American Speech-Language-Hearing Association (1989, March). Guidelines for audiologic screening of newborns infants who are at risk for hearing loss. *Asha* 31:89-92.

Bergman I, Hirsch RP, Fria TJ, Shapiro SM, Holzman I and Painter MJ (1985). Cause of hearing loss in the high-risk premature infant. *Journal of Pediatrics* 106:95-101.

Bess FH and Hall JW (Eds) (1992). *Screening children for auditory function.* Nashville, TN: Bill Wilkerson Center Press.

Bess FH (Ed) (1988). *Hearing loss in children.* Parkton, MD: York Press.

Brummett RE (1981). Ototoxicity resulting from the combined administration of potent diuretics and other agents. *Scandinavian Audiology Supplement* 14:215-224.

Eichwald J and Mahoney T (1993). Apgar scores in the identification of sensorineural hearing loss. *Journal of the American Academy of Audiology* 4:133-138.

Halpern J, Hosford-Dunn H and Malachowski N (1987). Four factors that accurately predict hearing loss in "high risk" neonates. *Ear and Hearing* 8:21-25.

Hendricks-Munoz KD and Walton JP (1988). Hearing loss in infants with persistent fetal circulation. *Pediatrics* 81:650-656.

Jones KL (1988). *Smith's recognizable patterns of human malformation* (4th ed). Philadelphia: W.B. Saunders.
Matz G (1990). Clinical perspectives on ototoxic drugs. *Annals of Otology, Rhinology, and Laryngology* 99:39-41.

Naulty CM, Weiss IP and Herer GR (1986). Progressive sensorineural hearing loss in survivors of persistent fetal circulation. *Ear and Hearing* 7:74-77.

Nield TA, Schrier S, Ramos AD, Platzker ACG and Warburton D (1986). Unexpected hearing loss in high-risk infants. *Pediatrics* 78:417-422.

Northern JL and Downs MP (1991). *Hearing in children* (4th ed). Baltimore: Williams and Wilkins.

Turner RG (1990, October). Analysis of recommended guidelines for infant hearing screening. *Asha* 32:57-61.

Turner RG (1992). Comparison of four hearing screening protocols. *Journal of the American Academy of Audiology* 3:200-207.

Early Intervention

A Report to the Congress of the United States: Toward equality: Education of the deaf (1988). The Commission on Education of the Deaf.

American Speech-Language-Hearing Association (1991). The use of FM amplification instruments for infants and preschool children with hearing loss. *Asha* 33 (Suppl. 5), 1-2.

Early intervention program for infants and toddlers with handicaps: Final regulations. *Federal Register* 54(119), 26306-26348, June 22, 1989.

Kramer S and Williams D (1993). The hearing-impaired infant and toddler: Identification, assessment and intervention. *Infants and Young Children* 6:35-49.

Levitt H, McGarr N and Geffner D (1987). *Development of language and communication skills in hearing impaired children* (ASHA

Monograph No. 26). Rockville, MD: American Speech-Language-Hearing Association.

Ling D (1989). *Foundations of spoken language for hearing-impaired children.* Washington, DC: Alexander Graham Bell Association for the Deaf.

McGonigel MJ, Kaufman RK and Johnson BH (Eds) (1991). *Guidelines and recommended practices for the IFSP* (2nd ed). Bethesda, MD: Association for the Care of Children's Health.

Infant Heairng Resource (1985). *Parent infant communication: A program of clinical and home training for parents and hearing impaired infants* (3rd ed). Portland, OR: Infant Hearing Resource.

Schuyler V and Rushmer N (1987). *Parent infant habilitation: A comprehensive approach to working with hearing impaired infants and toddlers and their families.* Portland, OR: Infant Hearing Resource.

Simmon-Martin A and Rossi K (1990). *Parents and teachers: Partners in language development.* Washington, DC: Alexander Graham Bell Association for the Deaf.

Diagnosis and Management

Bess FH (Ed) (1988). *Hearing loss in children.* Parkton, MD: York Press.

Calvert DR (1986). *Physician's guide to the education of hearing-impaired children.* Washington, DC: Alexander Graham Bell Association for the Deaf.

Diefendorf AO (Ed) (1990). Pediatric audiology. *Seminars in Hearing* 11:315-411.

Dodge P, Davis H, Feigin R, Homes S, Kaplan S, Jubeliere D, Stechenberg B and Hirsh S (1984). Prospective evaluation of hearing loss as a sequela of acute bacterial meningitis. *New England Journal of Medicine* 311:869-874.

Ross M (1992). Implications of audiologic success. *Journal of the American Academy of Audiology* 3:1-4.

Ross M (1990, February/March). Implications of delay in detection and management of deafness. *Volta Review* 92:69-79.

Roush J and McWilliams RA (1990). A new challenge for pediatric audiology: Public Law 99-457. *Journal of the American Academy of Audiology* 1:196-208.

United States House of Representatives 99th Congress, 2d session. Report 99-860. *Report accompanying the education of the handicapped act amendment of 1986.*

Watkins S and Clark T (1993). *The SKI-HI Model: A resource manual for family centered, home-based programming for infants, toddlers, and preschool-aged children with hearing loss.* Logan, UT: HOPE, Inc.

Index